Flying Up the Stairs!

What You Need to Know About Menopausal Arthritis to Break Free

Phyllis Rickel-Wong

Endover Press

Boston

Flying Up the Stairs!: What You Need to Know About Menopausal Arthritis to Break Free
Copyright © 2012 by Phyllis Rickel-Wong

Rickel-Wong, P. (2012). Flying up the stairs!: What you need to know about menopausal arthritis to break free. Boston, MA: Endover Press. Copyright: © 2012 by Phyllis Rickel-Wong. All rights reserved.

Exercise and anatomical illustrations by Matthew Gouig
Cover design and art by Matthew Gouig
Illustrations and art: Copyright © 2012 by Phyllis Rickel-Wong. All rights reserved.

Endover Press
1 International Place, Suite 1400
Boston, MA 02110

PUBLISHER'S CATALOGING-IN-PUBLICATION DATA

Rickel-Wong, Phyllis
        Flying up the stairs! : what you need to know about menopausal arthritis to break free /
Phyllis Rickel-Wong. -- First Edition
        p. cm.
    Includes bibliographical references and index.
    ISBN-13: 978-0985185701
    ISBN-10: 0985185708

1. Arthritis--Alternative treatment--Popular works. 2. Arthritis--Exercise therapy. 3. Menopause--Alternative treatment--Popular works. 4. Joint--Disease--Alternative treatment.
I. Rickel-Wong, Phyllis   II. Title.

RC933.R53 2012
616.7/2206 RIC

First printing, 2012
Printed in the United States of America

The information within this book is based upon the research and experience of the author, and contains the opinions and ideas of the author. It is intended to provide helpful informative material on the subjects addressed in the publication. It is sold with the understanding that the author and the publisher are not engaged in rendering medical, health, or any other kind of personal professional services in the book. It is not intended as a substitute for consulting with your physician or medical provider. The reader should consult his or her medical, health, or other competent professional before adopting any of the suggestions, preparations or procedures in this book or drawing inferences from it. Any attempt to diagnose and/or treat an illness or other medical condition should be done under the direction of a health-care professional. All matters that pertain to your health require medical supervision.

The author and the publisher specifically disclaim all responsibility for any liability, loss, or risk, personal or otherwise, which is incurred as a consequence, directly or indirectly, of the use and application of any of the contents of this book.

This book is dedicated to the two most important people in my life,

my husband and my daughter.

Acknowledgements

I extend my great appreciation to Dr. Herbert Wong for his important role in developing the exercise program for my healing plan. His unique exercise plan does not isolate groups of muscles, but rather uses whole chains of muscles and tendons to tone and strengthen them. As a result, these crucial muscles and tendons are able to serve as critical supports for the body's joints. Dr. Wong has created these unique and powerful exercises from his deep understanding of Asian exercise forms and the martial arts. However, the beauty of these exercises is that you do not need to know a thing about martial arts, nor ever have practiced any of them, to perform these beneficial exercises. Dr. Wong holds the teaching rank of Shihan (Master Teacher) and is an 8th Degree Black Belt in Okinawan and Japanese Karate. He has practiced in many forms of the Asian martial arts to include Chi Kung, Tai Chi, and Kung Fu health exercises. Dr. Wong is personally dedicated to demystifying the principles behind Asian exercise forms so that they can be better understood by all who might embrace them.

I would like to extend my gratitude to the very talented artist, Matthew Gouig. The exercises that Dr. Wong has developed have come alive in the energetic illustrations created and drawn by him. My feeling of "flying up the stairs!" has been captured so well by Matt Gouig in his book cover design. In addition to his work as a commercial and graphic designs artist, Matthew Gouig is an accomplished martial artist, holding the rank of 5th Degree Black Belt in Okinawan and Japanese Karate. Bringing this expertise to his artwork has allowed him to beautifully portray the essential components of my program's exercises.

I would also like to extend my great appreciation to the very gifted web developer and designer, Michele Wong. She has brought together her masterful technical skills and knowledge with her exceptional vision and talent as an artist, to provide an excellent website for my book and program for transforming the experience of

v

menopause (www.transformingmenopause.com). Her creative logo for my website truly captures the essence of transformation! Her background in web design and development, psychology, and the fine arts come together so beautifully; she is able to understand and feel a person's vision and then transform it into an exquisite blend of art and technology.

Contents

List of Illustrations

Preface

For a great number of women, menopause is accompanied by aching and stiff joints that seem to only get worse as we get further and further into menopause. We quit dancing, drop aerobics, cancel outings, shun stairs, stop gardening, and although we just chaired a meeting, we can't get up out of our chair! Menopausal arthritis is aggravatingly present as we attend school, run errands, and go about every aspect of our lives. The joint aches (especially in the knees) can distract us, or worse they can completely disable us. In fact, some of us with aches and pains at menopause can at times hurt so much that we may even think we are succumbing to fibromyalgia.

All too often, though, the only thing that we hear about menopausal arthritis in books or on websites on women's health issues is that it is probably the "wear and tear" disease of osteoarthritis brought on by a decline in estrogen during menopause. However, research has revealed some much-needed information about menopausal arthritis and osteoarthritis. For anyone trying to break free of menopausal arthritis this is what you need to know:

Menopausal arthritis pain is more complex than just osteoarthritis brought on by menopause, and osteoarthritis goes beyond just a "wear and tear" disease of aging.

Before we go on to talk about some of the new research, let's go back nearly one hundred years to when menopausal arthritis was first recognized in the medical literature. Two very insightful medical doctors, Dr. Russell Cecil and Dr. Benjamin Archer first brought this form of arthritis to light in their 1925 journal article. Unfortunately, the article pretty much has remained in the dusty archives of the Journal of the American Medical Association. But, they were on to something. They knew that the most common attribute of women with menopausal arthritis, other than menopause itself, was obesity. The joint most affected by menopausal arthritis was the knee joint, and it was usually the first in which this arthritis developed. Their patients complained of pain going up and down the stairs, and getting up out of a chair. Since the knee was the main joint afflicted, Drs. Cecil and Archer had wondered whether excess body weight load upon the knee was the root cause of menopausal arthritis. They reasoned, though, that it had to be more than just the mechanical weight upon the knee joint, since other non-weight-bearing joints were affected too. They speculated that it was most likely endocrine in nature. They discounted that it could be metabolic in nature; this was 1925, though, and insulin resistance wouldn't really become a topic in the medical literature until the 1930's.

We *now* know that women in menopause who become obese are more likely to have metabolic syndrome and insulin resistance, along with leptin resistance. Most of us are aware that visceral fat is a virtual endocrine organ that releases inflammation-causing proteins. Powerful hormones, such as leptin, are produced by visceral fat. Hormones such as leptin are associated with inflammation and the release of inflammatory cytokines (I'll talk more about cytokines in Chapter Two). Most of us are probably aware that leptin and other hormones produced by white adipose tissue have been linked to the risk for cardiovascular disease and type II diabetes.

What *wasn't* known until recently is that higher levels of leptin are *linked to osteoarthritis!* The proinflammatory cytokines that leptin promotes within the body are involved in breaking down cartilage! Osteoarthritis exists within a metabolic milieu! Moreover, brand new research out of Stanford University Medical School shows that the low-grade inflammation that has now been associated with osteoarthritis may actually play a *dynamic* role in how and why osteoarthritis develops. We'll be discussing the pioneering 1925 research of Drs. Cecil and Archer in Chapter One, and the cutting-edge 2011 research out of Stanford University Medical School in Chapter Twelve.

It is now clear that to beat osteoarthritis and menopausal arthritis you must fight low-grade inflammation! My healing plan includes a vast array of very effective inflammation-fighting foods, herbs, and supplements. I have described each of them along with the scientific evidence-based findings that support their use. These anti-inflammatory allies are a cornerstone of the natural healing program within this book, and they are your *first line of defense against menopausal arthritis*.

There are overlaps between menopausal arthritis and osteoarthritis, and that is why there will be an emphasis upon natural ways to fight the inflammation we now know exists within the disease process of osteoarthritis. However, what is also critical to know is that there are *other things* that are involved in the experience of menopausal arthritis pain. Many of these things have actually *nothing directly to do with the disease process of osteoarthritis*. For example, there are many physical ailments such as soft tissue disorders that are *more common in women* and can easily be mistaken for osteoarthritis knee pain. In fact, they can produce severe knee pain that feels just like arthritis pain! These ailments that "mimic" arthritis include several key forms of bursitis (such as pes anserine bursitis), and we'll take a look at them in Chapter Six.

To find the original research study on pes anserine bursitis, we return once again to the invaluable archives of the Journal of the American Medical Association. The pes anserine syndrome was first described in 1937 by Dr. Eli Moschcowitz who called this syndrome "bursitis of sartorius bursa." "For an unknown reason" he wrote, "the malady occurs almost exclusively in women." The primary disease characteristic? Pain in both knees only when going up and down the stairs. Importantly, Dr. Moschcowitz noted that the knee joint *did not show any arthritis* upon x-ray examination.

This brings up an interesting point about x-rays. Did you know that there is often a total *lack of connection* between symptoms of osteoarthritis pain and x-ray evidence of arthritis? X-ray findings that diagnose osteoarthritis *do not necessarily correspond to self-reported pain with osteoarthritis*. This means that *you could have deterioration of cartilage on an x-ray, but not have any pain*. Conversely, *you could have no deterioration of cartilage on an x-ray and have considerable joint pain*.

Current writings on osteoarthritis have not unraveled all of the reasons for the different experiences of men and women. In addition to soft tissue problems such as bursitis, there are also other problems of importance such as muscle imbalances and shortened muscles that may be more specific to women than to men. These muscle problems can cause women to adopt gait patterns that put tremendous strain on the knees. Oftentimes, this resulting knee pain may be identified as being arthritis pain, *when it is not!*

Women experience a rapid loss of muscle mass within the first few years right after menopause, whereas men lose muscle more gradually over time. There are significant differences between men and women in muscles, cartilage, and ligaments. These key differences are of much importance in developing an exercise program for women with menopausal arthritis. We'll look at physiological and biomechanical differences between men and women in Chapters Four, Five, and Seven.

The healing plan within this book includes a set of unique and effective exercises that will allow you to enhance and maximize the ability of your muscles and tendons to support your joints. The exercises have been developed using principles of modern sport training, kinetic muscle chain development, and principles of the integrative muscle-tendon unit found in the Asian martial arts. We describe the research and theoretical bases for our exercise program in Chapter Seven -- Part I, and in Chapter Seven Part II we present the exercises with illustrations and full descriptions of how to perform them, as well as exercise tips and check points.

Rather than isolated eccentric or concentric exercises that you may find in many exercise programs for arthritis, our exercises use whole chains of muscles. At once you will be exercising many muscles involving many joints (*no* solitary knee extensions with a burdensome weight at your ankle!). As you strengthen your muscles in ways that engage and use whole chains of muscles, you will increase muscle force. As these chains of muscles begin to work together in a coordinated and smooth fashion, you will build speed and generate increased power. These exercises have been expressly designed for women who are experiencing menopausal arthritis.

All of the exercises are done standing, so there is no need to disrupt the flow of your everyday activities by having to get down on the floor. It can hurt to have to lower your body into a floor position and then get back up off of the floor when you have painful joints. Nor is there any need to set up exercise props such as bands or weights. For menopausal women with arthritis, props such as bands can be uncomfortable or painful. So, in doing these exercises you benefit doubly -- through the exercises, *and* in not increasing problems in already painful or vulnerable joints.

Menopausal arthritis is far more complex than originally thought. But, what about estrogen loss? How *does* it fit into the picture? From my research, it is clear that estrogen loss matters, and it seems to be a trigger for the unfolding menopausal arthritis pain. I will discuss how estrogen relates to menopausal arthritis in the first half of this book. However, one of the appealing things about my natural healing plan for menopausal arthritis is that it is not dependent upon hormone supplementation. Moreover, my plan does not need to include pharmaceutical drugs nor NSAIDs (non-steroidal, anti-inflammatory drugs such as ibuprofen).

I am writing this book because women need to know about what may really be causing their menopausal arthritis. There is an impressive body of research with much needed information on the topic. Unfortunately by far, most of the findings from this body of research have not made their way out of the medical and other professional journals into the general public media.

I began my research with the classic studies that I have touched upon above. However, following this research and a handful of other early studies, there would be a dearth of empirical research on arthritis and the menopause for many decades. Perhaps it is no great coincidence that as the massive baby-boomer generation began to meet menopause head on, research on menopausal arthritis took a quick, upwards swing. By the end of the decade from 1985-1995 there were 130 articles related to menopause and arthritis accessible through PubMed. Then, from 1995 to January 2011 the research had burgeoned, with the number of scientific studies reaching 416!

In this book I have included findings from many diverse professional fields including rheumatology, orthopedics, sports medicine, biophysics, nutritional science, and many more. I have explored research that looks at why osteoarthritis and menopausal arthritis develop, and research that shows what you can do about it. With empirical research as my base and launching point, I have developed a plan with specific and effective ways to help heal from menopausal arthritis. I provide in my plan the basic and fundamental information that you need to fortify your body so that you can resist inflammation and develop strong and smoothly functioning joints. I am going to provide you with the exciting and fascinating research behind my healing plan throughout this book.

If you are a perimenopausal, menopausal or postmenopausal woman experiencing arthritis symptoms common to menopause, then this book is written for you. It is about getting back your pleasure in movement! It is about regaining your strength and ability to move with a body free of arthritis pain! After many years of pain going up and down the stairs that ultimately led to pain just in walking, I am now without menopausal arthritis pain. I am enthusiastic that my healing plan can help you, too!

Phyllis Rickel-Wong
San Francisco, California
January, 2012

Part One: *Menopausal Arthritis*

Chapter One

What is Menopausal Arthritis?

——— ▢ ———

Some may question whether there really is such a thing as menopausal arthritis. Isn't menopausal arthritis actually just osteo-arthritis or the so-called "wear and tear" disease of aging brought on by estrogen loss? Current research knowledge reveals that the answer is a definitive, "No!" Menopausal arthritis is much more complex than simply "osteoarthritis" brought on by declining estrogen, and osteoarthritis is much more than just a "wear and tear" disease of aging! First of all, there are many soft tissue conditions that can "mimic" arthritis pain, and that are far more common in older women than in older men. In fact, they can produce severe knee pain that feels just like arthritis pain; nevertheless, they have nothing directly to do with the disease process of osteoarthritis. We will take a look at these ailments in Chapter Six, as they may contribute greatly to the knee pain many menopausal women feel in going up and down the stairs.

Although osteoarthritis is no doubt part of the picture of menopausal arthritis, new research reveals that it is *not* just a disease of wear and tear on the joint. Rather, it develops and exists within a highly metabolic milieu characterized by inflammation! Women are at greater risk for experiencing the inflammation associated with osteoarthritis after menopause. There is a sharp increase in the incidence of metabolic syndrome in postmenopausal women, and this syndrome is connected with a biochemical profile that is associated with osteoarthritis. Metabolic syndrome is associated with insulin resistance, and insulin resistance is associated with leptin resistance. We now know that higher levels of leptin, as in leptin resistance, are associated with osteoarthritis. In Chapter Two we will look at why this is the case, and why leptin can no longer be considered just an energy regulator.

There are also differences between men and women in social and psychological factors that may contribute to women's unique experience of arthritis in older adulthood. We will explore all of these factors so important to the topic of menopausal arthritis in the chapters that follow. For now, though, let's take a look at the first, classic study of menopausal arthritis.

The Pioneering, Classic Medical Study

Historically, we have known about menopausal arthritis for a very long time. In 1925, two medical doctors, Dr. Russell Cecil and Dr. Benjamin Archer, established the connection between menopause and arthritis within the medical literature.[1] Their patients were women admitted to the Cornell clinic, and they found that one-third of them had arthritis that was connected to the menopause. Carefully examining fifty clinical cases, a clearer picture began to emerge. Besides the menopause, what did they find was the second most common characteristic of menopausal arthritis? It was obesity. Of the 20 cases for which they established a height-weight relationship, the women were on average 5'3" tall, 184 lbs., with an average age of 51 years. Nearly all of the women were overweight. Most seemed to have fairly well-distributed weight; however some of the women had excess abdominal fat and fat more concentrated in the hips and breasts.

Menopausal arthritis seemed to especially target the knees. Eight-four percent of the women had pain and stiffness, or both, first appearing in their knee joints. It might begin with pain on climbing the stairs or going down the stairs, or perhaps getting out of a chair. It would over time worsen and extend to more basic movements with discomfort experienced while walking or when bending the knees. In a small number of the women it started in their fingers (14%), and only a very small percentage of women (2%) said that it started in their back. Approximately three-quarters of the women also had "Heberden's nodes." These are small, fixed bumps that are seen on the last joint of the finger, and they contribute to a feeling of stiffness in the fingers. Approximately 10% of the women experienced arthritis of the feet, and in 12% of the women one shoulder was affected.

It is now nearly a century later, and the experience of arthritis pain associated with the menopause captured so long ago by Drs. Cecil and Archer rings true today. In a large study, the Framingham Osteoarthritis Study, women succumbed to knee osteoarthritis nearly twice as often as men.[2] Looking at women over a period of eight years during the menopausal transition, a large Australian study found that aches and stiff joints were the most common symptoms during this time. In fact, the aching and stiff joints increased as the women got further and further into menopause.[3] Similarly, in a large multi-ethnic study within the United States (Women's Health Across the Nation), menopausal women reported experiencing a high prevalence of aches and pains. Postmenopausal women reported significantly more pain than premenopausal women. For one in six of these women, aches and pains were a daily occurrence.[4]

My Own Story

When I first read the article by Dr. Cecil and Dr. Archer I was astonished and shocked! They seemed to be describing me. At about 53 years of age, I began to experience knee pain that was centered in one knee. I also had nearly the same body dimensions as the women in Dr. Cecil's and Dr. Archer's study with a height of 5'4" and body weight of 185 lbs. I was obviously also what medical doctors would consider "obese," and I was menopausal. By the time I was 57 years of age, the pain in my right knee had intensified. To top it off, I had also developed a small, but definite Heberden's node on the last joint of a finger on my right hand! Just like Dr. Cecil's and Dr. Archer's patients, my experience of menopausal arthritis was centered decisively upon my knee. I fit the classic profile of menopausal arthritis to a "T."

Another classic study resonated, too, with what I was experiencing. In an article published in 1937 in the Journal of the American Medical Association, Dr. Eli Moschcowitz described a syndrome that he found occurred almost singularly in women. His patients complained about pain in the knees upon walking up or down the stairs. They didn't have pain when simply walking on level ground. The knee joint itself was not sore or tender to the touch. Rather, what was sore or tender to the touch was a spot on the inner tibia (shinbone) where the sartorius, gracilis and semitendinosus muscles conjoin (See Figure 5 in Chapter Four). Importantly, x-ray examination of the knee joint did not show any arthritis.[5] Upon reading this, I checked for any tender spots on and around my knee. My knee itself was not sore to the touch; however, there was indeed a very tender and painful spot at the pes anserinus. I would not even have thought to look there, had I not come across the article by Dr. Moschcowitz. This area on my leg was very painful when pressed on with my fingers. Could this have been associated with my problems with pain going up and down the stairs, just as it had been for Dr. Moschcowitz's patients? What I ended up learning through my research was that my muscles that were attached to the tendons at the pes anserinus had developed many problems such as shortening. Muscle shortening can create an excessive pull upon the tendons. Friction upon the bursa or soft tissue beneath the tendons results, and this causes pain. I will discuss this more in Chapter Four. So, it was becoming very clear to me that my problem with knee pain didn't have to do just with the knee joint itself. The experience of aches and pains for women at menopause, though, can sometimes be even more pervasive than just knee pain.

The odd thing about these aches and pains is that, along with the menopausal arthritis as described by Drs. Cecil and Archer and bursitis conditions such as described by Dr. Moschcowitz, the pain can sometimes flare into a more global experience over many joints. I had been working very hard to prepare the house for a large, holiday, family get-together last year. After the dinner, and after every last family member had left, I found that my whole body ached, muscles and joints. It was not the same kind of "whole body ache" that one might get after a good exercise workout. Rather, it was a penetrating, debilitating ache that made me think that I might even be succumbing to fibromyalgia. Interestingly, in a very large study of older adults, the Framingham Study, widespread pain that affects all parts of the body was more common in women than in men.[6]

Could it just be that more of my joints were becoming involved in my menopausal arthritis? One large research study found that middle aged women were prone to developing osteoarthritis involving several joints, and that in postmenopausal women the pattern seemed to point toward a systemic cause.[7] In addition, although many women begin with arthritis in just one knee, a study found that over one-third of the middle-aged women (mean age of 57 years) with osteoarthritis in one knee will go on to develop arthritis in the other knee within two years.[8] However, that couldn't be what was happening here after my preparation for the family event. A day earlier I had knee joint pain and the usual "over-exercised muscle" pain. What could have caused this sudden and dramatic change in my experience of joint and muscular pain?

Psychological stress can trigger inflammatory processes in the body involved in the onset and progression of many illnesses (such as rheumatoid arthritis and cardiovascular disease). In fact, stress that has to do with our social relationships has been shown to be especially potent in stimulating inflammation.[9] Stress produces an increase in immune and inflammatory responses that nature intended to be protective against whatever harmful agent or intruder may be threatening us (as in the "fight or flight" response). Sometimes, though, we aren't really in danger but our bodies react as if we were. Dr. Hans Selye explained that this is because we may not have been able to use interventions to correct inappropriate defenses. They remain "automatic." The adaptive defense response kicks in (even when it doesn't need to) and brings with it the full-blown consequences such as disease.[10]

In addition to psychological stress, the phenomenon of "central sensitization" can also result in hypersensitivity to pain. What is central sensitization? This occurs when harmful or potentially harmful stimulation to the body repeatedly occurs, and the body responds by increasing sensitivity to the stimulation. The nerve cells become *too* reactive, and this results in an overblown perception of pain. Even a relatively harmless (or completely non-injurious) stimulation can be perceived as painful.[11] Some of us may think of this as occurring mainly in diseases such as fibromyalgia. However, current research suggests that it occurs in many other disorders and diseases, to include osteoarthritis.[12]

Could stress have caused my all-over body ache experience? Yes, say researchers! Dr. Pamela Lyon, of the University of Australia, Adelaide, and her colleagues have suggested that this form of chronic pain experienced throughout the whole body results from a "whole-organism stress response" in which central sensitization to pain is controlled within the brain. They explained this as being a general stress response that has continued through our evolution as human beings.[13] In fibromyalgia, the whole body is made excruciatingly sensitive to pain (the pain is turned up - it is amplified, and the pain signals are dispersed widely). In my case, fortunately the stress subsided, the family guests left, and with them so did my overall body aches (not instantly, of course, but over the next day or so). My body went back to its usual, more localized pain syndrome. Stress and its association with arthritis is an exceptionally fascinating area, and we will come back to it in Chapter Six and in Chapter Eleven.

So what was going on with me? In perimenopause I was completely different -- dancing, exercising, stair-climbing with no knee problems. My attempts at weight loss, however, were dismal failures as the scale simply would not budge. Hence, I gained 45 lbs. en route to menopause and thus fit the "obese" aspect of the classic menopausal arthritis.

It was not until about six years after menopause, though, that things really began to take a distinct turn for the worse. Although right after menopause my muscles and my joints were beginning to hurt more than they had after work and exercise, they always recovered within a day or so. Now, however, my muscles just did not heal the same way after house or garden work or aerobic exercise. For example, I would work for hours in my garden, and then find that I was unable to get up out of my chair. Driving a car to the grocery store was completely out of the question; a monumental and impossible task!

My joints would not recover either. My knees, that used to hurt after physical work, had always gotten better. Not now. I also had the surprising addition of a "snapping" sound as I extended my right knee. Worse yet, a persistent, gnawing, aching pain had invaded the center of my knee. I had thought that all of the gardening work had been good for me; with the digging, and the hoeing I had thought that I was getting a pretty good exercise work-out. I was using my whole body in weight-bearing exercise. What's more, gardening has always been recommended as a good non-aerobic activity. So, this was good for me, right?

Well, as no doubt you've already guessed, "No!" At this point I had already begun my research on menopausal arthritis. A very large study of 1,025 people in Wuchuan County in China proved to be illuminating. These researchers found that heavy physical levels of work, such as digging or cycling, were associated with the risk of developing medial compartment knee osteoarthritis.[14] This occurs in the inner middle side of the knee, and where I was feeling that aching pain. Digging! Just exactly what I had been spending hours upon hours doing. Nevertheless, while my recent landscaping efforts may have made my knee pain worse, my knee pain was there long before I began the intensive gardening. So, what was causing it?

Research into the Heart of the Metabolic Matter

Perhaps, what was most surprising to me about what was causing my menopausal arthritis was the connection with the hormone, leptin. I had worked on a couple of dieting attempts post menopause. One of the weight loss books I was using as a guide had referred to leptin as the hormone that would signal to us that our appetite was satisfied, that we were "full." In contrast, ghrelin was the hormone that would signal to us that we were hungry, that we needed to eat. So, why would leptin be in any way related to arthritis?

I found out that the metabolic processes that were making me stubbornly fat were producing a whole legion of inflammatory chemicals called "cytokines," which I will talk about in greater detail in Chapter Two. The presence of these cytokines within the body is linked to chronic inflammatory diseases. Researchers had begun to question whether leptin was actually the connection between obesity and arthritis. What they discovered was that leptin was found in the joint fluid of people with knee osteoarthritis, and that the levels of leptin *did* correspond to body mass index. Moreover, although only a small number of cartilage cells produced leptin in normal knees, there was a *great presence of leptin in the cartilage of osteoarthritic knees.*[15]

Entering Menopause into the Equation

Have you noticed how common it is for women to gain weight, sometimes a considerable amount of it, in menopause? Weight gain targeting the abdomen as a primary fat depot markedly increases. So too does the prevalence of metabolic syndrome.[16] For example, in a study of 6,044 adults it was found that metabolic syndrome occurred in approximately 10% of premenopausal women as compared to approximately 28% of postmenopausal women.[17] Moreover, in another study of 940 women, the incidence of metabolic syndrome was approximately 18% in premenopausal women and approximately 54% in postmenopausal women.[18] These are dramatic increases in metabolic syndrome in postmenopause!

So, if metabolic syndrome sharply increases in women after menopause then it must be the decline in estrogen that is causing it, right? Apparently *not*, at least not directly! New research shows that the decline in estrogen at menopause is only *indirectly* responsible for the greater prevalence of metabolic syndrome. The findings of a large longitudinal study of midlife women (The Study of Women's Health Across the Nation) showed that changes in estradiol, per sé, were not associated with the occurrence of metabolic syndrome. Rather, it was the level of *free androgen* (as well as total testosterone) that was related to the prevalence of metabolic syndrome at the beginning of the menopausal transition. Indeed, across the whole menopausal transition, it was the proportion of testosterone to estradiol, the ratio and its rate of change, that predicted the increased incidence of metabolic syndrome.[19] An excess of androgen as compared with estrogen is associated with metabolic syndrome. As women go through the menopausal transition, estrogen levels decrease and androgen levels become predominant. Thus, metabolic syndrome sets in. I was beginning to see that the flood of hormonal change that had arrived at my doorstep at menopause had brought with it metabolic syndrome and menopausal arthritis, both swept in with the tide.

Arthritis and the Unique Experiences of Women

Women and men have different profiles with regard to the incidence and severity of osteoarthritis. The incidence of osteoarthritis is higher in women than in men, and it increases markedly at menopause.[20, 21] In addition, knee osteoarthritis is more prevalent in women than men no matter how it is defined (e.g., through x-ray, self-reports, symptoms plus x-ray).[22] There are metabolic, hormonal, and physiological factors that are different in women and in men that influence muscle, ligaments, cartilage, and other soft tissues. There are even gender differences in psychological and social factors that influence the experience of arthritis pain. These wide-ranging factors contribute to the unique experience of arthritis in menopause and after. These are the topics that will be of concern to us as you read on within this book. Menopausal arthritis is a unique form of arthritis, and in the following chapters I will show you why.

Notes for Chapter One

[1]Cecil, R. L., & Archer, B. H. (1925) Arthritis of the menopause: A study of fifty cases. *The Journal of the American Medical Association, 84* (2), 75-79.1

[2]Felson, D. T., Zhang, Y., Hannan, M. T., Naimark, A., Weissman, B. N., Aliabadi, P., & Levy, D. (1995). The incidence and natural history of knee osteoarthritis in the elderly. The Framingham Osteoarthritis Study. *Arthritis & Rheumatism, 38*(10), 1500-1505.

[3]Szoeke, C.E., Cicuttini, F. M., Guthrie, J. R., & Dennerstein, L. (2008). The relationship of reports of aches and joint pains to the menopausal transition: A longitudinal study. *Climacteric, 11*(1), 55-62.

[4]Dugan, S. A., Powell, L. H., Kravitz, H. M., Everson Rose, S. A., Karavolos, K., & Luborsky, J. (2006). Musculoskeletal pain and menopausal status. *Clinical Journal of Pain, 22(*4), 325-331.

[5]Moschcowitz, Eli. (1937). Bursitis of Sartorius bursa: An undescribed malady simulating chronic arthritis. *Journal of the American Medical Association, 109*(17), 1362.

[6]Leveille, S. G., Zhang, Y., McMullen, W., Kelly-Hayes, M., & Felson, D. T. (2005). Sex differences in musculoskeletal pain in older adults. *Pain, 116*(3), 332-338.

[7]Cooper, C., Egger, P., Coggon, D., Hart, D. J., Masud, T., Cicuttini, F., Doyle, D. V., & Spector, T. D. (1996). Generalized osteoarthritis in women: Pattern of joint involvement and approaches to definition for epidemiological studies. *Journal of Rheumatology, 23*(11), 1938-1942.

[8]Spector, T., D., Hart, D. J., & Doyle, D. V. (1994). Incidence and progression of osteoarthritis in women with unilateral knee disease in the general population: The effect of obesity. *Annals of the Rheumatic Diseases, 53*, 565-568.

[9]Slavich, G. M., Way, B. M., Eisenberger, N. I., & Taylor, S. E. (2010). Neural sensitivity to social rejection is associated with inflammatory responses to social stress. *Proceedings of the National Academy of Sciences of the United States of America, 107*(33), 14817-14822. doi: 10.1073/pnas.1009164107

[10]Selye, H. (1976). Forty years of stress research: Principal remaining problems and misconceptions. *Canadian Medical Association Journal, 115*, 53-56.

[11]Meeus, M., & Nijs, J. (2007). Central sensitization: A biopsychosocial explanation for chronic widespread pain in patients with fibromyalgia and chronic fatigue syndrome. *Clinical Rheumatology, 26*, 465-473. doi: 10.1007/s10067-006-0433-9

[12]Woolf, C. J. (2011). Central sensitization: Implications for the diagnosis and treatment of pain. *Pain, 152*(3 Suppl), S2-S15.

[13]Lyon, P., Cohen, M., & Quintner, J. (2011). An evolutionary stress-response hypothesis for chronic widespread pain (fibromyalgia syndrome). *Pain Medicine, 12*(8), 1167-1178. doi: 10.1111/j.1526-4637.2011.01168.x

[14]Lin, J., Li, R., Kang, X., & Li, H. (2010). Risk factors for radiographic tibiofemoral knee osteoarthritis: The Wuchuan osteoarthritis study. *International Journal of Rheumatology, 2010*, 1-6. doi: 10.1155/2010/385826

[15]Pottie, P., Presle, N., Dumond, H., Terlain, B., Mainard, D., Leuille, D., & Netter, P. (2004) Is leptin the link between obesity and osteoarthritis? *Arthritis Research and Therapy, 6*(Suppl. 3), 8. doi: 10.1186/ar1342.

[16]Chedraui, P., Jaramillo, W., Pérez-López, F. R., Escobar, G. S., Morocho, N., & Hidalgo, L. (2011). Pro-inflammatory cytokine levels in postmenopausal women with metabolic syndrome. *Gynecological Endocrinology, 27*(9), 685-691.

[17]Jehn, M., Clark, J. M., & Guallar, E. (2004). Serum ferritin and risk of metabolic syndrome in U.S. adults. *Diabetes Care, 27*(10), 2422-2428.

[18]Eshtiaghi, R., Esteghamati, A., & Nakhjavani, M. (2010). Menopause is an independent predictor of metabolic syndrome in Iranian women. *Maturitas, 65*(3), 262-266.

[19]Torréns, J. I., Sutton-Tyrrell, K., Zhao, X., Matthews, K., Brockwell, S., Sowers, M., & Santoro, N. (2009). Relative androgen excess during the menopausal transition predicts incident metabolic syndrome in midlife women: SWAN. *Menopause, 16*(2), 257-264. doi: 10.1097/gme.0b013e318185e249

[20]Maleki-Fischbach, M., & Jordan, J. M. (2010). Sex differences in magnetic resonance imaging-based biomarkers and in those of joint metabolism. *Arthritis Research & Therapy, 12*, 212. doi: 10.1186/ar3091

[21]O'Connor, M. I. (2007). Sex differences in osteoarthritis of the hip and knee. *Journal of the American Academy of Orthopaedic Surgeons, 15*(1), 522-525.

[22]Pereira, D., Peleteiro, B., Araújo, J., Branco, J., Santos, R. A., & Ramos, E. (2011). The effect of osteoarthritis definition on prevalence and incidence estimates: A systematic review. *Osteoarthritis and Cartilage, 19*(11), 1270-1285,

Chapter Two

Leptin – More Than Just an Energy Regulator

At the time of Dr. Cecil's and Dr. Archer's classic menopausal arthritis study, little was known about visceral fat as a virtual endocrine "organ" in the body capable of producing potent hormones.[1] However, these doctors were certain that it was not solely the mechanical weight of the body on the knee joints that caused the arthritis (after all, non-weight-bearing joints were also affected). At that time, though, they were not able to discover what the hormonal or endocrine connections were. It was not until 1994, nearly 70 years later, that the hormone leptin was discovered and its role in the regulation of body weight revealed.[2] As the next decade unfolded, leptin would prove to be a vital endocrine connection to osteoarthritis; leptin was linked to *both* obesity and osteoarthritis.

Most of us have heard of leptin with regard to its role in dieting and energy expenditure. Leptin resistance, which is essentially a chemical imbalance, prevents the body from naturally regulating appetite. Leptin is blocked in delivering its message that appetite has been satisfied. Not only does leptin communicate to the hypothalamus in the brain to signal that one is satiated or "full," but it also inhibits the production of insulin by the pancreas.

There is a complementary (or "yin and yang") relationship with regard to the two hormones, insulin and leptin. Researchers from Mount Sinai School of Medicine noted that both hormones control the energy balance within the body and are active in maintaining it.[3] They are both involved in regulating the release of fatty acids from white adipose tissue (WAT) for energy and the formation of fat cells. Leptin and insulin have been viewed as having a "yin and yang" relationship because they regulate energy balance in opposing ways. Insulin helps prevent the breakdown of fat and increases its formation within the body. Leptin, on the other hand, opposes insulin's effects by speeding up fat breakdown and helping to prevent the formation of fat.[4]

This is a beautifully orchestrated system through which white adipose tissue metabolism is regulated. However, when leptin metabolism is altered, insulin metabolism is also altered. In the majority of people who are markedly overweight, leptin's ability to regulate energy metabolism has been thwarted. This leads to "leptin resistance" and higher levels of leptin. With leptin resistance, one produces excessive amounts of insulin, too. Increased insulin leads to insulin resistance and this, in turn, leads to more leptin production from the fat cells. This vicious cycle in obese persons can ultimately result in type 2 diabetes.[5]

What we *didn't know* until this past decade is *that high levels of leptin are associated with osteoarthritis!* Leptin is highly involved in immune and inflammation responses within the body. Studies have shown leptin to be part of the disease process in many disorders. For example, these would include autoimmune conditions that affect the bowel, and type 1 diabetes. Now we know that *osteoarthritis is affected too.*[6]

So, how exactly is leptin connected with osteoarthritis? Basically, leptin causes a release of cytokines that in turn causes cartilage breakdown. Cytokines are powerful cell-to-cell messengers within the body. Whether you experience arthritis or the stubborn metabolic syndrome that keeps you obese, may all depend to a large extent upon which cytokines are the key players in your body. In contrast, if you have smoothly working joints and an efficiently working metabolism that keeps you lean, this may also be a result of which cytokines predominate within your body. Cytokines can increase inflammation or decrease it depending upon whether they are proinflammatory or anti-inflammatory cytokines. In the case of osteoarthritis, leptin causes the release of proinflammatory cytokines.

These proinflammatory cytokines have a role in breaking down cartilage cells and in decreasing the production of collagen in the joint cartilage. The collagen acts to provide structure and shape to the cartilage; its breakdown is part of the destructive process of osteo-arthritis. The process begins with proteoglycans lost first, and then the joint is further damaged through collagen degradation.[7] Proteo-glycans are essential for smooth joint movement. They exist in the extracellular matrix of cartilage cells. This matrix contains collagen and a ground substance that is composed of proteoglycans and elastin (which is a connective tissue elastic in nature). The main function of proteoglycans is to hydrate the tissue and to help them swell so that the tissue can stand up to the force of compression.[8]

You have probably heard of chondroitin if you are one of the many people who have tried glucosamine/chondroitin supplements. Well, chondroitin sulfate is a proteoglycan. Hyaluronic acid is part of what is called a proteoglycan aggregate; this is basically a group of proteoglycans collected together to form a whole, bound to a long hyaluronic acid molecule. You can picture this by thinking of a delicate branch off of a shrub with the stem itself representing the hyaluronic acid molecule and the attached offshoots to the main stem, the proteoglycans. The bulk of hyaluronic acid that is present in carti-lage is associated with these proteoglycan aggregates. Non-aggregat-ed proteoglycans, those not combined together, do not intermingle with hyaluronic acid in the same way.[9]

So, basically proteoglycans form proteoglycan aggregates which come together with hyaluronic acid. Hyaluronic acid plays a vital role in assisting the cartilage to withstand friction, obtain ade-quate lubrication, and prevent wear.[10] Many of you reading this who have arthritis may have heard of hyaluronic acid which is what is injected into the knee joint in the "rooster comb injections" (which, by the way, may not be a good idea -- please see "Topic of Interest #1" below). The proteoglycans and collagen (the main protein providing structure and shape to the cartilage tissue) are degraded in osteoarthritis. Cartilage is broken down, and it is insufficiently repaired or regenerated. Cartilage destruction is the result of this process. Proinflammatory cytokines are go-betweens that foster inflammatory processes and induce breakdown and loss of joint cartilage.[11] Essentially, leptin is capable of stimulating these proinflammatory cytokines that cause cartilage breakdown. Leptin also promotes nitric oxide synthesis which, along with the actions of the proinflammatory cytokines, can become destructive to cartilage.[12]

Topic of Interest #1

Why You Might Want to Reconsider "Rooster Comb Injections"

Some research has shown that hyaluronic acid injections derived from the comb of the rooster can have therapeutic effects on pain in knee osteoarthritis.[13,14] There are many people with knee joint pain trying out these injections and hoping to obtain relief from their pain. Nevertheless, some studies do not show significant treatment effects.[15,16] In addition, some studies suggest that it may work best for those with early osteoarthritis, rather than those whose disease has progressed.[17] What's more, other studies have actually found accelerated cartilage destruction associated with hyaluronic acid injections![18,19]

For example, a large experimental study out of Denmark followed 337 people with osteoarthritis over a period of one year. It was found that for people with moderate to severe osteoarthritis of the knee, there was *no difference* between the treated group that had received intra-articular hyaluronan injections to the knee once a week for five weeks and a placebo group that had received saline injections, instead.[20]

In a ground-breaking study out of Baylor College of Medicine, researchers found the shocking result that hyaluronic acid injections may actually *accelerate* cartilage breakdown in patients with knee osteoarthritis. This was the first study to look at changes in biomarkers (or indicators of disease progression) of osteoarthritis after intra-articular hyaluronic acid injections in people with knee osteoarthritis. Contrary to what these researchers had predicted, the biomarkers showed *increased cartilage breakdown*.[21] Research from another study found that medial joint loading on the knee increased in those who responded to intra-articular hyaluronic acid injection of the knee. The researchers' concluded that the pain relief may spur people to increase their loading onto the vulnerable medial compartment of the knee, resulting in *more accelerated joint deterioration.*[22]

Instead of hyaluronic acid injections that may possibly lead to greater joint deterioration, why not try something non-invasive that may protect your cartilage instead? For example, researchers at Case Western Department of Medicine have found that pomegranate inhibits cartilage breakdown, protects cartilage, and may have an inhibitory effect on arthritis.[23] Indeed, in at least one study of short term pain relief and functional improvement of knee osteoarthritis, even the non-invasive technique of mud pack therapy worked just as well as a "rooster comb shot"![24]

Drawing the Connection Between Leptin and Arthritis

The important association of leptin with "metabolic syndrome" and insulin resistance ushered in the considerations that along with type 2 diabetes, perhaps *other* chronic diseases such as degenerative joint disease might also be related to leptin. In the decade 2000-2010, research studies established vital linkages between leptin and osteoarthritis.[25] Obese individuals have been found to have significantly higher leptin levels than non-obese individuals.[26] Clearly the association between obesity as a key factor in the clinical syndrome of menopausal arthritis, and obesity and its connection to higher leptin levels, proves to be a vital connection of leptin to menopausal arthritis.

Dr. Cecil and Dr. Archer were correct; it was not just weight on the joints from increased mechanical load that caused menopausal arthritis, but rather something endocrine or hormonal in nature. However, they had discounted the idea that it might be "metabolic" in nature, stating that the metabolism of the women they had studied showed no real deviation from normal. Problem was, though, that when they had written this article, "insulin resistance" had not even really surfaced in the medical literature as of yet! This would not be a substantial topic of discussion until about the 1930's, with greater discussion beginning in the 1940's.[27,28] Moreover, the hormone, leptin, would not be discovered until the 1990's, when Jeffrey A. Friedman and colleagues discovered a gene that codes for leptin; the lack of the expression of this gene was the cause of a particular strain of obese mice.[29] Menopausal arthritis was indeed *both* hormonal and metabolic in nature, but at the time that Drs. Cecil and Archer did their research, the nature of these connections were as yet unknown.

The Surprising Role of Leptin

The recent research linking leptin to the disease process of osteoarthritis is ground-breaking! Again, most of us have heard of leptin as being important in signaling to our bodies that we have enough energy resources and supply and that it is okay to stop eating. However, this surprising connection with arthritis would not be one that many of us would have ever suspected! This new body of know-ledge revealed that leptin (and adiponectin) secrete biologically active chemicals that modify and in part control inflammatory processes.[30] The new focus was upon these adipokines. We talked earlier about cytokines; well, adipocytokines (also referred to as adipokines) are cytokines that are produced by adipose tissue such as leptin and adiponectin. Leptin and adiponectin have also been considered to be hormones that act upon other cytokines such as interleukin-6, for example.

These exciting connections between leptin and arthritis have only unfolded over the last decade or so. Presenters at the Global Arthritis Research Network: Fourth World Congress on Arthritis in Montreal in 2004 shared research that showed that leptin might possibly be the link between obesity and arthritis. These research findings showed that leptin levels in joint fluid corresponded to body mass index. The *greater the body mass, the greater the leptin levels in knee osteoarthritis* patients. They explained that leptin is not ordinarily produced by cartilage in normal knees, but in the cartilage from osteoarthritic knees there was a striking presence of leptin.

Moreover, the greater the expression of leptin in cartilage tissues, the greater the amount of cartilage destruction that was found.[31] There is even a difference between men and women with regard to leptin within the joint. Women have been shown to have higher levels of free leptin in the joint cavity. This, of course, points toward a possible reason why there may be a higher occurrence of osteoarthritis among women.[32] Dr. Cecil's and Dr. Archer's hunch that there must be something endocrine in nature proved true.

Also at the Fourth World Congress on Arthritis, researchers from the University of Michigan reported additional findings linking leptin with osteoarthritis. Their research showed that the osteoarthritis which is associated with obesity may partly be a result of leptin's capacity to increase a potent fatty acid found in body fat, arachidonic acid.[33] This is important because arachidonic acid facilitates the production of some of the inflammatory chemicals (such as leukotrienes and prostaglandins) that produce allergic and inflammatory reactions. Leukotrienes, for example, can cause immediate, powerful reactions to something to which you are allergic. You may be quite familiar with the association of leukotrienes to seasonal allergies, with some medications blocking the production of leukotrienes, not just blocking histamine (as in the action of antihistamines). So, countering the overproduction of leptin in the body may be a potential way of countering allergies, as well!

I had suffered from intense hay fever every spring for several years after returning to San Francisco from Boston. My eyes would begin to itch intensely, and then my eyelids would swell up so much that my eyes were barely visible. This would last for several months each year during the allergy season. When I went on my program to rid myself of my arthritis, I was amazed to find that for the first time in three years the allergy season had passed without any of my eye itching and irritation, or swelling! Apparently, I had decreased the inflammatory response through my herbs and supplements! It appears that my inflammation may have possibly been caused by high arachidonic acid (perhaps resulting from leptin resistance) that led to leukotriene secretion and allergies. Also, with the typical Western diet, human cells are predisposed to having a rather high content of arachidonic acid. Supplementation with the omega 3 fatty acids EPA and DHA can help to modify this oversupply of arachidonic acid in the cells.[34] I had also been taking fish oil supplements abundant with omega 3 fatty acids. We will take a closer look at these invaluable anti-inflammatory and balancing nutritional supports in Chapter Ten.

During this groundbreaking decade of research on leptin, it had indeed become clear that the inflammation associated with obesity, leptin resistance, and insulin resistance, had yet another manifestation -- arthritis. In 2010, researchers out of George Washington University went so far as to declare that "…osteoarthritis deserves a seat at the Metabolic Syndrome 'table' of disorders."[35] They emphasized that calling osteoarthritis a "degenerative" disease *was simply inaccurate*. The unique proteins and genes involved in osteoarthritis indicated inflammation as being highly involved. They stressed that osteoarthritis and metabolic syndrome have related bio-chemical profiles and similar inflammatory responses.[36]

Cytokines and Inflammation

So what are some of the inflammatory responses that are common to both metabolic syndrome and to osteoarthritis? How is leptin involved in ways that could contribute to menopausal arthritis? To understand the similar inflammatory responses one must look at cytokines. As noted earlier, cytokines are proteins with an enormous power to influence how your body's cells will operate. These small but commanding proteins can determine how your cells interact with one another. Cytokines are released by a variety of cells within the body (such as T cells that are key immune cells). They can actually change the communication and behavior between cells within your body. Your cells carry on elaborate communications with each other, and cytokines are the controlling mediators. The directives that they deliver to waiting cells (such as those in your joint cartilage) can determine whether the joint cartilage will be attacked and degraded or conversely, protected and maintained.

Recall as I had mentioned earlier, that your body has *both* proinflammatory cytokines and anti-inflammatory cytokines, and ulti-mately your overall health has a lot to do with which ones are acti-vated. Acquiring ways of intervening in this intense interchange between cytokines and cells within your body is a *primary* means of healing from menopausal arthritis! Although the number of cytokines that influence arthritis is rather daunting, a large number of them belong to a family of cytokines known as interleukins.

Interleukins are vital to the immune and inflammatory responses within the body. The interleukins (similar to all cytokines) are not stockpiled within cells. Instead, when prompted by a stimulus such as bacteria, for example, they are then rapidly produced and released. After interleukins are secreted, they attach to their target cell. This initiates a series of signals to occur (called a signaling cascade) that proceeds to affect the cell's actions. There is a dizzying array of numbered interleukins (e.g., IL-1, IL-4, IL-6, IL-8, IL-10, etc.). Some are proinflammatory such as IL-1; some are anti-inflammatory such as IL-10; and some can have both functions such as IL-6 (although it seems to be proinflammatory in many arthritis processes).

Another important cytokine is tumor necrosis factor. Tumor necrosis factor (necrosis meaning "death") is another proinflammatory cytokine. It is named as such because when it is working in its most beneficial sense, it destroys tumor cells. Tumor necrosis factor (TNF) is involved in a whole variety of biological processes from fat metabolism, blood clotting, and insulin resistance, to the functioning of the cells that line the blood vessels. It is also highly involved within the inflammation process.

The inflammatory cytokine, interleukin-6 (IL-6) along with C-reactive protein (CRP), a plasma protein (one of many proteins found in blood), are two inflammatory chemicals connected with metabolic syndrome.[37] The unusual nature of IL-6, though, is that it can sometimes be proinflammatory, and other times anti-inflammatory. Its double-sided nature makes its significance in disease processes somewhat confusing. It appears, though, that its actions in arthritis are primarily proinflammatory, although it can even play different roles within the same disease process. For example, in an animal research study, IL-6 had a dual role with respect to its actions on connective tissue. IL-6 reduced the loss of proteoglycans (needed for the lubrication of the joint) in the *beginning* during the acute phase. However, IL-6 *promoted osteophyte (abnormal bony outgrowths) formation* in the *chronic* phase of the disease.[38] This promotion of osteophytes is important, as they are associated with how severe the arthritis is, and the extent of cartilage breakdown and destruction that occurs. The presence of a greater number of osteophytes is associated with more advanced arthritis.

Knee Osteoarthritis and the Commanding Cytokines

Now that you have a brief introduction to the key cytokine players, let us look at knee osteoarthritis which is the primary joint problem in menopausal arthritis. In a study of radiographic knee osteoarthritis, both IL-6 and CRP were elevated.[39] Additionally, in another recent study it was found that obese women had significantly higher IL-6 levels and higher levels of both IL-6 and tumor necrosis factor if they had high blood pressure. Levels of both of these proinflammatory cytokines increased as time since menopause increased.[40]

It is very clear that obesity and the disorders of insulin resistance, metabolic syndrome, and arthritis have common indicators of inflammation; these disorders are involved in complex and interactive ways! If one lowers leptin resistance, for example, one might find that insulin resistance lessens as well. Or, if one lowers leptin resistance, one might find that arthritis symptoms diminish and blood pressure is reduced. In fact, research has shown that leptin may provide a link between obesity and high blood pressure. Higher leptin levels are related to higher blood pressure in both men and women.[41]

BMI was also significantly higher in the people with knee osteoarthritis.[42] This brings us back to the point that obesity (a factor in metabolic syndrome) is significantly associated with osteoarthritis. Nevertheless, not all obesity is equal! Researchers at the University of Michigan stressed that not all types of obesity have the same effects upon knee osteoarthritis. Endocrine and other processes initiated by fat cells affect the knee joint, demonstrating that osteoarthritis exists in an *extremely metabolic milieu.* Within this dynamic environment, inflammation is imposed upon the knee joints by adipokines (also called adipocytokines) from body fat. As discussed earlier, adipocytokines are cytokines that are secreted by adipose, or fat cells; thus, they are also cell-to-cell communicators. It is not just *any body fat,* however, that will produce this particular cytokine mix and effect upon knee osteoarthritis. As Dr. Sowers and colleague wrote, ". . . pound-for-pound, not all obesity is equivalent for the development of knee osteoarthritis; development appears to be strongly related to the coexistence of disordered glucose and lipid metabolism."[43] Disturbed glucose and lipid metabolism seem to go hand-in-hand with the obesity that is associated with knee osteoarthritis. Moreover, as we saw earlier when talking about the yin and yang nature of insulin and leptin, disturbed glucose metabolism (such as in insulin resistance) is associated with higher leptin levels.

Increased abdominal fat in women during the menopausal transition leads to abnormal adipokine production. Leptin, an adipokine and a hormone, increases in postmenopausal women. High levels of leptin, as in the case of leptin resistance (and low levels of adiponectin), have been associated with the risk for type 2 diabetes, cardiovascular disease and metabolic syndrome.[44] Visceral adipose tissue is believed to increase the production of proinflammatory cytokines. It appears to be the *ratio* of adiponectin to leptin within the synovial fluid of the knee that predicts knee osteoarthritis, however. A greater adiponectin to leptin ratio is associated with *less* pain among people with severe knee osteoarthritis.[45]

Discussing white adipose tissue (WAT) as an endocrine organ brings to mind the "omentum" (that apron-like fatty organ that everyone trying to diet recently has no doubt heard about). However, apparently it is not the *only* fat pad that should concern you if you are suffering from menopausal arthritis (See Topic of Interest #2).

Topic of Interest #2

Why the Omentum Is Not the Only Fat Pad You May Need to Worry About

Remarkably, the infrapatellar fat pad (the little pad of fat that rests just under and behind your knee cap) is an active, joint tissue which can secrete inflammatory cytokines such as IL-6! What's more, it contains macrophages and lymphocytes that can further the disease process.[46,47] This is similar to what the visceral white adipose tissue (WAT) does within your omentum! Research has found that both the joint lining (synovium) and the infrapatellar fat pad have been shown to release *large amounts of leptin*.[48]

The low-grade inflammation that comes with obesity is associated with increased adipokines or cytokines. Could this fat pad on top of the knee be a contributing cause in knee osteoarthritis? In one study it was found that for people with osteoarthritis, the volume of their fat pad was associated with their age; that is, it enlarged with age. Are people with knee osteoarthritis more disposed to an enlarging knee fat pad, or do some of the processes in knee osteoarthritis cause the knee fat pad to get larger? Researchers do not know at this point. We will just have to await further research to find some of the ways that fat in local areas (such as this one on top of the knee) may contribute to osteoarthritis.[49] If it is at all like the omentum, then one could guess that a larger fat pad might mean more proinflammatory cytokines being released.

Speaking of white adipose tissue, we sometimes do not think about the fact that it is not only made up of adipocytes (fat cells). The non-fat cells, such as connective tissues cells and those that line the blood vessels, for example, are not always thought of when we think of "adipose tissue." Moreover, there are also macrophages (large, white blood cells) that are present in fat tissue, as well. In fact, obesity is linked with the buildup of macrophages in white adipose tissue. It has also been found that these macrophages are responsible for nearly all of the production of tumor necrosis factor-alpha and a significant amount of IL-6, as well.[50]

We *should indeed* be focusing on these non-fat cells in fatty tissue! It turns out that over 90% of the release of adipokines such as tumor necrosis factor-alpha (TNF-α), IL-6, IL-8, IL-10, to name just a few, are directly released by *non-fat cells* in the adipose tissue! In a study of 12 adipokines released from the adipose tissue of obese women, it was found that only leptin and lipoprotein lipase (LPL) were released almost exclusively by fat cells.[51] The rest of the destructive lot, such as tumor necrosis factor-alpha and other very active proinflammatory cytokines in osteoarthritis, are produced by non-fat cells in adipose tissue!

Going back to the adipokines and their role in arthritis, we have heard a lot about leptin. However, what is adiponectin's role in osteoarthritis? One of the functions of adiponectin in the body is to boost insulin sensitivity by cutting the amount of circulating fatty acids and reducing triglycerides in the muscle and liver.[52] Similar to leptin, adiponectin has multiple functions within the body not directly related to arthritis. Adiponectin is the most plentiful protein in white adipose tissue, and it does have very strong anti-inflammatory effects (such as helping to prevent atherosclerosis).[53] It also reduces proinflammatory TNF-alpha and IL-6.[54] However, in arthritis, the role that adiponectin plays is unclear at this point. On the negative side, this critical adipokine has been implicated in stimulating proinflammatory cytokines in cartilage cells. Some research shows that adiponectin increases nitric oxide (NO) and metalloproteinases (MMPs) which lead to degradation of osteoarthritis cartilage.[55,56] Matrix metalloproteinases have the ability to break down protein such as collagen, the fundamental building block of connective tissues.

On the positive side, other research has shown a protective effect of adiponectin in osteoarthritis. For example, it had been found that adiponectin may positively contribute to preservation of cartilage by increasing TIMP-2 (which inhibits destructive metalloproteinases that break down cartilage). It may also decrease MMP-13 (a type of metalloproteinase) related to cartilage degradation in osteoarthritis.[57] Some researchers have argued that adiponectin has a role merely in insulin and fat metabolism, not a role in promoting inflammation. Its effects are seen as metabolic, not proinflammatory.[58] It may, however, be more a matter of the ratio of adiponectin to leptin that is most important. Recall that in the study of knee osteoarthritis cited earlier, that the severity of pain was less with a higher adiponectin to leptin ratio.[59]

More Recently Discovered Adipokines and Their Roles in Arthritis

What about other more recently discovered adipokines that may have a role in arthritis such as resistin and newly identified visfatin? Both of these proinflammatory adipokines have a role in altering insulin sensitivity although it has not been determined just exactly how they affect it. With regard to osteoarthritis, it has been found that knee osteoarthritis patients had higher levels of visfatin in their synovial fluid than those without knee osteoarthritis; a worsened grade of knee osteoarthritis was associated with higher visfatin levels. Visfatin also correlated with the markers for cartilage matrix degradation.[60] The role of these critical adipokines in menopausal women's health appears to extend into areas that had not previously been known. For example, originally resistin was thought to be a risk factor for insulin resistance, but the current research shows some contradictory findings in this regard.[61] It appears, though, that resistin may have a role in the risk of ischemic stroke (lack of adequate blood circulation to the brain) in postmenopausal women. In a current 2011 report on the results from the Women's Health Initiative, resistin (but neither leptin nor adiponectin) was associated with an increased risk of ischemic stroke in postmenopausal women. This result still held, even when obesity and other cardiovascular risk factors were taken into consideration.[62]

Cartilage cells in osteoarthritis patients have been found to produce visfatin, and synovial fluid visfatin is associated with carti- lage degradation.[63] Importantly, visfatin was found to be a trigger for the secretion of heightened and excessive amounts of prostaglandin E2.[64] We saw earlier that leptin increases arachidonic acid leading to the production of prostaglandins. Prostaglandin E2 is a primary factor in the process of osteoarthritis; it promotes cartilage destruction (as do the metalloproteinases). So, visfatin's ability to promote excessive amounts of prostaglandin E2 is important.[65] Moreover, it helped met- alloproteinases to be produced and set into motion.[66] Clearly, leptin is not the *only* adipokine associated with arthritis. It appears that a variety of adipokines and cytokines come together in specific ways to provide fertile ground for arthritis to develop and worsen. The re- search over the past decade or so that was described earlier, however, has provided a strong link among leptin, obesity and osteoarthritis.[67]

Leptin Resistance, Metabolic Syndrome and Menopause

Metabolic syndrome is highly associated with insulin resistance, as well as with high blood pressure and abdominal obesity. Metabolic Syndrome is also often referred to as Metabolic Syndrome X, or Insulin Resistance Syndrome. It has been recently defined on a National Institutes of Health website as a grouping of medical conditions that heighten one's risk for cardiovascular disease and diabetes to include the risk factors of: High blood pressure; high blood sugar, or insulin levels; high levels of triglycerides (a type of circulating fat) in your blood; low levels of HDL (high density lipoprotein, the "good" cholesterol); and excess fat around the waist (central or abdominal obesity). Although the cause is not agreed upon, insulin resistance is thought to be a condition that may be central to metabolic syndrome.[68]

So, is leptin resistance also associated with metabolic syndrome? Using similar parameters or biomarkers of the metabolic syndrome, researchers from the University of Verona found significant associations between leptin resistance and metabolic syndrome in postmenopausal, elderly women. Their research showed that leptin was significantly related to adiposity, insulin levels, insulin resistance, and cholesterol levels.[69] Thinking back to the "yin and yang" relationship between insulin and leptin, this makes sense. Moreover, it has been found that the increase in obesity among postmenopausal women resulted in increased production of leptin.[70] In fact, leptin is directly correlated with fat mass in both men and women. However, you might find it interesting to know that with regard to a given percentage of fat mass, women have been found to have *three times the level of leptin compared with men!*[71] Very importantly, the prevalence of metabolic syndrome increases greatly after menopause, as had been noted in Chapter One.[72,73,74] The increased leptin has the effect of producing increased insulin and insulin resistance, thought to be possibly central to metabolic syndrome.

Leptin and Menopausal Arthritis: Vital Connections

This research on leptin, obesity and osteoarthritis is important in shedding light on why women who gain abdominal weight in menopause may also be at higher risk for arthritis. The connection of osteoarthritis with obesity is, of course, extremely important to menopausal arthritis. As we saw in the classic medical study of Drs. Cecil and Archer, obesity was the *second most associated factor with menopausal arthritis following the state of being in menopause.* As noted earlier, obesity results in higher leptin levels. The linkage of abdominal obesity and leptin, and leptin and arthritis is clear.

With these things in mind: *Overcoming leptin resistance is one of the key factors in combatting menopausal arthritis*! We will discuss ways to lower leptin levels associated with leptin resistance in Part II of this book. What is critical to understand is that research has shown that the effects of leptin within the body go *beyond* just energy regulation: *Leptin is a key player in the process of osteoarthritis.*

Notes for Chapter Two

[1]Ahima, R. S., & Flier, J. S. (2000). Adipose tissue as an endocrine organ. *Trends in Endocrinology and Metabolism, 11*(8), 327-332.

[2]Zhang, Y., Proenca, R., Maffei, M., Barone, M., Leopold L., & Friedman, J. M. (1994). Positional cloning of the mouse obese gene and its human homologue. *Nature, 372*(6505), 425-432.

[3]Scherer, T., & Buettner, C. (2011). Yin and yang of hypothalamic insulin and leptin signaling in regulating white adipose tissue metabolism. *Reviews in Endocrine and Metabolic Disorders, 12*(3), 235-243. doi: 10.1007/s11154-011-9190-4

[4]Ibid.

[5]Seufert, J. (2004). Leptin effects on pancreatic ß-cell gene expression and function. *Diabetes, 53*(Suppl.1), S152-S158.

[6]Lago, R., Gómez, R., Lago, F., Gómez-Reino, J., & Gualillo, O. (2008). Leptin beyond body weight regulation – Current concepts concerning its role in immune function and inflammation. *Cellular Immunology, 252*(1-2), 139-145.

[7]Oohashi, T., & Nishida, K. (2011). Cutting edge on research of cartilage metabolism. Recent progress in bio-molecular imaging of articular cartilage. *Clinical Calcium, 21*(6), 896-902.

[8]Yanagishita, M. (1993). Function of proteoglycans in the extracellular matrix. *Acta Pathologica Japonica, 43*(6), 283-293.

[9]Hardingham, T. E., & Muir, H. (1974). Hyaluronic acid in cartilage and proteoglycan aggregation. *Biochemical Journal, 139*(3), 565-581.

[10]Greene, G. W., Banquy, X., Lee, D. W., Lowrey, D. D., Yu, J., & Israelachvili, J. N. (2011). Adaptive mechanically controlled lubrication mechanism found in articular joints. *Proceedings of the National Academy of Sciences of the United States of America, 108*(13), 5255-5259.

[11]Abramson, S. B. , & Attur, M. (2009). Developments in the scientific understanding of osteoarthritis. *Arthritis Research & Therapy, 11*(3). doi: 10.1186/ar2655

[12]Otero, M., Lago, R., Gomez, R., Dieguez, C., Lago, F., Gómez-Reino, J., Gualillo, O. (2006). Towards a pro-inflammatory and immunomodulatory emerging role of leptin. *Rheumatology (Oxford), 45*(8), 944-950.

[13]Wang, C. T., Lin, J., Chang, C. J., Lin, Y. T., & Hou, S. M. (2004). Therapeutic effects of hyaluronic acid on osteoarthritis of the knee. A meta-analysis of randomized controlled trials. *Journal of Bone and Joint Surgery. American Volume, 86-A*(3), 538-545.

[14]Brzusek, D., & Petron, D. (2008). Treating knee osteoarthritis with intra-articular hyaluronans. *Current Medical Research and Opinion, 24*(12), 3307-3322.

[15]Zhang, W., Nuki, G., Moskowitz, R. W., Abramson, S., Altman, R. D., Arden, N. K., Bierma-Zeinstra, S., Brandt, K. D., Croft, P., Doherty, M., Dougados, M., Hochberg, M., Hunter, D. J., Kwoh, K., Lohmander, L. S., & Tugwell, P. (2010). OARSI recommendations for the management of hip and knee osteoarthritis: Part III: Changes in evidence following systematic cumulative update of research published through January 2009. *Osteoarthritis and Cartilage, 18*(4), 476-499. doi: 10.1016/j.joca.2010.01.013

[16]Jørgensen, A., Stengaard-Pedersen, K., Simonsen, O., Pfeiffer-Jensen, M., Eriksen, C., Bliddal, H., Pedersen, N. W. Bødtker, S., Hørslev-Petersen, K., Snerum, L. Ø., Egund, N., & Frimer-Larsen, H. (2010). Intra-articular hyaluronan is without clinical effect in knee osteoarthritis: A multicentre, randomised, placebo-controlled, double-blind study of 337 patients followed for 1 year. *Annals of the Rheumatic Diseases, 69*(6), 1097-1102.

[17]Hasegawa, M., Nakoshi, Y., Tsujii, M., Sudo, A., Masuda, H., Yoshida, T., & Uchida, A. (2008). Changes in biochemical markers and prediction of effectiveness of intra-articular hyaluronan in patients with knee osteoarthritis. *Osteoarthritis and Cartilage, 16*(4), 526-529.

[18]Gonzalez-Fuentes, A.M., Green, D. M., Rossen, R. D., & Ng, B. (2010). Intra-articular hyaluronic acid increases cartilage breakdown biomarker in patients with knee osteoarthitis. *Clinical Rehumatology, 29*(6), 619-624.

[19]Briem, K., Axe, M. J., & Snyder-Mackler, L. (2009). Medial knee joint loading increases in those who respond to hyaluronan injection for medial knee osteoarthritis. *Journal of Orthopaedic Research, 27*(11), 1420-1425.

[20]Jørgensen et al. (2010). Op. Cit.

[21]Gonzalez-Fuentes et al. (2020). Op. Cit.

[22]Briem et al. (2009). Op. Cit.

[23]Rasheed, Z., Akhtar, N., & Haqqi, T. M. (2010). Pomegranate extract inhibits the interleukin-1ß-induced activation of MKK-3, p38_-MAPK and transcription factor RUNX-2 in human osteoarthritis chondrocytes. *Arthritis Research & Therapy, 12*(5), R195.

[24]Bostan, B., Sen, U., Güne, S, T., Sahin, S.A., Sen, C., Erdem, M., & Erkorkmaz, U. (2010). Comparison of intra-articular hyaluronic acid injections and mud-pack therapy in the treatment of knee osteoarthritis, *Acta Orthopaedica et Traumatologica Turcica, 44*(1), 42-47.

[25]Presle, N., Pottie, P., Mainard, D., Netter, P., & Terlain, B. (2007). Adipokines in osteoarthritis. In L. Sharma and F. Berenbaum (Eds.) *Osteoarthritis: A companion to rheumatology* (pp. 85-103). Philadelphia, PA: Mosby Elsevier.

[26]Considine, R.V., Sinha, M. K., Heiman, M. L., Kriauciunas, A., Stephens, T. W., Nyce, M. R., Ohannesian, J. P., Marco, C. C., McKee., L. J., Bauer, T. L., & Caro, J. F. (1996). Serum immunoreactive-leptin concentrations in normal-weight and obese humans. *New England Journal of Medicine, 334*, 292-295.

[27]Root, H. F., & Carpenter, T. M. (1940). Studies of carbohydrate metabolism in cases of insulin resistance. *Transactions of the American Clinical and Climatological Association, 56*, 1-11.

[28]Axelrod, A. R., Lobe, S., Orten, J. M., & Myers, G. B. (1947). Insulin resistance. *Annals of Internal Medicine, 27*(4), 555-574.

[29]Zhang, Y. et al. (1994). Op. Cit.

[30]Gómez, R., Conde, J., Scotece, M. Gómez-Reino, J. J., Lago, F., & Gualillo, O. (2011). What's new in our understanding of the role of adipokines in rheumatic diseases? *Nature Reviews Rheumatology, 7*(9), 528-536. doi:10.1038/nrrheum.2011.107

[31]Pottie, P., Presle, N., Dumond, H., Terlain, B., Mainard, D., Leuille, D., & Netter, P. (2004) Is leptin the link between obesity and osteoarthritis? *Arthritis Research and Therapy, 6*(Suppl. 3), 8. doi: 10.1186/ar1342

[32]Presle, N., Pottie, P., Dumond, H., Guillaume, C., Lapicque, F., Pallu, S., Mainard, D., Netter, P., & Terlain, B. (2006). Differential distribution of adipokines between serum and synovial fluid in patients with osteoarthritis. Contribution of joint tissues to their articular production. *Osteoarthritis and Cartilage, 14*(7), 690-695. doi:10.1016/j.joca.2006.01.009

[33]Mancuso, P., Mehta, H. H., Canetti, C., Peters-Golden, M., Roessler, B. J., & Crofford, L. J. (2004). Regulation of eicosanoid synthesis by leptin. *Arthritis Research & Therapy, 6* (Suppl. 3), 9. doi: 10.1186/ar1343

[34]Calder, P. C. (2012). Mechanisms of action of (n-3) fatty acids. *Journal of Nutrition*. Advance online publication. PMID: 22279140

[35]Katz, J. D., Agrawal, S., & Velasquez, M. (2010). Getting to the heart of the matter: Osteoarthritis takes its place as part of the metabolic syndrome. *Current Opinions in Rheumatology, 22*(5), 512-519.

[36]Ibid.

[37]Kirilmaz, B., Asgun , F., Alioglu, E., Ercan, E., Tengiz, I., Turk, U., Saygi, S., & Ozerkan, F. (2010). High inflammatory activity related to the number of metabolic syndrome components. *Journal of Clinical Hypertension, 12*(2), 136-144.

[38]van de Loo, F. A., Kuiper, S., van Enckevort, F. H., Arntz, O. J., & van den Berg, W. B. (1997). Interleukin-6 reduces cartilage destruction during experimental arthritis. A study in interleukin-6-deficient mice. *American Journal of Pathology, 151*(1), 177-191.

[39]Livshits, G., Zhai, G., Hart, D. J., Kato, B. S., Wang, H., Williams, F. M., & Spector, T. D. (2009). Interleukin-6 is a significant predictor of radiographic knee osteoarthritis: The Chingford Study. *Arthritis and Rheumatism, 60*(7), 2037-2045.

[40]Chedraui et al. (2011). Op. Cit.

[41]Shankar, A., & Xiao, J. (2010). Positive relationship between plasma leptin level and hypertension. *Hyptertension, 56*(4), 623-628.

[42]Livshits et al. (2009). Op. Cit.

[43]Sowers, M. R., & Karvonen-Gutierrez, C. A. (2010). The evolving role of obesity in knee osteoarthritis. *Current Opinion in Rheumatology, 22*(5), 533-537.

[44]Lecke, S. B., Morsch, D. M., & Spritzer, P. M. (2011). Leptin and adiponectin in the female life course. *Brazilian Journal of Medical and Biological Research, 44*(5), 381-387.

[45]Gandhi, R., Takahashi, M., Smith, H., Rizek, R., & Mahomed, N. N. (2010). The synovial fluid adiponectin-leptin ratio predicts pain with knee osteoarthritis. *Clinical Rheumatology, 29*(11), 1223-1228.

[46]Klein-Wieringa, I. R., Kloppenburg, M., Bastiaansen-Jenniskens, Y. M., Yusuf, E., Kwekkeboom, J. C., El-Bannoudi, H., Nelissen, R. G., Zuurmond, A., Stojanovic-Susulic, V., Van Osch, G. J., Toes, R. E., & Ioan-Facsinay, A. (2011). The infrapatellar fat pad of patients with osteoarthritis has an inflammatory phenotype. *Annals of the Rheumatic Diseases, 70*(5), 851-857.

[47]Clockaerts, S., Bastiaansen-Jenniskens, Y. M., Runhaar, J., Van Osch, G. J., Van Offel, J. F., Verhaar, J. A., De Clerck, L. S., & Somville, J. (2010). The infrapatellar fat pad should be considered as an active osteoarthritic joint tissue: A narrative review. *Osteoarthritis and Cartilage, 18*(7), 876-882.

[48]Presle et al. (2006). Op. Cit.

[49]Chuckpaiwong, B., Charles, H. C., Kraus, V. B., Guilak, F., & Nunley, J. A. (2010). Age-associated increases in the size of the infrapatellar fat pad in knee osteoarthritis as measured by 3T MRI. *Journal of Orthopaedic Research, 28*(9), 1149-1154.

[50]Weisberg, S. P., McCann, D., Desai, M., Rosenbaum, M., Leibel, R. L., & Ferrante, Jr., A. W. (2003). Obesity is associated with macrophage accumulation in adipose tissue. *Journal of Clinical Investigation, 112*(12), 1796-1808. doi: 10.1172/JCI200319246

[51]Fain, J. N., Tagele, B. M., Cheema, P., Madan, A. K., & Tichansky, D. S. (2010). Release of 12 adipokines by adipose tissue, nonfat cells, and fat cells from obese women. *Obesity, 18*(5), 890-896. doi: 10.1038/oby.2009.335

[52]Presle et al. (2006). Op. Cit.

[53]Brochu-Gaudreau, K., Rehfeldt, C., Blouin, R., Bordignon, V., Murphy, B. D., & Palin, M. F. (2010). Adiponectin action from head to toe. *Endocrine, 37*(1), 11-32.

[54]Weigert, J., Neumeier, M., Schäffler, A., Fleck, M., Sch_lmerich, J., Schütz, C., & Buechler, C. (2005). The adiponectin paralog CORS-26 has anti-inflammatory properties and is produced by human monocytic cells. *FEBS Letters, 579*(25), 5565-5570.

[55]Lago, R., Gomez, R., Otero, M., Lago, F., Gallego, R., Dieguez, C., Gomez-Reino, J. J., & Gualillo, O. (2008). A new player in cartilage homeostasis: Adiponectin induces nitric oxide synthase type II and pro-inflammatory cytokines in chondrocytes. *Osteoarthritis and Cartilage, 16*(9), 1101-1109. doi: 10.1016/j.joca.2007.12.008

[56]Kang, E . H. , Lee, Y. J., Kim, T. K., Chang, C. B., Chung, J-H, Shin, K., Lee, E. Y., & Lee, E. B., & Song, Y. W. (2010). Adiponectin is a potential catabolic mediator in osteoarthritis cartilage. *Arthritis Research & Therapy, 12*, R231. doi:10.1186/ar3218.

[57]Chen, T. H., Chen, L., Hsieh, M. S., Chang, C. P., Chou, D. T., & Tsai, S. H. (2006). Evidence for a protective role for adiponectin in osteoarthritis. *Biochimica et Biophysica Acta, 1762*(8), 711-718.

[58]Schäffler, A., Ehling, A., Neumann, E., Herfarth, H., Tarner, I., Sch_lmerich, J., Müller-Ladner, U., & Gay, S. (2003). Adipocytokines in synovial fluid. *Journal of the American Medical Association, 290*(13), 1709-1710.

[59]Gandhi et al. (2010). Op. Cit.

[60]Stofkova, A. (2010). Resistin and visfatin: Regulators of insulin sensitivity, inflammation and immunity. *Endocrine Regulations, 44*(1), 25-36.

[61]Ibid.

[62]Rajpathak, S. N., Kaplan, R. C., Wassertheil-Smoller, S., Cushman, M., Rohan, T. E., McGinn, A. P., Wang, T., Strickler, H. D., Scherer, P. E., Mackey, R., Curb, D., & Ho, G. Y. (2011). Resistin, but not adiponectin and leptin, is associated with the risk of ischemic stroke among postmenpausal women: Results from the Women's Health Initiative. *Stroke, 42*(7), 1813-1820.

[63]Duan, Y., Hao, D., Li, M. Wu, Z., Li, D., Yang, X., & Qiu, G. (2011). Increased synovial fluid visfatin is positively linked to cartilage degradation biomarkers in osteoarthritis. *Rheumatology International*, In Press. doi: 10.1007/s00296-010-1731-8

[64]Gosset, M., Berenbaum, F., Salvat, C., Sautet, A., Pigenet, A., Tahiri, K., & Jacques, C. (2008). Crucial role of visfatin/pre-B cell colony-enhancing factor in matrix degradation and prostaglandin E2 synthesis in chondrocytes: possible influence on osteoarthritis. *Arthritis & Rheumatism, 58*(5), 1399-1409.

[65]Pallu, S., Francin, P. J., Guillaume, C., Gegout-Pottie, P., Netter, P. , Mainard, D., Terlain, B., & Presle, N. (2010). Obesity affects the chondrocyte responsiveness to leptin in patients with osteoarthritis. *Arthritis Research & Therapy, 12*(3), R112.

[66]Gossett et al. (2008). Op. Cit.

[67]Pallu et al. (2010). Op. Cit.

[68]MedlinePlus (U.S. National Library of Medicine) (2011, August 31). Metabolic syndrome. Retrieved from: http://www.nim.nih.gov/medlineplus/metabolicsyndrome.html

[69]Zamboni, M., Zoico, E., Fantin, F., Panourgia, M. P., Di Francesco, V., Tosoni, P., Solerte, B., Vettor, R., & Bosello, O. (2004). Relation between leptin and the metabolic syndrome in elderly women. *Journals of Gerontology. Series A, Biological Sciences and Medical Sciences, 59*(4), 396-400.

[70]Hong, S. C., Yoo, S. W., Cho, G. J., Kim, T., Hur, J. Y., Park, Y., K., Lee, K. W., & Kim, S. H. (2007). Correlation between estrogens and serum adipocytokines in premenpausal and postmenopausal women. *Menopause, 14*(5), 835-840.

[71]Nicklas, B. J., Katzel, L. I., Ryan, A. S., Dennis, K. E., & Goldberg, A. P. (1997). Gender differences in the response of plasma leptin concentrations to weight loss in obese older individuals. *Obesity Research, 5*(1), 62-68.

[72]Chedraui, P., Jaramillo, W., Pérez-López, F. R., Escobar, G. S., Morocho, N., & Hidalgo, L. (2011). Pro-inflammatory cytokine levels in postmenopausal women with metabolic syndrome. *Gynecological Endocrinology, 27*(9), 685-691.

[73]Jehn, M., Clark, J. M., & Guallar, E. (2004). Serum ferritin and risk of metabolic syndrome in U.S. adults. *Diabetes Care, 27*(10), 2422-2428.

[74]Eshtiaghi, R., Esteghamati, A., & Nakhjavani, M. (2010). Menopause is an independent predictor of metabolic syndrome in Iranian women. *Maturitas, 65*(3), 262-266.

Chapter Three

Estrogen and Menopausal Arthritis

—— ◼ ——

Estrogen's Role in Menopausal Arthritis

What exactly is estrogen's role in menopausal arthritis? How does estrogen fit into the picture? We have seen in the previous chapter how cytokines can either promote the disease process of osteoarthritis or help prevent it depending upon whether they are pro-inflammatory or anti-inflammatory cytokines. Estrogen seems to play a role in the back and forth communication between these cellular messengers. We also saw that insulin and leptin were involved. Disorders of energy metabolism are associated with the metabolic syndrome, and the prevalence of metabolic syndrome increases in women after menopause. How exactly is estrogen involved in these processes? In this chapter we will explore the effects of estrogen on the many factors associated with menopausal arthritis. We will also take a look at whether estrogen replacement therapy helps stem osteoarthritis in menopausal and postmenopausal women.

Dr. Jorge Roman-Blas and colleagues conducted a review of the literature on osteoarthritis and estrogen deficiency. They noted that many studies, both experimental and observational, have linked estrogen levels with joint health. As discussed earlier, there is a sharp rise in the prevalence of osteoarthritis in postmenopausal women. This rise in osteoarthritis post menopause has been associated with estrogen decline. Since estrogen receptors have been found in the joint tissues, this would point toward an association between estrogen depletion in menopause and osteoarthritis. These researchers stressed that not only does estrogen have an impact upon joint cartilage in osteoarthritis, but it also affects many *other* joint tissues such as the synovial lining (the lining within the capsule of the whole joint), the ligaments of the joint, the subchondral bone (the bone just below the cartilage), as well as surrounding muscles.[1] Important research findings include the discovery that estrogens may help prevent the synthesis of proinflammatory cell messengers or cytokines, such as tumor necrosis factor-alpha (TNF-α) and interleukin-12 (IL-12). Moreover, estrogen may stimulate the production of anti-inflammatory cytokines, such as interleukin-10 (IL-10) and interleukin-4 (IL-4).[2]

As discussed earlier, menopause seems to be associated with the increased incidence of metabolic syndrome, and estrogen may be pivotal here. For example, in a very interesting animal study, researchers "silenced" or blocked the ability of estrogen receptors to work in a part of the hypothalamus critical to energy homeostasis or balance. These animals gained *visceral fat but not subcutaneous fat*. In fact, they exhibited characteristics associated with metabolic syndrome such as impaired glucose tolerance and elevated glucose levels.[3] In another animal study in which the estrogen receptors in the hypothalamus gland were silenced, it was found that estrogen receptor-alpha (ERalpha) was found to interact with both leptin and insulin signaling pathways (the chain of chemical reactions involving leptin and insulin use).[4] Clearly, estrogen and its loss are involved in processes in which leptin and insulin have important roles.

Let's not leap too fast to the conclusion that the lack of estrogen is the primary problem, though, in bringing on metabolic syndrome in menopausal women. Research shows that we need to consider the critical role of testosterone, as well. Women of course have lower levels of testosterone than men, but their bodies do produce testosterone. As a woman's estrogen levels begin to decline, the presence of testosterone becomes more visible and pronounced. Visceral fat increases in menopause, and this rise has been found to be directly associated with testosterone levels. In a very large research study, the "Study of Women's Health Across the Nation" (SWAN) it was found that bioavailable testosterone was significantly associated with visceral fat even after the researchers had adjusted for insulin resistance. Testosterone was clearly shown to play a critical role in determining where fat would be stored in these midlife women (ages 42-60 years). It was the testosterone, *not estrogen* (estradiol) that was significantly related to waist circumference.[5] Moreover, as testosterone increased and the hormonal profile became increasingly dominated by androgens in the transition from perimenopause to postmenopause, metabolic syndrome in women increased. This was found to be independent of aging itself.[6]

The Many Faces of Estrogen

It is commonly thought that estrogen has anti-inflammatory protective benefits in preventing arthritis as was noted above. However, some studies have shown estrogen to actually heighten or promote some autoimmune diseases. Whether it helps or hinders a particular disease seems to depend upon which type of T cell (along with related cytokines) is predominant. T cells, of course, are white blood cells active within the immune system to fight off disease. For example, estrogen has been found to worsen or heighten the symptoms of systemic lupus erythematosus (SLE) whereas it has been found to help or slow down rheumatoid arthritis. With pregnancy and the rise in estrogen, rheumatoid arthritis has been found to recede and symptoms greatly lessen. On the other hand, in the postpartum period when there is a rapid drop in estrogen levels, rheumatoid arthritis has been found to flare up, the body once again left without the additional protection afforded by estrogen.[7] However, it is important to note here that "menopausal arthritis" has usually been associated with *osteoarthritis, not rheumatoid arthritis*, and so our focus will be on the role of estrogen loss at the onset and progression of osteoarthritis during and after menopause. Whether this association with osteoarthritis is actually as clear-cut as it may have initially seemed will be discussed in Chapter Six.

With regard to osteoarthritis, Dr. Herrero-Beaumont and colleagues came to the conclusion that primary osteoarthritis (that which occurs in previously undamaged joints) can no longer be considered "primary." Where there is no obvious cause for the arthritis, these researchers have argued that there are three clear groupings: *genetically* controlled, *estrogen* regulated, and *aging* related. Which osteoarthritic changes occur as a result of aging and which as a result of estrogen loss? Dr. Herrero-Beaumont and colleagues noted that tendon stiffness and decreased thickness and density of the bone directly under the joint cartilage were found to be specific to aging, rather than to estrogen loss. Conversely, high turnover of the bone directly under the joint cartilage, and increased body fat associated with higher secretion of cytokines by fat tissue were associated with loss of estrogen, not aging.[8]

Estrogen loss does matter in promoting menopausal arthritis. In a review of the literature on aromatase inhibitors and arthralgia (joint pain) to include musculoskeletal symptoms, estrogen deprivation seemed to be highly linked with the syndrome of arthralgia and musculoskeletal pain. The findings from this review indicated that women who had taken medication (e.g., aromatase inhibitors) to lower estrogen levels to essentially postmenopause levels in the treatment of breast cancer also had a rapid onset of arthritis-like pain symptoms.[9]

In this review of the aromatase inhibitors and arthralgia mentioned above, it was explained that estrogen does not have any known direct effect on the cartilage structure of the joints that would contribute to the experience of joint pain. What it does affect is inflammation and the processing of pain that is registered by the nerve cells. Estrogen has the effect of countering the processing of pain by the nerve cells, and so women deprived of estrogen may experience increased pain as a result. Women have higher pain thresholds (i.e., able to withstand more pain) during pregnancy when estrogen levels are high. Also in research with non-pregnant animals, there were higher pain thresholds when pregnancy levels of estrogen and progesterone were simulated.[10]

However, the effects of estrogen are not relegated to just the effects of estradiol alone. This is the primary estrogen in premenopause in a woman's fertile years, and it is often in the spotlight. What can be overlooked though are the breakdown products of estrogen. For example, estradiol and estrone (the primary estrogen, post menopause) do not remain in the body in their exact forms without undergoing any changes. Rather, they embark on a physiological journey in which they are broken apart, both changing their character and their actions. There are some other interesting possibilities for why estrogen might in some instances help promote health and in others hamper it, and it has to do with these metabolites of estrogen. It appears that some forms that estrogen takes when it is broken down into its new entities may help ward off inflammation, and some may increase it.

Research has found that women with knee osteoarthritis were more likely to be high in one estrogen metabolite (16 alpha-hydroxyestrone) in comparison to another estrogen metabolite (2-hydroxyestrone). These are both products of the breakdown of estradiol and estrone that occurs within metabolism. In fact, obese women had significantly less 2-hydroxyestrone. This metabolite is associated with moderating the effects of prostaglandins and arachidonic acid. Recall that as we had noted in the last chapter, both prostaglandin E2 and arachidonic acid can promote inflammation. As BMI (body mass index) increased, the "good" estrogen metabolite 2-hydroxyestrone -- *the one that helps to ward off the effects of inflammation-causing prostaglandins and arachidonic acid* -- decreased.[11] Remember, aside from menopause the next strongest predictor of menopausal arthritis was obesity, as found within the classic study by Drs. Cecil and Archer.

Loss of estrogen during menopause and the metabolic changes occurring post menopause do matter in setting up the stage for a body more prone to menopausal arthritis. So, wouldn't estrogen replacement therapy help prevent and/or reverse menopausal arthritis, then? Maybe not.

Does Estrogen Supplementation Counter Menopausal Arthritis? – The Verdict's Still Out But the Case Isn't Very Convincing

Very early in the identification of menopausal arthritis, small trials of estrogen were attempted as it had appeared to be a hormonally mediated disease. Estrogen supplementation did not seem to have any significant effects, though, in lessening the arthritis symptoms.[12] Since those earlier times, many large-scale, controlled experimental studies have been conducted on the effects of estrogen supplementation on arthritis and the findings are mixed. Studies have assessed whether the chances of the onset of arthritis, the lessening of symptoms, and the prevention of the worsening of arthritis in post-menopausal women are affected by estrogen replacement therapy (ERT). What we do know so far is that the effects of ERT on arthritis are far from conclusive, showing different findings in different studies.

Some studies have found a decreased risk of radiographic knee osteoarthritis with hormone replacement therapy (HRT). The Chingford Study is one such trial in which 1,003 women aged 45-64 (mean age of 54.2 years) provided information on their HRT use which was then compared with x-rays of their hands and knees for the presence of osteoarthritis. The researchers used data for their analysis from 606 women who were definitely of postmenopausal status. These researchers found that HRT seemed to have provided a pro-tective effect against radiographically determined osteoarthritis of the knee. There was not a significant effect for the hand joints.[13]

Other large-scale studies have shown no statistically signifi-cant relationship between HRT and osteoarthritis. In the Heart and Estrogen/Progestin Replacement Study (HERS), for example, partici-pants with coronary heart disease (postmenopausal women under age 80, with a mean age of 66 years) were randomly assigned to an HRT group or non-HRT (placebo) group. They were then studied for a period of four years. In this trial group of post-menopausal women, no differences were found between the two groups (HRT or control/placebo) in terms of experience of knee pain or related disability. Hormone replacement therapy had no significant effect on women's self-reported symptoms.[14] Similarly, in a very large-scale population study of osteoarthritis with an elderly sample (mean age of the parti-cipants was 71 years) the Framingham Osteoarthritis Study, there was no statistically significant relationship found between estrogen use and knee osteoarthritis symptoms. The findings did show a trend for current users of estrogen replacement therapy (as opposed to "never users" or "past users") to have a decreased risk of their knee osteoarthritis worsening. Because of this moderate (although statis-tically non-significant) effect for current users, the authors interpreted their results as pointing toward a possible protective effect against worsening of the disease.[15]

Still other large studies have even shown an *increased* relationship between knee osteoarthritis and ERT. In a longitudinal study conducted out of the National Center for Health Statistics, the association between estrogen replacement therapy and arthritis in 2,416 postmenopausal women was examined. The risk of the occurrence of arthritis was found to be significantly *higher* among ERT users than among non-ERT users, and this risk *increased* the longer ERT was used. In fact, the risk for self-reported, physician-diagnosed arthritis among estrogen replacement users increased by 30% for 1-4 years of use, and by *96% for 4-10 years of use.* If the estrogen replacement therapy continued for 10 or more years, *the risk for arthritis was increased by 104%.*[16]

In just this simple illustration of four large studies, I am sure that you can see some of the problems with this body of research. Across studies, the women were of different ages, different types of hormonal therapy were used, and the health status of participants differed. In addition, they did not even measure the same things in terms of outcome; radiographic evidence of osteoarthritis is very different from self-reported symptoms or reported physician diagnosis.

Another problem is that in studies using hormone replacement therapy in which a progestin is added to estrogen, it isn't possible to disentangle the different effects of the two hormones. Research methodologies were not the same either with one study (the HERS Study) using an experimental research design allowing for greater certainty with regard to the meaning of the results obtained. The other studies were not experimental in nature; they simply measured the participants' symptoms and hormone use and then drew associations or correlations between these factors (which cannot be interpreted in any causal way).

Another complicating factor is that the effect of estrogen may be related to the body site of the osteoarthritis. For example, in a study of 1,001 postmenopausal women aged 43-97 years (mean age of 72) the effects of estrogen on hip, knee, and hand osteoarthritis were assessed. The evaluations were based upon history of pain plus a clinical examination. These researchers conducted analyses that would take into consideration the factors of age, BMI, exercise, smoking, and type of menopause (natural, or through hysterectomy and/or removal of the ovaries). This way they could control for these factors and separate them out from the effect of estrogen on osteoarthritis. What they found was that there were no differences among women who had used postmenopausal estrogen for at least one year and those who had not used it in the proportion of women with knee osteoarthritis. However, among women who had used postmenopausal estrogen, a greater proportion had hip and hand osteoarthritis in comparison to nonusers of postmenopausal estrogen.[17]

Overall, reviews of the association between estrogen (or estrogen plus progestin) supplementation and its effect upon arthritis do not offer strong evidence for the use of estrogen therapy. The conclusion from one research review was that the hormonal changes at menopause do seem to modulate or in some ways regulate changes seen in osteoarthritis (such as changes in cartilage). This would also be altered by the current state of the woman's cartilage and her own particular genes. Although it was concluded that there is evidence that HRT use reduces the progression of osteoarthritis and may have a preventative effect, they pointed out a major problem: *randomized, controlled studies* (such as the experimental study that I have described above) *are needed.*[18]

As a side note with regard to the influence of genes in osteoarthritis, research reveals some interesting connections. In a study of estrogen and androgen receptors and knee osteoarthritis, there were significant differences in combinations of long and short alleles (alternative forms of a gene in a pairing) for two different estrogen receptor types. For example, women with the long (contrasted with short) alleles for the estrogen receptor beta (ER-beta) along with androgen receptor genes, had a significantly greater risk for developing osteoarthritis.[19]

A more recent review on the effects of estrogen replacement therapy by some of the same researchers as the review above was conducted out of the Jean Hailes Foundation in 2004. They concluded that there is only weak evidence for the use of estrogen therapy for joint health in postmenopausal women. They did find that the results of the studies overall seemed to suggest a trend toward estrogen replacement therapy as protective against large joint osteoarthritis. There did seem to be a protective effect of long-term estrogen use on knee cartilage. There was little support for any protective effect on hand osteoarthritis, though. What these researchers concluded was that although estrogen replacement therapy might help in preserving joint health after menopause, *all of these data were from non-experimental studies.* Importantly as well, they noted that the viability of estrogen replacement therapy for knee osteoarthritis would seem unlikely given the reported risks and results from the Women's Health Initiative (WHI) study.[20]

Correlational studies simply cannot provide us with any conclusive information about whether estrogen use *caused* any of the observed effects. That is why these researchers emphasized that all of the findings were from non-experimental studies. Additionally, as most people are aware, the Women's Health Initiative trial of postmenopausal supplementation with estrogen and progestin was halted. This was due to the fact that more cases of breast cancer were being found than was expected, and the risks exceeded the benefits in continuing the trial. Estrogen plus progestin therapy may increase the risk of coronary heart disease among healthy postmenopausal women. It was concluded that the risk-benefit profile did not support estrogen and progestin as a practicable therapeutic intervention for chronic diseases.[21,22] The findings of this very large study, of course, changed the way in which estrogen replacement therapy and hormone replacement therapy are considered and approached as possible therapies for menopause and after.

Does Estrogen Replacement Therapy Prevent Muscle Loss and Deterioration?

Are women's muscles affected by estrogen replacement therapy in postmenopause? The research findings are mixed, and many questions still remain. For example, in one large research study of 840 postmenopausal women (ages 70-79), there was a significant difference between the current users of estrogen replacement therapy and non-users in quadriceps muscle size (cross-sectional area) and density. The estrogen users were found to have increased muscle size and density. Take notice, though, because here's what is really important in this study: the increases in muscle size and density for the quadriceps among estrogen users *did not result in improved strength and physical functioning.* There were no differences between the two groups with regard to lower extremity physical functioning such as in walking, chair stands, and balance while standing. The researchers concluded that estrogen replacement therapy in postmenopausal women may not be indicated in order to maintain muscle composition and functioning.[23]

So, if you are one of hundreds of older women working out in the gym to build muscles, take heed! Don't expect that your increased muscle mass in singularly worked muscles is necessarily going to translate into strength in physical tasks. That is what Chapter Seven in this book is all about. Although estrogen may help increase the muscle mass, if the muscle mass doesn't help with functioning then how is it really related to our goal of breaking free from the hold of arthritis? Moreover, research just published in 2011 in the journal, *Menopause,* revealed findings that do not support the use of hormone therapy for preserving long-term, lean-body mass in postmenopausal women. The researchers reported the six-year results from the Women's Health Initiative study of hormone trials. It was found that although hormone therapy did provide *early* preservation of lean-body mass (at three years through the trials), it did not affect the *long-term* loss of lean body mass (at six years through the trials).[24] What you will find out in Chapter Seven is that strength is not only dependent upon muscle mass!

A very important focus of the exercise program within this book is upon the muscle-tendon unit. I will emphasize the strengthening of this unit as primary in preventing much of the physical dysfunction associated with menopausal arthritis. So, does hormone replacement therapy affect the muscle-tendon unit? In a study of ninety-three postmenopausal women, stiffness in the muscle-tendon unit was assessed. There were no statistical differences in muscle-tendon unit stiffness between the group that used hormone therapy and the group that did not use hormone therapy. The researchers concluded that their data suggested no relationship between hormone therapy in postmenopausal women and muscle-tendon unit stiffness.[25] With muscle-tendon stiffness you don't want either too much or too little stiffness. Too much can lead to increased risk of bone injuries, and too little can lead to soft tissue injuries.[26] Soft tissue injuries would include those to ligaments and tendons. The important take-away point here is that, at least within this research, hormone therapy use did not affect muscle-tendon stiffness.

As we noted earlier, research has found that there are differential effects for aging versus estrogen loss on joint and surrounding soft tissues. However, with regard to estrogen depletion, it could be that it is the diminished number and quality of estrogen receptors among older postmenopausal women that may be of greatest importance. With fewer available estrogen receptors, estrogen replacement therapy will obviously not work as well.

In a Swedish study out of the Karolinska Institutet it was found that both estrogen receptor-alpha and estrogen receptor-beta are found in human skeletal muscle tissue. Postmenopausal women had *fewer of these estrogen receptors* when compared with young adult women (with a mean age of 24 years). Sections from muscle biopsies had been triple-stained for ER-alpha and ER-beta and collagen IV. In a very clear and striking depiction of the differences among these older and younger women, dramatic differences in the concentrations of estrogen receptors were shown in their skeletal muscle tissue. [27] Perhaps the findings of this next review study make sense, then, if you think about the plummeting number of estrogen receptors in postmenopausal women. Within this review, although a positive effect for estrogen was found upon muscle strength, this was seen primarily in women aged 50-60. In contrast, when studies showed no effect of hormone replacement therapy, the women were 60 years of age and older.[28]

Clearly, there are many factors at play that have to do with why hormone and estrogen replacement therapy may or may not have a positive effect upon osteoarthritis symptoms. Same thing with muscle mass, strength, and physical functioning -- there seems to be much more involved than just the hormones or the supplementation of them! At this point, it is simply not clear whether estrogen supplementation helps prevent or ease menopausal arthritis. Nevertheless, in light of the Women's Health Initiative (WHI) study findings it would seem wise to look for other means of easing arthritis symptoms than supplementation with estrogen. In a follow-up of the WHI trial of estrogen plus progestin versus a placebo (three years after stopping the trial due to poor health outcomes), the researchers found the following: the increased cardiovascular risks in women who had been in the estrogen and progestin use group were not seen after the intervention was discontinued. However, a greater risk of fatal and non-fatal malignancies was found in the estrogen and progestin use group in comparison with the placebo/control group, post-intervention. Their results showed that the risks of estrogen plus progestin use may exceed the benefits in terms of the prevention of chronic diseases.[29]

There are non-hormonal interventions that, for many women, can counter some of the effects of estrogen loss at menopause. In Part II, I will discuss what research shows is helpful in this regard with the focus upon countering proinflammatory cytokines caused by estrogen loss. For now, though, let's move on to why the health and functioning of your muscles (and tendons) may be of central importance to healing from menopausal arthritis, and how they, too, can be affected by the metabolic milieu of menopause.

Notes for Chapter Three

[1]Roman-Blas, J. A., Castañeda, S., Largo, R., & Herrero-Beaumont, G. (2009). Osteoarthritis associated with estrogen deficiency. *Arthritis Research & Therapy, 11,* 241. doi:10.1186/ar2791

[2]Salem, M. L. (2004). Estrogen, a double-edged sword: Modulation of TH1- and TH2- mediated inflammation by differential regulation of TH1/TH2 cytokine production. *Current Drug Targets – Inflammation & Allergy, 3,* 97-104.

[3]Musatov, S., Chen, W., Pfaff, D. W., Mobbs, C. V., Yang, X.-J., Clegg, D. J., Kaplitt, M. G., & Ogawa, S. (2007). Silencing of estrogen receptor _ in the ventromedial nucleus of hypothalamus leads to metabolic syndrome. *Proceedings of the National Academy of Sciences, 104*(7), 2501-2506. doi: 10.1073/pnas.0610787104

[4]Zhang, Q. H., & Yao, Y. M. (2010). The central mechanism for estrogen receptor to mediate nutrients and energy metabolism. *Sheng Li Ke Xue Jin Zhan, 41*(5), 347-351.

[5]Janssen, I., Powell, L. H., Kazlauskaite, R., & Dugan, S. A. (2010). Testosterone and visceral fat in midlife women: The Study of Women's Health Across the Nation (SWAN) fat patterning study. *Obesity (Silver Spring), 18*(3), 604-610.

[6]Janssen, I., Powell, L. H., Crawford, S., Lasley, B., & Sutton-Tyrrel, K. (2008). Menopause and the metabolic syndrome: The Study of Women's Health Across the Nation. *Archives of Internal Medicine, 168*(14), 1568-1575.

[7]Salem (2004). Op. Cit.

[8]Herrero-Beaumont, G., Roman-Blas, J. A., Castañeda, S., & Jimenez, S. A. (2009). Primary osteoarthritis no longer primary: Three subsets with distinct etiological, clinical, and therapeutic characteristics. *Seminars in Arthritis and Rheumatism, 39*(2), 71-80.

[9]Felson, D. T., & Cummings, S. R. (2005). Aromatase inhibitors and the syndrome of arthralgias with estrogen deprivation. *Arthritis & Rheumatism, 52*(9), 2594-2598. doi: 10.1002/art.21364

[10]Ibid.

[11]Sowers, M. R., McConnell, D., Jannausch, M,, Buyuktur, A. G., Hochberg, M. & Jamadar, D. A. (2006). Estradiol and its metabolites and their association with knee osteoarthritis. *Arthritis & Rheumatism, 54*(8), 2481-2487. doi: 10.1002/art.22005

[12] Spector, T. D., & Campion, G. D. (1989). Generalised osteoarthritis: A hormonally mediated disease. *Annals of the Rheumatic Diseases, 48,* 523-527.

[13]Spector, T. D., Nandra, D., Hart, D. J., & Doyle, D. V. (1997). Is hormone replacement therapy protective for hand and knee osteoarthritis in women? The Chingford Study. *Annals of the Rheumatic Diseases, 56*(7), 432-434.

[14]Nevitt, M. C., Felson, D. T., Williams, E. N., & Grady, D. (2001). The effect of estrogen plus progestin on knee symptoms and related disability in postmenopausal women: The Heart and Estrogen/Progestin Replacement Study, a randomized, double-blind, placebo-controlled trial. *Arthritis & Rheumatism, 44*(4), 811-818.

[15]Zhang, Y., McAlindon, T. E., Hannan, M. T., Chaisson, C. E., Klein, R., Wilson, P. W., & Felson, D. T. (1998). Estrogen replacement therapy and worsening of radiographic knee osteoarthritis: The Framingham Study. *Arthritis & Rheumatism, 41*(10), 1867-1873.

[16]Sahyoun, N. R., Brett, K. M., Hochberg, M. C., & Pamuk, E. R. (1999). Estrogen replacement therapy and incidence of self-reported physician-diagnosed arthritis. *Preventative Medicine, 28*(5), 458-464.

[17]Von Mühlen, D., Morton, D., Von Mühlen, C. A., & Barrett-Conner, E. (2002). Postmenopausal estrogen and increased risk of clinical osteoarthritis at the hip, hand, and knee in older women. *Journal of Women's Health and Gender-Based Medicine, 11*(6), 511-518.

[18]Wluka, A. E., Cicuttini, F. M., & Spector, T. D. (2000). Menopause, oestrogens and arthritis. *Maturitas, 35*, 183-199.

[19]Fytili, P., Giannatou, E., Papanikolaou, V., Stripeli, F., Karachalios, T., Malizos, K., & Tsezou, A. (2005). Association of repeat polymorphisms in the estrogen receptors alpha, beta, and androgen receptor genes with knee osteoarthritis. *Clinical Genetics, 68*(3), 268-277.

[20]Hanna, F. S., Wluka, A. E., Bell, R. J., Davis, S. R., & Cicuttini, F. M. (2004). Osteoarthritis and the postmenopausal woman: Epidemiological, magnetic resonance imaging, and radiological findings. *Seminars in Arthritis and Rheumatism, 34*(3), 631-636. doi: 10.1016/j.semart.2004.07.007

[21]Rossouw, J. E., Anderson, G. L., Prentice, R. L., LaCroix, A. Z., Kooperberg, C., Stefanick, M. L., Jackson, R. D., Beresford, S. A., Howard, B. V., Johnson, K. C., Kotchen, J. M., & Ockene, J.; Writing Group for the Women's Health Initiative Investigators (2002). Risks and benefits of estrogen plus progestin in healthy postmenopausal women: Principal results from the Women's Health Initiative randomized controlled trial. *Journal of the American Medical Association, 288*(3), 321-333.

[22]Manson, J. E., Hsia, J., Johnson, K. C., Rossouw, J. E., Assaf, A. R., Lasser, N. L., Trevisan, M., Black, H. R., Heckbert, S. R., Detrano, R., Strickland, O. L., Wong, N. D., Crouse, J. R., Stein, E., & Cushman, M.; Women's Health Initiative Investigators (2003). Estrogen plus progestin and the risk of coronary heart disease. *New England Journal of Medicine, 349*(6), 523-534.

[23]Taaffe, D. R., Newman, A. B., Haggerty, C. L., Colbert, L. H., De Rekeneire, N., Visser, M., Goodpaster, B. H., Nevitt, M. C., Tylavsky, F. A., & Harris, T. B. (2005). Estrogen replacement, muscle composition, and physical function: The

Health ABC Study. *Medicine & Science in Sports & Exercise, 37*(10), 1741-1747. doi: 10.1249/01.mss.0000181678.28092.31

[24]Bea, J. W., Zhao, Q., Cauley, J. A., LaCroix, A. Z., Bassford, T., Lewis, C. E., Jackson, R. D., Tylavsky, F. A., & Chen, Z. (2011). Effect of hormone therapy on lean body mass, falls, and fractures: 6-yr results from the Women's Health Initiative hormone trials. *Menopause, 18*(1), 44-52.

[25]Faria, A., Gabriel, R., Abrantes, J., Brás, R., Sousa, M., & Moreira, H. (2010). Ankle stiffness in postmenopausal women: Influence of hormone therapy and menopause nature. *Climacteric, 13*(3), 265-270.

[26]Faria, A., Gabriel, R., Abrantes, J., Brás, R., & Moreira, H. (2009). Triceps-surae musculotendinous stiffness: Relative differences between obese and non-obese postmenopausal women. *Clinical Biomechanics, 24*(10), 866-871.

[27]Wiik, A., Ekman, M., Johansson, O., Jansson, E., & Esbjornsson, M. (2009). Expression of both oestrogen receptor alpha and beta in human skeletal muscle tissue. *Histochemistry and Cell Biology, 131*(2), 181-189.

[28]Jacobsen, D. E., Samson, M. M., Kezic, S., & Verhaar, H. J. (2007). Postmenopausal HRT and tibolone in relation to muscle strength and body composition. *Maturitas, 58*(1), 7-18.

[29]Heiss, G., Wallace, R., Anderson, G. L., Aragaki, A., Beresford, S. A., Brzyski, R., Chlebowski, R. T., Gass, M. LaCroix, A., Manson, J. E., Prentice, R. L., Rossouw, J., & Stefanick, M. L.; WHI Investigators (2008). Health risks and benefits 3 years after stopping randomized treatment with estrogen and progestin. *Journal of the American Medical Association, 299*(9), 1036-1045.

Chapter Four

Muscles, Tendons, and Menopausal Arthritis

—— ▣ ——

Muscle Decline -- It Happens Sooner Than You May Think

I never dreamed that I would have to actually "develop" muscles to simply walk upstairs. I thought that everyday movement such as this just came naturally. However, the rapid decline in muscle mass and in physical functioning after menopause occur quickly and much sooner than expected. As discovered in research out of the University of Michigan, impaired physical functioning to include gait and stair climbing performance began to decline much earlier than was thought. How well people were functioning was determined by factors such as their speed in walking, the amount of support used through handrails, and the time it took to ascend and descend the stairs. A large number of the middle-aged women within this research study (with a mean age of 47 years) already had compromised or diminished functioning. Nearly 31% of the middle-aged women in the study walked at speeds that were too slow. In fact, 12% of these middle-aged women walked at speeds that might compromise their safety in pedestrian situations, and which could qualify them as being *"frail"* if they were older.[1]

Stair Climbing Aspirations -- Stair Ascent, Descent, and Menopausal Arthritis

I had not anticipated any rapid change in my body mechanics as I entered menopause. I didn't know that I had been unconsciously altering my posture to avoid knee pain as I climbed up the stairs, though. So when I realized this I began to try to ascend in a correct position using the full strength of my buttocks, quadriceps, hamstrings, and hip flexors. Instead of my usual leaning forward to allow gravity to help propel me up the stairs, I was now standing straight up vertically and forcing my upper and lower legs and buttocks muscles to do the work of ascent. My legs wobbled on the stairs as I attempted to do this. Stair descent was even worse. I had found that it had become so painful that I ended up walking sideways down the stairs taking each step slowly, one by one. It was only through the results of my healing program that I could finally descend the stairs without pain and ascend the stairs with strength and ease.

When I was still in the throes of stair climbing with its resultant pain, I had learned something about myself that I had not known; *every muscle* in my lower body was weak! This would include my thighs and buttocks muscles (quadriceps and gluteus maximus, medius and minimus), my calf muscles (gastrocnemius, soleus), and ankle flexion muscles (soleus, tibialis posterior), to name just a few.

I had been thinking only about how my knee joint hurt without much of a thought toward any of my muscles. I was aware that I did have weakness and some pain in my quadriceps; nevertheless, it never even occurred to me to actually try to strengthen my muscles. The reason was that I was so singularly focused on my knee joint pain. Moreover, I had no idea that my muscles were in rapid decline. Plus, I had been fairly sedentary for most of menopause. Exercise was slipping further and further away from my mindset and from my usual daily routines.

Now, I use *every* muscle as I ascend the stairs, muscles from my hips to my toes! They are *linked* . . . all of the muscles. It is not just a matter of strengthening the quadriceps or stretching your hamstrings. Only when you begin to see the powerful unity of the extensive muscular system in your body will you be on your way to freeing yourself from menopausal arthritis!

Topic of Interest #3

Stair-Climbing Inspirations!

     I am not sure how I stumbled upon this website, "Stair ClimbingSport.com,"[2] but it turned out to be inspirational! The purpose of the website is to promote stair climbing as a sport since, as is said on the website, it really constitutes a total body workout (if you use handrails to pull yourself up the stairs), and it is a great cross-training exercise. However, unlike the middle-aged women that we noted at the beginning of the Chapter (who may have used the hand-rails as a prop or support), those engaged in a full-body workout in stair climbing do so in order to utilize *all* of their muscles *fully*. This website was inspirational to me, not because I plan on entering any stair climbing races in the near future, but because it was motivating to read about people who are strong at this physical feat. The point here for women suffering from menopausal arthritis is that *stair climbing is hard physical exercise*. I am not suggesting that you should aspire to be part of the Empire State Building Run-Up (that is, unless you want to of course)! On this website, that memorable scene in the now classic film, "Rocky," was featured. As you may recall, Sylvester Stallone, as Rocky, ran up the stairs of the Philadelphia Museum of Art in his final triumphant exercise training for the big fight (to the popular recording hit "Gonna Fly Now"). Stair climbing is indeed good exercise! To put things into perspective for all of us who are not athletes, and you want something to bring a smile to your face, click onto one of this website's links, "Stairs made fun" which takes you to a YouTube segment: *Piano stairs -- TheFunTheory.com – Rolighetsteorin.se!*[3]

The Basic Muscle Group Twosome

In my quest to strengthen the muscles supporting my knees, I began by looking at just the quadriceps and hamstrings muscle groups. These were the ones that were emphasized in most of the books that I had been reading at the time. There was really not a great deal of information, though, as to how these two muscle groups worked together. I did learn that if there was an imbalance between these two muscle groups (that is, if one were weaker or conversely stronger than the other), then this could create problems with knee function.[4] In fact, some findings suggest that it is an imbalance (both in strength and endurance) between these two muscle groups that can lead to knee problems. Female athletes have been found to experience a greater incidence of muscle imbalances compared to male athletes. Some of the injuries that women sustain in sports may stem from weakened hamstrings strength and endurance relative to quadriceps strength and endurance.[5]

Quadriceps and hamstrings imbalance may be of particular importance in osteoarthritis. Researchers have found higher co-contraction of the two muscle groups in walking among osteoarthritis patients as compared with those without osteoarthritis. Osteoarthritis patients develop greater antagonistic (i.e., hamstrings) muscle activity.[6] In fact, increased activation of the hamstrings muscles has been found to occur in osteoarthritis patients while they are performing other activities of daily living in addition to walking. In a study out of East Carolina University, muscle activation was examined for level walking, stair ascent, and stair descent. In all three activities, the osteoarthritis patients used less knee flexion and more hip flexion. Because they are underusing their quadriceps, they compensate with increased hip extensor muscle, or hamstrings use. In the face of impaired quadriceps function, co-activation of hamstrings and quadriceps is used to increase overall knee stability.[7]

In addition, slower walking speeds in people with osteoarthritis are most likely related to changes in the lower extremity kinetic chains of muscles. We will take a closer look at these chains of muscles in a moment, because along with the muscle-tendon unit, their importance is fundamental to our exercise program. Muscle weakness and joint pain cause changes in the way the muscles should work together. For example, in a study of walking speeds and gait, those with osteoarthritis changed their gait quite dramatically when walking faster. They used significantly more ankle motions and significantly less hip motions.[8] I thought of my own fast-walking gait, and I was doing that, too! I had been completely mystified as to how I could weigh the same as I had a decade ago but not be able to keep up a walking pace with my husband and daughter anymore. At that time, I thought it must be the distribution of my weight or something, as my physique was increasingly becoming more of an "apple-shape." In fact, one day when we were late to meet someone on UC Berkeley's vast campus, they sped "miles" ahead of me even though I was walking as fast as I could! I now know that I was working my ankles into a frenzy, while my idle hip muscles took a cat nap!

The alterations in muscle balance in knee osteoarthritis go beyond just the two muscle groups, the hamstrings and quadriceps -- they do not just remain localized around the knee! In fact, activation of the gastrocnemius (calf muscle) in relation to the tibialis anterior (muscle near the shin bone) was also higher in patients with knee osteoarthritis than in those without the disease. These altered neural mechanisms related to muscle balance are not confined to just those of the problem joint. With regard to clinical biomechanics, it has been stressed that strengthening exercises should focus on *all* muscles that cross the knee joint, and *should also include the hip and ankle joints.*[9]

Remember that I had said in the beginning of this chapter that my knees hurt on stair climbing but there was also quadriceps weakness and some muscle pain? Well, research shows that this pain in my quadriceps may have caused me to take on a gait that actually *avoided* the use of my quadriceps. In an experimental study of twenty healthy young adults, Danish researchers investigated the effect of quadriceps muscle pain on knee joint control. With the informed consent of all participants and approval by the local ethics committee, two groups were compared: one in which quadriceps pain was induced and a control group without induced muscle pain. They found that when the vastus medialis quadriceps muscle was injected with a solution to bring on muscle pain, the control and stability of the knee joint during walking was impaired. One fifth of the participants who had the pain-inducing hypertonic saline injection (as opposed to a non-pain-inducing isotonic saline injection) began to completely avoid any use of their quadriceps. Participants with muscles that were induced to feel pain had significantly reduced quadriceps usage. *Pain* had a *powerful effect* in controlling the way in which these people walked. What was perhaps *more surprising* was that even *after* the pain subsided, the muscle pattern did not change for at least 20 minutes. Even with the pain stimulus gone, the avoidance continued. Importantly, the continued non-use of the quadriceps muscle, even after the pain had subsided, could render the unstable knee to greater risk of injury and chronic knee problems.[10]

Beyond the Quadriceps and the Hamstrings: Muscle Loops

How do you strengthen the muscles to optimally support your knee joint? As mentioned earlier, many exercise books seem to focus on the thigh muscles and in particular the quadriceps. Some also focus on addressing the imbalance between the quadriceps and the hamstrings. It is clear from the studies above, though, that there is a synergistic effect among the muscle groups. What's more, the neural mechanisms promoting muscle balance are not limited to the muscles surrounding the knee itself. Muscles work together to support joint function and include muscles that are not confined to the immediate joint.

In Europe there has been recognition of muscle loops since the 1930's. Muscle loops are muscular chains in which groups of muscles work together and influence each other. Most important in strengthening muscles for stair climbing, and other physical movement, is what is called a "muscle sling." In the Janda approach to the assessment of muscle imbalance, a muscle sling is a group of muscles that work together in a particular pattern of movement that involves *more than one joint*. "Synergists," on the other hand, are muscles that work with another muscle to generate movement of a *specific joint*. Muscle slings work across *multiple* joints to provide stability and movement of the body. The hamstrings and the hip flexors, for example, would constitute one such muscle sling. This muscle sling has the femur (thigh bone) as its stability point (called a "keystone') for these two muscle groups. Another sling would be the quadriceps and the plantar flexors, with the tibia (shinbone) as the keystone. (See Figure 1 for a diagram of the hip flexor and extensor slings.)

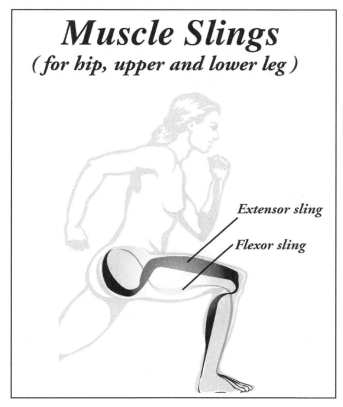

Muscle Slings
(for hip, upper and lower leg)

Extensor sling

Flexor sling

Figure 1: Muscle Slings

In a muscle sling the muscle groups work together for the total *functional movement pattern*, such as in walking up the stairs. They do not work together for the *isolated* movement of a joint.[11] This is important! It is not just one or two muscle groups that you use when you walk up the stairs, but rather, many, many muscles involving multiple joints. If you want to stair climb well, then you must exercise all of the muscles in each muscle sling as they work together. Let's look at some of the muscles within muscle slings for a moment that are so important to stair climbing. When I walk up the stairs now

I am aware of muscles contracting in the hip area, my iliacus muscle, and psoas minor and major which flex the thigh at the hip. The iliacus and the psoas are commonly thought of as the hip flexors. As they function so closely together, they have been termed the "iliopsoas" (See Figure 2).

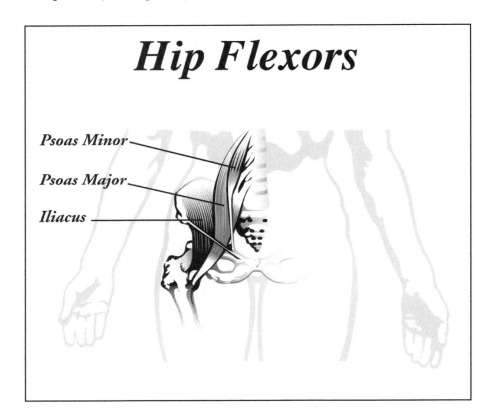

Hip Flexors

Psoas Minor

Psoas Major

Iliacus

Figure 2 - Hip Flexors

Although the iliopsoas are of primary importance in hip flexion, there are other muscles, too, that are involved in hip flexion. I am aware of rectus femoris (one of the quadriceps muscles) that both flexes the thigh at the hip and also extends the leg at the knee. The other quadriceps muscles act as extensor muscles. Vastus lateralis, vastus intermedius and vastus medialis (See Figure 3) all extend the leg at the knee.

Notice that within the vastus medialis is a portion of muscle called the vastus medialis oblique (VMO). Weakness in this muscle area has been associated with knee pain. Also notice in Figure 3 the muscles, sartorius and gracilis. These adjacent muscles to the

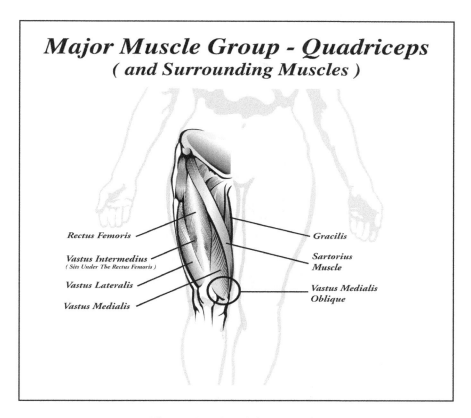

Major Muscle Group - Quadriceps
(and Surrounding Muscles)

Rectus Femoris

Vastus Intermedius
(Sits Under The Rectus Femoris)

Vastus Lateralis

Vastus Medialis

Gracilis

Sartorius
Muscle

Vastus Medialis
Oblique

Figure 3 - Quadriceps Group

quadriceps are vitally important with regard to menopausal arthritis. They work in opposing ways to abduct and adduct the thigh at the hip (that is to move it outward and away from the body and inward back toward the body). They also both work to flex the leg at the knee. If they are not strong, or have become shortened through trauma or muscle imbalances, this can lead to soft tissue problems such as pes anserine bursitis (which I will discuss shortly).

The back of your thighs as well as your gluteal muscles are also being extensively used in stair climbing. Semimembranosus, semitendinosus, and biceps femoris-long head flex the leg at the knee and also extend the thigh at the hip, and biceps femoris-short head flexes the leg at the knee. (These muscles comprise the hamstrings group - See Figure 4).

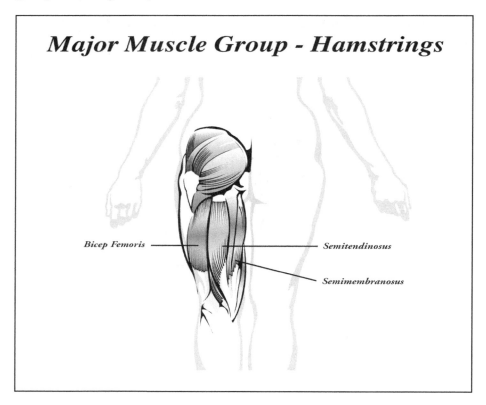

Figure 4 – Hamstrings Group

Gluteus maximus, the primary buttocks muscle, extends the thigh at the hip. The gluteal muscles (or, informally the "glutes"), are increasingly underused as we age. They are critical in helping to prevent knee pain on walking up and down the stairs. If the gluteus maximus is weak, then there will be extra strain put on the legs, knees, and feet. This is intensified going down the stairs with the added force of gravity. Gluteus maximus (along with tensor fasciae latae, a muscle that stems from the iliac crest and iliac spine at the front of the body) assist in stabilizing the hip and the knee when standing and walking and in movements like ascending and descending the stairs.

Critical Two-Joint Muscles: Sartorius, Gracilis, and Semitendinosus

Sartorius, gracilis, and semitendinosus muscles are vitally important in coordinated, large movements of the body since they all cross two joints, the hip and the knee. By acting upon the thigh at the hip and the leg at the knee all of these muscles are able to help produce fluid and robust movements of the lower body. Their lengths are impressive, and in fact, sartorius, which is a thin, ribbon-like band, is the longest muscle in the human body. Injury can occur through overuse or when muscles are not activated correctly. This can

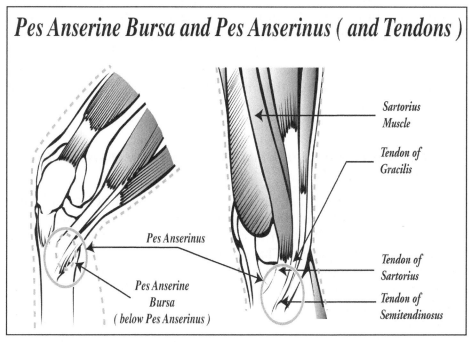

Figure 5 - Pes Anserine Bursa and Pes
Anserinus (and Tendons)

cause excessive pulling upon the tendons of these muscles. As a result, the bursa (a fluid-filled sac) which is positioned just below the point where the tendons of gracilis, sartorius, and semitendinosus meet (pes anserinus) can become inflamed and subject to excruciating pain (See Figure 5 - Pes Anserine Bursa and Pes Anserinus).

In menopausal arthritis, I suspect that it may often be a shortening of the gracilis and sartorius muscles (and hamstrings) that causes irritation at the tendons. Muscles can shorten as a result of many things such as sports injuries, repetitive motions performed at work, or direct trauma to the muscle such as in a fall or a car accident.[12] With shortened muscles there is excessive pull on the tendons, and the underlying bursae becomes inflamed. The pes anserine bursa has a protective function in that it decreases the friction between the tendons and the bone. It can become inflamed, though, if there is a continual source of irritation, and this can cause knee pain. When muscles are injured or traumatized in some way they can develop myofascial trigger points. These are hypersensitive spots in the muscle that usually feel painful when stimulated.[13] We'll go into this more fully in Chapter Nine, on "Healing from the Outside." Also, we'll take a closer look at pes anserine bursitis pain within Chapter Six. This is a very important factor to consider in the experience of menopausal arthritis, since it is a source of knee pain that is much more common in women than in men. It is also often mistaken for osteoarthritis pain.

The Calf Muscle (and Other Leg Muscles): Often Overlooked Sources of Knee Pain

Did you know that weak and/or tight calf muscles can cause pain in the front of your knee? As you plant your foot down on the stair step and then lift it up to climb the stairs you are calling into action your calf muscles. This is especially the case with the soleus muscle which if tight can cause you to rely more on the front of your foot. Instead of planting your whole foot down in an efficient and complete motion, the heel is underused and the weight goes toward the toes. This action puts strain on the tibialis anterior muscle and may cause shin pain. This was a major problem for me; the shinbone area (of my leg with menopausal knee arthritis) was a constant additional source of pain. Your calf muscle (gastrocnemius) flexes the leg at the knee and at the foot. Activation of the medial gastrocnemius muscle when walking may be significantly reduced in people with osteoarthritis as compared with those without osteoarthritis. Moreover, it was found that those people *without* osteoarthritis had a *highly activated* medial gastrocnemius muscle when walking.[14]

Popliteus, which is a small muscle at the back of the knee, flexes the leg at the knee, but it also medially rotates it. So, if you had a staircase that made some turns (instead of a vertical path up) you would engage all of the functions of this muscle going up the stairs. Plantaris (which works with gastrocnemius), is a small muscle at the back of your knee which flexes the leg at the knee, but it amazingly also flexes the foot. This occurs because of its extremely long tendon; the foot action happens at its tendinous end. In fact, the tendon of plantaris stretches all the way from the back of the knee to the foot. Tendons are often overlooked in their actions and movements within the body. The multitude of muscles and tendons that are used in activities requiring you to flex your knees is truly quite amazing! So too are the ways in which tendons work together with muscles to move your upper and lower legs and other parts of your body.

Kinetic Muscle Chains and Muscle Loops -- What Can Go Wrong

Earlier in this chapter I had described muscle loops based in the Janda approach. These muscle slings have also been referred to as kinetic muscle chains. As described in a book published by the American Physical Therapy Association, the knee is part of a "kinetic chain." In the case of the knee, the kinetic chain (or the chain of motion) begins with the pelvis, hip and upper leg (i.e., thigh) and moves on to the lower leg, ankle, and the foot. The muscles within these different parts of the body are interrelated, and the movement of the body and the proper functioning of the knees are governed by how the muscles in this kinetic chain work together.[15]

If a problem within a kinetic chain is not fixed, the pain and inflammation will persist and altered gait patterns can develop. If there is muscular weakness in the muscles at the beginning of a muscle chain, then the next strongest muscle will be forced to over-exert itself. For example if the gluteus muscles are not strong, the hamstrings will take on extra work. This causes muscle strain in the hamstrings, and perhaps a shortening of the hamstring muscle, too. If one takes on an improper gait (for example, due to weak quadriceps or hip muscles), knee pain may develop. It does not take a trauma to the knee (such as a fall or sports injury) to cause knee pain; just the accumulated stress and strain from poor body mechanics can result in knee pain. Many things can go wrong with the muscles within the chain including "tightness" which can restrict your knee's range of motion. Also, repetitive stress can cause inflammation of the muscles and shortening of the muscles, as discussed above. Excess lactic acid and other chemicals can build up causing inflammation and pain. Microscopic tears in the muscles can occur. When this happens it is referred to as "muscle strain," and it occurs when muscles are over-used or overexerted. The most severe form would be an actual "muscle tear" in which the muscle is torn partially or completely usually resulting from a direct trauma to the muscle.[16]

The coordinated effort of muscles and ligaments working together to generate the forces to move the body and change its po-sition is called the "biomechanical moment of force."[17] During level walking, the knee joint does not have nearly the amount of muscle and ligament exertion (or flexor moment) that it has when one is ascending or descending the stairs. Flexor moments have been found to be much higher for stair ascent and descent compared with those experienced during walking on a level surface. For example, a study of knee kinetics during stair ascent found that the peak patellofemoral force was *eight times* higher during stair climbing than it was during level walking. These researchers suggested that the pain that people with early osteoarthritis feel upon stair ascent may be due to this increased force on the patella (kneecap).[18]

Stair descent can really cause considerable pain for people with osteoarthritis. People with knee osteoarthritis have been found to use less knee flexion during their early stance upon going down stairs. If one has less strength in the quadriceps, one might adopt this stance as a way of reducing the forces upon the knee. Weak quadri-ceps muscles are not capable of absorbing the mechanical load and forces during descent. This may render other musculoskeletal tissues (e.g., surrounding muscles, bones, and cartilage) vulnerable to damage from the considerable forces that have not been dissipated or dispersed.[19] The brunt of the mechanical load is placed upon the knee joint because the quadriceps are not able to act as a buffer and reduce some of this force.

The importance of the kinetic chain working properly cannot be overemphasized. For example, in both men and women, motor control of the quadriceps has been found to be significantly associated with hip strength. This would suggest an important connection between hip muscle control and neuromotor control of the quadriceps group.[20]

Are Muscles Mechanically Independent of Each Other?

In a very fascinating line of research, evidence was provided to suggest that muscles may *not* be mechanically independent! It has been found that muscle fibers transmit force not just over the length of the muscle to their attached tendons, but also across the muscle along adjoining muscle fibers. Some studies have suggested that force is transmitted, not only from muscles to tendons, but also from muscles to other muscles. The myofascial connective tissue that surrounds each muscle and connects it with others may possibly be a route for the transmission of force from one muscle to another. Fascia or fascial tissue consists of bands or sheets of connective tissue that provide support to muscles and to organs within the body. (Please See Figure 6 -- Muscle Fascia).

Another possible transmission route would be tendons if they are shared by muscles. The evidence is still mixed in terms of how this transmission may occur.[21] However, it does make sense in terms of the close relationship between muscles in muscle chains, and it would provide scientific evidence for what seems intuitive in effective exercise.

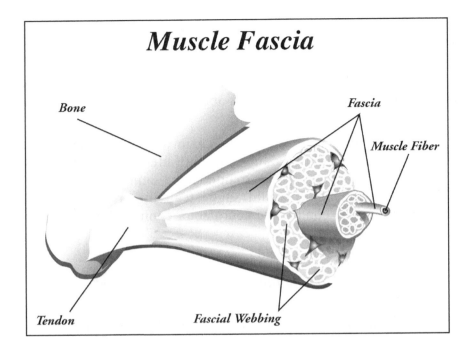

Muscle Fascia

Bone

Fascia

Muscle Fiber

Tendon

Fascial Webbing

Figure 6 - Muscle Fascia

Tendons - More than Just Connectors of Muscle to Bone

The tendons, like muscles, are also subject to similar micro-scopic tears due to stress. If a tendon is stretched too far beyond its capacity it can cause tendinitis. The tendon itself does not have the network of nerve fibers of surrounding joint tissues. So, pain may not be felt until the bursa that cushions the tendon becomes irritated or the lining of the sac that encloses the knee joint becomes inflamed. With tendon irritation, there may be an aching of an area of the knee that feels non-specific, and seems deeply imbedded within the joint.[22] This type of pain will be discussed using many examples of it in Chapter Six. The actual rupture of a tendon due to osteoarthritis rarely occurs. However, if it did it would probably be a result of lim-ited or constrained joint movement and atrophy of the tendon. This wasting away of the tendon could result, for example, from over engaging in routine activities which require little physical exertion (e.g., watching TV, sitting at the computer, etc.).[23]

Tendons and Elastic Energy

We sometimes think of tendons as simply a band of connective tissue attaching muscle to bone. However, they are much more dynamic than this! They possess the capacity to store and use what is called "elastic energy." Elastic energy could be explained as the potential of the tendon to hold and use energy upon stretching such as the elastic energy of a rubber band. When you pull it, it exerts an energy force to go back to its original position. As a muscle lengthens, elastic energy is stored within the tendon, and then this stored elastic energy is used in muscle flexion. Moreover, tendons are not just flexible and elastic in nature; they are also extremely strong. Tendons can resist high forces as they transmit force from muscle to bone; they can absorb shock which helps to prevent damage to the muscle.[24]

There are changes in human tendons and ligaments with the aging process to include some alterations in the amounts of trace elements within tendons and ligaments. Some of the most abundant minerals in tendons are calcium, sulphur and phosphorous.[25] Interestingly, different tendons and ligaments show variations in the amounts of minerals present. The tendon of the iliopsoas muscle group, for example, was found to have an increase in phosphorous and magnesium content with aging; conversely, the Achilles tendon was found to have a significant decrease in magnesium and phosphorous.[26]

Could a lack of some minerals affect the functioning of the tendons? In a study of trace elements in tendon collagen it was found that copper may be a vital element to collagen. Copper atoms may be importantly involved in the molecular organization of the collagen, or in the organization of the collagen fibrils that compose the tendon collagen.[27] This finding is interesting, as copper supplementation has been suggested as a remedy to help with arthritis in some complementary and alternative medicine therapies.[28] In addition, animal research has also suggested that nutritional supplementation with copper may have an anti-arthritic effect.[29] Nevertheless, there is no solid evidence to support supplementation with copper or the use of copper jewelry as an effective treatment for arthritis. There are few studies on the efficacy of copper jewelry, and those that do exist show conflicting results.[30,31]

The importance of minerals within tendon is clearly seen in the research conducted out of Robert Wood Johnson Medical School. In animal research it was found that elastic tendon energy may indeed be related to tendon mineral content. Both the elastic spring content and elastic energy of the tendon were proportionately related to the mineral content of the tendon. So, increased minerals in the tendon meant increased elastic strength to bear loads on the tendon.[32] If true for humans too, then finding out how to ensure that needed minerals are within our tendons is of prime importance!

Perhaps this could be at least in part why the age-old practice of using mineral-rich mud packs and mud baths to alleviate the symptoms of osteoarthritis have garnered so much popular support. Research does provide evidence for the effectiveness of these practices. In a very comprehensive review of the scientific research on spa therapies, there are studies that show beneficial effects of the trace minerals in the treatments of rheumatic diseases.[33] The effects of heat (which can be relaxing and alleviate pain) were even separated out from the effects of the minerals themselves in controlled experimental research. The therapeutic effect was attributed to the minerals, not to the heat.[34] We will discuss treatments such as mineral rich mud packs in Chapter Nine.

In addition to changes in the mineral content of tendons with aging, tendons show age-related changes in physical functioning. Older people have less capacity to store and use elastic energy compared with younger people.[35] Considering the above research on elasticity of tendons and mineral content, could a decrease in the mineral content in older people's tendons be one of the causes? It would certainly be of much benefit in physical functioning of older people if increasing the mineral content of tendons could increase elastic energy and hence the ability to take on greater mechanical loads on the joints.

Because people often limit the physical demands on their body as they age, this reduces their muscle strength, as well. Decreased muscle strength, in turn, degrades the biomechanical properties of the tendons. Overall, tendons become drier, with less ability to stretch and they become stiffer as we age. Rehabilitation usually emphasizes appropriate and non-strenuous stretching exercises.[36]

Tendons and Soft Tissue Stretching

Physical therapist, Carol D. Figuers, advises that soft tissue stretching in older active adults should involve increased time and decreased speed. The force of the stretch should be mild, and there should be no pain. She emphasizes that in older people, low-intensity and longer duration stretching is vital to promote elasticity. This has been theorized to help counteract some of the effects of muscle stiffness experienced in older adults. Also, the flexibility of soft tissues around the joint may be impaired through the disease process of arthritis. When the soft tissue is not as flexible, muscular attachments must be able to compensate and to extend the range of motion. When muscles, too, have lost their flexibility then there is a much greater risk of injury.[37] In building muscles and muscle-tendon units to alleviate menopausal arthritis, it is essential to avoid injury. It is important to stretch in ways that encourage tendons to become more flexible, but do not involve stretches that are beyond your tendons' current capability (or your muscles' ability to compensate for stiff tendons). If one begins an exercise program later in one's life, it may not be as possible to reverse some of the degenerative changes in tendons. Be aware of your limitations with regard to tendon stretching. It is critical to avoid a tendon tear, as the ability and potential to heal is limited in age-related injuries of this nature.[38] This is why our exercise program within this book works your muscles and tendons through holistic and progressive movements that begin gently. You stretch and strengthen muscles slowly but extremely effectively. You *do not* isolate muscles and muscle-tendons and subject them to weights or mechanical exercise machines -- you do not have to be a weight lifter to increase muscle power!

Changes to our muscles and tendons as we age can be challenging to alter, and the decreased strength and functioning can be difficult to correct. However there are some things, along with the exercises in this book, which can be of help. Sometimes supplements might make a difference, as we talk about in Topic of Interest #4 below.

Topic of Interest #4

Three Supplements that May Help Muscle Strength and Functioning

I have come across three supplements that seem to have significantly helped my muscles: glutamine, taurine, and coenzyme Q10. Two of them, glutamine and taurine, I had discovered during the end of perimenopause.[39] However, although glutamine was discussed in terms of helping muscles, taurine was highlighted for other benefits such as being a natural diuretic. I had accidentally discovered the benefits of taurine on muscle functioning, as I did, too, with coenzyme Q10.

Research had shown that glutamine was helpful in recovery from intense exercise. Glutamine levels were found to decrease significantly with exercise stress.[40] Other research found that available glutamine following exercise promoted production of muscle glycogen.[41] Muscle glycogen is of course important as an immediate source of energy for muscles. We have all heard of the phenomenon of endurance athletes such as marathon runners "hitting the wall," where the athletes simply cannot continue, their bodies unable to keep moving. This is when nearly all of the athletes' glycogen stores have been used up. The ability of the body to increase glycogen synthesis after exercise is important in recovery from intense exercise stress. I have found glutamine supplementation to be enormously helpful in recovery from sore muscles and in alleviating muscle fatigue. I have been using glutamine following exercise, and other physical workouts such as heavy gardening, for many years now.

Taurine's effects upon muscle came as a surprise to me. I had decided to try taurine once more for water retention, and it seemed to help somewhat. However, what was astonishing was that I seemed to have acquired increased strength in my quadriceps and calf muscles for uphill walking! How did this happen? I realized that the only new thing that I had added to the supplements that I was taking was the taurine.

I began to research it, and to my surprise taurine may be very involved in muscle strength. One animal study showed that the taurine content of muscles could affect the changes in contractile strength that occur in the aging process. The researchers concluded that using taurine as a supplement may help to preserve normal muscle function in elderly individuals.[42] In addition, in new animal research conducted by Dr. Diana Conte Camerino of the University of Bari, Italy, and her colleagues, further benefit of taurine supplementation was found. In atrophied soleus muscles, taurine restored the functioning of an atrophy-related gene that could provide early protective effects to the muscle. These researchers concluded that taurine may be of benefit in the treatment of muscle dysfunction due to lack of use such as in bed rest.[43] Moreover, another animal study showed that taurine supplementation improved running performance and protected the cells from muscle injury after exercise.[44] My experience is that it did improve muscle strength!

I had found the effects of coenzyme Q10 on muscle purely by accident, as well. I had begun to take coenzyme Q10 as a general supplement, not for my muscles or arthritis, per sé. To my surprise, it seemed to help take away some of the persistent pain below my knee! From my research, it seemed likely that this pain was due to bursitis as a result of shortened muscles (which I discussed earlier). Perhaps, too, the remaining pain was due to weakness in my vastus medialis oblique muscle that I had discussed as a source of knee pain. It certainly could have been caused by both of these and other things as well. However, exactly how might the coenzyme Q10 have produced such an unexpected positive effect upon my menopausal arthritis pain?

It has been known for some time that coenzyme Q10 has been involved as a key player in mitochondrial energy production.[45] The mitochondria of course are considered to be the powerhouses of the cell. In addition to coenzyme Q10's role in cellular energy production, it has more recently been found that it plays a role in cellular signaling and in metabolism.[46] How, though, would it help in reducing the pain below my knee? It seems that it might have had an effect either upon the functioning of the muscle itself or perhaps on the nerves, or both.

Researchers out of Baylor University and colleagues discussed study findings on supplementation with coenzyme Q10 and exercise. Within their research study, they did find positive effects of coenzyme Q10 supplementation. Among their results, they found lowered oxidative stress, and a tendency toward an increased time before exhaustion.[47]

In another study in which a group taking coenzyme Q10 was compared with a control group, positive effects upon exercise performance were also found. Those who had taken coenzyme Q10 had an increase in anaerobic muscle power during supramaximal exercise.[48] Research has found that coenzyme Q10 supplementation prior to exercise lowers oxidative stress and also stops the over-expression of TNF-α after exercise. This and other positive effects upon inflammation help to reduce muscle damage after exercise.[49] Could it also have an effect upon the oxidative stress and inflammation within the disease process of arthritis? As you may recall from Chapter Two, tumor necrosis factor-alpha (TNF-α) is a primary regulator of joint inflammation. Perhaps, this important substance might be effective in preventing the over-expression of TNF-α in arthritis inflammation, as well.

Moreover, research into the age-related loss of muscle mass is beginning to point toward the importance of more than just muscle size in affecting weakness. The motor neuron (neuron that affects the control of the muscles) and motor unit (neuron plus the affected muscle fibers) are gaining recognition as critical contributors to muscle weakness.[50] Coenzyme Q10 has been used as a treatment in a broad range of neurodegenerative and neuromuscular disorders.[51] It seems, then, that it might possibly be useful in alleviating the irritated tissues in bursitis where there are many nerve endings, or in helping to strengthen weak muscles.

The Paramount Importance of Tendons

Attention to the health of one's tendons is critical to maintaining strength at older ages. In the animal world, cheetahs, gazelles, and antelopes are considered to be some of the fastest running creatures on this earth. If you look at their legs, you will see that they are composed mainly of tendons rather than heavy, bulky muscles. Their legs are examples of strong muscle-tendon units. For these animals, the kinetic muscle chains and interconnectedness of tendons, bones, ligaments, and muscles allow for maximum performance; they are able to develop great speed and sustain power over long distances without tiring. Similarly, if you have observed some of the world-class marathon runners such as those competing in the Olympics, New York Marathon, Boston Marathon, or San Francisco Bay to Breakers, you will notice that these runners depend greatly upon tendon strength (within the interconnected fascia of tendons, bones, ligaments, and muscles) to achieve power and strength for their distance running. You will notice that these runners' legs tend to be composed of very strong tendons and less bulky muscles.

The authors of an article in the journal, *Nature*, reported that in the animal world there are catapult mechanisms at work to allow for rapid acceleration and speed. For example, the horse uses a biceps muscle which contains within it a large tendon. This is a very elastic muscle, due to the power of the tendon to store and use elastic energy to propel the horse in a gallop. In contrast, in non-elastic muscles which lack substantial tendons, the elastic energy is greatly reduced. For example, a horse would need 50 kg. of non-elastic muscle to obtain the same elastic power generated in the small, 0.4 kg. elastic biceps muscle. The authors suggested that similar mechanisms to this tendon-driven muscle mechanism probably exist in other animals, as well.[52]

Indeed, research published in the *Journal of Applied Physiology* has found just that; and, in fact, they determined that catapult mechanisms occur in the activity of *walking*! Consider this: The pattern of how the muscles and tendons work together in walking did not follow the commonly held notion that tendons store energy in the first phase of stepping, and return the energy ("spring-like") in the second stepping phase. Rather, these researchers found that the medial gastrocnemius (medial calf muscle) and the soleus (muscle deeper in beneath the medial calf muscle) act as a *catapult mechanism* to strengthen and intensify muscle power![53]

This is especially interesting if you think back to what was noted earlier in the chapter about the use of the medial gastrocnemius muscle among people with osteoarthritis versus those without osteoarthritis. Recall that the activation of the medial gastrocnemius muscle when walking is *significantly reduced in people with osteoarthritis* as compared with those without osteoarthritis. In fact, in those *without* osteoarthritis, the medial gastrocnemius was found to be *highly activated!* Is it possible that people with osteoarthritis are not effectively using the catapult mechanism, that they have somehow lost this vital function? In Chapter Seven, you will find an exercise called "Stepping and Holding Your Ground" that is designed to build energy in the first phase of stepping and then use it in the second phase as you walk. This exercise is exceptionally helpful in retraining your ability to garner muscle power!

The researchers who uncovered the catapult mechanism in walking emphasized that it is the *interaction between the muscle fascicles and the tendon tissues* that is critically important in the storing and release of this elastic energy.[54] If you want to develop your ability to function well physically, you must focus on the muscles and tendons together -- the muscle-tendon unit!   That is a fundamental premise of our exercise program within this book!

By the way, if you return to Figure 6, the protruding small muscle fiber is within a tubular bundle of other fibers which comprises the muscle fascicle (which along with other muscle fascicles make up the inner structure of the muscle itself). As you begin to gain an appreciation for the amazing complexity of your muscles and their tendons, you will probably never think of a concentric muscle contraction (or any type of muscle contraction) in the same way again!

When you look at both the muscles and tendons *together*, you can see that losing muscle mass (or having a smaller muscle mass) that comes with aging does not necessarily mean a decline in the ability to effectively perform both basic and complex movements. Legendary are Asian martial arts masters such as Keiko Fukuda in Judo (at age 98, she still teaches three nights each week in San Francisco), Morihei Uyeshiba in Aikido, Kyuzo Mifune in Judo, Chosin Chibana in Karate, etc. who maintained their power and strength into their 70's, and 80's through cultivating their tendon strength (even though their muscle mass had diminished greatly).

As you will see in our Exercise Program, described and illustrated within Chapter Seven, we will be using principles of modern sport, kinetic muscle chain development exercises, and principles of the integrative muscle-tendon unit exercises found in the Asian martial arts. The exercises within this program are designed to build strong and interconnected tendons, muscles, ligaments, and bones. Through focusing upon the muscle-tendon units and muscle-tendon-bone units (not just the muscles), one will be able to develop well-coordinated and effective muscle chains that optimally will last you throughout your lifespan. When these kinetic muscle chains are smoothly and efficiently working, you should find that you are well on your way to healing from menopausal arthritis!

Notes for Chapter Four

[1] Sowers, M., Jannausch, M. L., Gross, M., Karvonen-Gutierrez, C. A., Palmieri, R. M., Crutchfield, M., & Richards-McCullough, K. (2006). Performance-based physical functioning in African-American and Caucasian women at midlife: Considering body composition, quadriceps strength, and knee osteoarthritis. *American Journal of Epidemiology, 163*(10), 950-958. doi: 10.1093/aje/kwj109

[2] Snyder, D. N. (2011, September 8). Stair climbing sport. Retrieved from www.stairclimbingsport.com/

[3] Ibid.

[4] Baratta, R., Solomonow, M., Zhou, B. H., Letson, D., Chuinard, R., & D'Ambrosia, R. (1988). Muscular coactivation. The role of the antagonist musculature in maintaining knee stability. *American Journal of Sports Medicine, 16*(2), 113-122.

[5] Devan, M. R., Pescatello, L. S., Faghri, P., & Anderson, J. (2004). A prospective study of overuse knee injuries among female athletes with muscle imbalances and structural abnormalities. *Journal of Athletic Training, 39*(3), 263-267.

[6] Zeni, J. A., Rudolph, K., & Higginson, J. S. (2010). Alterations in quadriceps and hamstrings coordination in persons with medial compartment knee osteoarthritis. *Journal of Electromyography and Kinesiology, 20*(1), 148-154. doi: 10.1016/j.jelekin.2008.12.003

[7] Hortobágyi, T., Westerkamp, L., Beam, S., Moody, J., Garry, J., Holbert, D., & DeVita, P. (2005). Altered hamstring-quadriceps muscle balance in patients with knee osteoarthritis. *Clinical Biomechanics, 20*, 97-104. doi: 10.1016/j.clinbiomech.2004.08.004

[8] Zeni, J. A., & Higginson, J. S. (2011). Knee osteoarthritis affects the distribution of joint moments during gait. *Knee, 18*(3), 156-159.

[9] Hortobágyi et al. (2005). Op. Cit.

[10] Henriksen, M., Alkjær, T., Lund, H., Simonsen, E. B., Graven-Nielsen, T., Danneskiold-Samsøe, B., & Bliddal, H. (2007). Experimental quadriceps muscle pain impairs knee joint control during walking. *Journal of Applied Physiology, 103*: 132-139. doi: 10.1152/japplphysiol.01105.2006

[11] Page, P., Frank, C. C., & Lardner, R. (2010). Assessment and treatment of muscle imbalance: the Janda approach. Champaign, IL: Human Kinetics.

[12] Magown, V. L., & Pellegrino, G. S. (2011, September 21). Myofascial Trigger Point Articles: Beware the Itis of Bursa. Retrieved from http://www.myorehab.net/articles/beware-the-itis-of-bursa.htm.

[13] Ibid.

[14]Hubley-Kozey, C. L., Hill, N. A., Rutherford, D. J.., Dunbar, M. J., & Stanish, W. D. (2009). Co-activation differences in lower limb muscles between asymptomatic controls and those with varying degrees of knee osteoarthritis during walking. *Clinical Biomechanics, 24*, 407-414. doi: 10.1016/j.clinbiomech.2009.02.005

[15]Moffat, M., & Vickery, S. (1999). *The American Physical Therapy Association book of body maintenance and repair.* New York: Round Stone Press, Henry Holt & Co.

[16]Ibid.

[17]Thomas, S. S., & Supan, T. J. (1990). A comparison of current biomechanical terms. *Journal of Prosthetics and Orthotics, 2(*2), 107-114.

[18]Costigan, P. A., Deluzio, K. J., & Wyss, U. P. (2002). Knee and hip kinetics during normal stair climbing. *Gait & Posture, 16*, 31-37.

[19]Sowers et al. (2006). Op. Cit.

[20]Cowan, S. M., & Crossley, K. M. (2009). Does gender influence neuromotor control of the knee and hip? *Journal of Electromyography and Kinesiology, 19*(2), 276-282.

[21]Herbert, R. D., Hoang, P. D., & Gandevia, S. C. (2008). Are muscles mechanically independent? *Journal of Applied Physiology, 104*, 1549-1550. doi: 10.1152/japplphysiol.90511.2008

[22]Moffat et al. (1999). Op. Cit.

[23]Józsa, L. G., & Kannus, P. (1997). Human tendons: Anatomy, physiology, and pathology. Champaign, IL: Human Kinetics.

[24]Kirkendall, D. T., & Garrett, W. E. (1997). Function and biomechanics of tendons. *Scandinavian Journal of Medicine & Science in Sports, 7*(2), 62-66.

[25]Kumai, T., Yamada, G., Takakura, Y., Tohno, Y., & Benjamin, M. (2006). Trace elements in human tendons and ligaments. *Biological Trace Element Research, 114*(1-3), 151-161.

[26]Yamada, M., Tohno, Y., Takakura, Y., Tohno, S., Moriwake, Y., & Minami, T. (2003). Age-related changes of element contents in human tendon of the iliopsoas muscle and the relationship among elements. *Biological Trace Element Research, 91*(1), 57-66.

[27]Ellis, E. H., Spadaro, J. A., & Becker, R. O. (1969). Trace elements in tendon collagen. *Clinical Orthopaedics and Related Research, 65*, 195-198.

[28]Herman, C. J., Allen, P., Hunt, W. C., Prasad, A., & Brady, T. J. (2004). Use of complementary therapies among primary care clinic patients with arthritis. *Preventing Chronic Disease, 1*(4), A12.

[29]Milanino, R., Marrella, M., Crivellente, F., Benoni, G., & Cuzzolin, L. (2000). Nutritional supplementation with copper in the rat. I. Effects on adjuvant arthritis development and on some in vivo- and ex vivo-markers of blood neutrophils. *Inflammation Research, 49*(5), 214-223.

[30]Richmond, S. J., Brown, S. R., Campion, P. D., Porter, A. J., Moffett, J. A., Jackson, D. A., Featherstone, V. A., & Taylor, A. J. (2009). Therapeutic effects of magnetic and copper bracelets in osteoarthritis: A randomized placebo-controlled crossover trial. *Complementary Therapies in Medicine, 17*(5-6), 249-256.

[31]Walker, W. R., & Keats, D. M. (1976). An investigation of the therapeutic value of the 'copper bracelet' - dermal assimilation of copper in arthritic/rheumatoid conditions. *Agents and Actions, 6*(4), 454-459.

[32]Silver, F. H., Freeman, J. W., Horvath, I., & Landis, W. J. (2001). Molecular basis for elastic energy storage in the mineralized tendon. *Biomacromolecules, 2*(3), 750-756.

[33]Fioravanti, A., Cantarini, L., Guidelli, G. M., & Galeazzi, M. (2011). Mechanisms of action of spa therapies in rheumatic diseases: what scientific evidence is there? *Rheumatology International, 31*, 1-8. doi: 10.1007/s00296-010-1628-6

[34]Ibid.

[35]Speer, K. P. (Ed.). (2005*). Injury prevention and rehabilitation for active older adults*. Champaign, IL: Human Kinetics.

[36]Ibid.

[37]Figuers, C. C. (2005). Soft tissue care: Flexibility, stretching and massage. In K. P. Speer (Ed.), *Injury prevention and rehabilitation for active older adults* (pp. 59-70). Champaign, IL: Human Kinetics.

[38]Speer (2005). Op. Cit.

[39]Atkins, R. C. (1998). *Dr. Atkins' vita-nutrient solution: Nature's answers to drugs*. New York: Simon & Schuster.

[40]Keast, D., Arstein, D., Harper, W., Fry, R. W., & Morton, A. R. (1995). Depression of plasma glutamine concentration after exercise stress and its possible influence on the immune system. *Medical Journal of Australia, 162*(1), 15-18.

[41]Varnier, M., Leese, G. P., Thompson, J., & Rennie, M. J. (1995). Stimulatory effect of glutamine on glycogen accumulation in human skeletal muscle. *American Journal of Physiology, 269*(2, Pt. 1), E309-E315.

[42]Pierno, S., De Luca, A., Camerino, C., Huxtable, R. J., & Camerino, D. C. (1998). Chronic administration of taurine to aged rats improves the electrical and contractile properties of skeletal muscle fibers. *Journal of Pharmacology and Experimental Therapeutics, 286*(3), 1183-1190.

[43]Pierno, S., Liantonio, A., Camerino, G. M., De Bellis, M., Cannone, M., Gramegna, G., Scaramuzzi, A., Simonetti, S., Nicchia, G. P., Basco, D., Svelto, M., Desaphy, J. F., & Camerino, D. C. (2011). Potential benefits of taurine in the prevention of skeletal muscle impairment induced by disuse in the hindlimb-unloaded rat. *Amino Acids*. Advance online publication. PMID: 21986958

[44]Dawson, R., Jr., Biasetti, M., Messina, S., & Dominy, J. (2002). The cytoprotective role of taurine in exercise-induced muscle injury. *Amino Acids, 22*(4), 309-324.

[45]Littarru, G. P., & Tiano, L. (2007). Bioenergetic and antioxidant properties of coenzyme Q10: Recent developments. *Molecular Biotechnology, 37*(1), 31-37.

[46]Ibid.

[47]Cooke, M., Iosia, M., Buford, T., Shelmadine, B., Hudson, G., Kerksick, C., Rasmussen, C., Greenwood, M., Leutholtz, B., Willoughby, D., & Kreider, R. (2008). Effects of acute and 14-day coenzyme Q10 supplementation on exercise performance in both trained and untrained individuals. *Journal of the International Society of Sports Nutrition, 5*, 8. doi: 10.1186/1550-2783-5-8

[48]Gökbel, H., Gül., I., Belviranli, M., & Okudan, N. (2010). The effects of coenzyme Q10 supplementation on performance during repeated bouts of supramaximal exercise in sedentary men. *Journal of Strength and Conditioning Research, 24*(1), 97-102.

[49]Díaz-Castro, J., Guisado, R., Kajarabille, N., García, C., Guisado, I. M., de Teresa, C., & Ochoa, J. J. (2011). Coenzyme Q(10) supplementation ameliorates inflammatory signaling and oxidative stress associated with strenuous exercise. *European Journal of Nutrition*. Advance online publication. PMID: 21990004

[50]Berger, M. J., & Doherty, T. J. (2010). Sarcopenia: Prevalence, mechanisms, and functional consequences. *Interdisciplinary Topics in Gerontology, 37*, 94-114.

[51]Mancuso, M., Orsucci, D., Volpi, L., Calsolaro, V., & Siciliano, G. (2010). Coenzyme Q10 in neuromuscular and neurodegenerative disorders. *Current Drug Targets, 11*(1), 111-121.

[52]Wilson, A. M., Watson, J. C., & Lichtwark, G. A. (2003). A catapult action for rapid limb protraction. *Nature, 421*, 35-36.

[53]Ishikawa, M., Komi, P. V., Grey, M. J., Lepola, V., & Bruggemann, G-P. (2005). Muscle-tendon interaction and elastic energy usage in human walking. *Journal of Applied Physiology, 99*, 603-608. doi: 10.1152/japplphysiol.00189.2005

[54]Ibid.

Chapter Five

Cartilage, Ligaments, and Menopausal Arthritis

■

Cartilage breakdown is a primary characteristic of osteoarthritis, and osteoarthritis is the form of the disease that is most associated with menopausal arthritis. In this Chapter, I will discuss what is known about cartilage (and ligament) differences in men and women and how these differences may be related to osteoarthritis. Most importantly, we'll look at what is known about cartilage and osteoarthritis in women after menopause. First, though, let's look at the nature of cartilage itself, and also at some aspects of cartilage within the disease process of osteoarthritis.

Cartilage - Critical Bone Protector

Cartilage is a wonderful, tough, flexible tissue that covers and protects the ends of your bones so that they can move smoothly within your joint without harm or damage due to friction. In the historical development of the species of vertebrates, cartilage is ancient tissue. In humans, the majority of the skeleton in early fetal development is formed from cartilage. In adults, cartilage covers the moving surfaces of synovial joints such as the knee (as well as being a component of other body parts such as the ears, nose, larynx, trachea, etc.).[1]

Did you know that within cartilage, actual cartilage cells (chondrocytes) are relatively scarce? Cartilage is primarily made up of the extracellular matrix.[2] The chondrocytes exist within this matrix which is composed of a formless gel-like "ground substance" surrounded by collagen fibers.[3] The solitary cartilage cells have the huge task of producing, maintaining and breaking down the extracellular matrix.[4] The resilient gel structure of the cartilage matrix is characterized by the many macromolecules in residence such as proteoglycans, the primary type of macromolecule. The large proteoglycan aggregates give the cartilage matrix much of its resiliency. Collagen makes up 40-70% of the "dry" weight of the matrix, and tissue fluid makes up 65-80% of the "wet" weight of the matrix.[5] Collagen acts as a reinforcement of the matrix providing strength and resisting stretch. The tissue fluid is vitally important to the cartilage matrix as it provides the nutrients to it. Since cartilage has no blood capillaries that can do this, nourishment is brought to the chondrocytes through diffusion into the matrix. Likewise, there are no lymph vessels, and the metabolic waste products are ushered out of the matrix in the reverse direction, again through diffusion.[6] The processes that keep the flexible, tough cartilage vital, are indeed quite complex.

Cartilage -- A Scarce Commodity Even in Normal Joints!

Many of us would probably be surprised by how scarce a commodity cartilage is within the average knee joint! The joint cartilage in the knee of the average adult is only about 3 to 4 mm thick, that is, at most about one-sixth of an inch! On top of the articular cartilage are two discs called menisci (the width of the medial meniscus is about 10 mm, or about two-fifths of an inch). The lateral meniscus is larger in size by about 2-3 additional millimeters or at most by one-eighth of an inch or less).[7] Each meniscus is made of fibrocartilage which makes it strong and flexible. They are movable "buffers" and are responsible for helping to distribute the force exerted from the femur or thigh bone to the tibia or shinbone. The contribution of the menisci allows the knee joint to be more "elastic." Stability is also needed, so the menisci team up with the ligaments that bind the joint together to form a working unit.[8] (Please See Figure 7 below.)

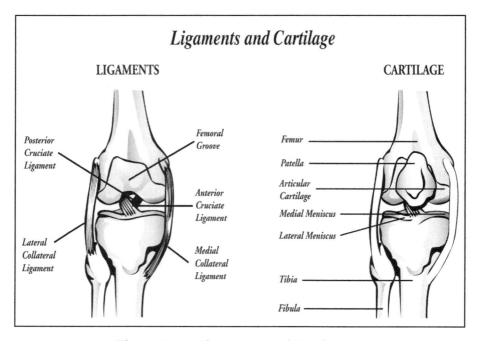

Figure 7 -- Ligaments and Cartilage

Changes involving deterioration or degeneration of the menisci can begin to occur in people as early as the age of 30. These changes alter the structure of the menisci, and they become less elastic and less able to help distribute the pressure from the thigh bone. There are great individual variations in how the menisci fare over time. Some people in their 30's or 40's may have considerable degeneration. On the other hand, there have been almost normal menisci found in some very old people. Extensive work involving kneeling or squatting can speed up degenerative changes within the menisci.[9]

In people who have beginning osteoarthritis where there may be little visible changes on x-ray, it is sometimes hard to tell if pain in the knee joint is coming from a meniscus problem or from arthritis-related symptoms. In people with early stage arthritis, a minor trauma to the knee or overuse of the knee joint may make the knee hurt in ways that are similar to a meniscus tear when indeed there is not one. Diagnosing knee pain is, to be sure, often quite complicated. Actual degeneration of the menisci that involves small tears in these structures does not usually occur until the later stages of osteoarthritis. The early stages involve the loss of the joint cartilage covering the bone.[10]

There are many problems that can occur with joint cartilage to include tears and injuries such as from an accidental slip or fall in everyday activity. Genetic differences can also contribute to cartilage problems. For example, one might be genetically predisposed to form a defective cartilage matrix, the important ground substance of cartilage cells. Because of the expression of certain genes in cartilage cells, an abnormal cartilage matrix could result. This could then put an individual at heightened risk for developing osteoarthritis.[11]

However, even the normal homeostasis of cartilage relies on complex processes that could be vulnerable to breakdown. As discussed earlier, without capillaries to provide nutrients to the matrix, cartilage depends upon diffusion of tissue fluids into the matrix. The diffusion taking place is a spontaneous movement of particles from inside of the matrix to outside of the matrix and vice versa; this is due to the balance of molecules inside and outside of the matrix. Because the chondrocytes need to depend upon this lengthy diffusion pathway to obtain vital nutrients, this can be a perilous state for them. This is especially so when proteoglycans, displaced from the matrix, are replaced by calcium salts which do not dissolve.[12] Recall back to our discussion in Chapter Two of the importance of proteoglycan aggregates to the smooth movement of the joint; through their hydration of the cartilage, it is able to withstand compression.

The role of calcium-containing crystals in the joints in osteoarthritis patients is not something that is clear as of yet. There is controversy within the field of rheumatology as to whether they have any role in advancing osteoarthritis, or rather they are just deposited as

part of the aging process. Advanced osteoarthritis is frequently associated with a cartilage matrix that contains calcifications. In early
osteoarthritis, however, it is hard to pinpoint and understand the process of calcification, because the calcium-containing crystals are often
in amounts that are too small to assess. At least in the end-stage of
osteoarthritis, there does appear to be some evidence suggesting that
cartilage calcification is involved in the breakdown of cartilage.[13]

What triggers cartilage break down is really a matter of debate
in the field of rheumatology. Although it had been thought that it was
propelled by processes within the cartilage itself, current research in
the study of osteoarthritis points toward the roles of surrounding
tissues as well. The bone, synovial or joint lining, and inflammation
in the joint lining all seem to have roles in cartilage breakdown.
Some research even suggests that the subchondral bone, or bone that
is underneath the joint cartilage, may play a role in initiating cartilage
breakdown.[14] Of much interest to us in our discussion of menopausal
arthritis is the role of inflammation. Research shows that inflammation is involved in the early and the late stages of osteoarthritis.[15] In
Chapter Two, we had looked at some of the inflammatory processes
that are connected with leptin and the production of cytokines which
promote cartilage breakdown. This is, of course, of critical importance to us in our discussion of menopausal arthritis.

In this chapter we will focus upon another topic of importance
to menopausal arthritis: gender differences in cartilage and ligaments
that may make women more vulnerable than men to osteoarthritis.
Before we move on to this area, another aspect of cartilage would be
important to bring up within our discussion. Cartilage is an avascular
tissue as noted earlier, and it has generally been thought that once it
has broken down that it cannot be regenerated. Some surprising findings follow in Topic of Interest #5.

Topic of Interest #5

Degeneration of Cartilage: A One-Way Street?

Degradation or breakdown of cartilage in osteoarthritis may not occur in just the way it was originally thought to occur. It has been commonly thought that cartilage in osteoarthritis is on a "one-way road of cartilage loss."[16] However, research has found that cartilage changes can go in both directions! Over the course of the disease, cartilage can be thickened *or* thinned in osteoarthritic knees. Although the proportion of thickened to thinned cartilage favors thinned cartilage in more advanced knee osteoarthritis (Grade 3), those with less severe osteoarthritis (Grade 2) had very similar percentages of thickened and thinned cartilage.[17]

Does this mean that some of the cartilage is actually regenerating? Is this even possible? In a very interesting animal study, researchers at the Oregon Health and Science University found a strain of mice that appears to be able to "regenerate" joint cartilage! Cartilage wound sites in these animals were abundant with the tools for cartilage repair; they were rich with the needed proteoglycans and collagens. This abundance in cartilage-building materials was particularly apparent after 12 weeks when these mice far surpassed the control group mice in terms of their healing response.

This special strain of mice had a superior supply of cartilage cells and rich extracellular matrix whereas the control group mice had far fewer of the vital proteoglycans and collagen II (the primary form of collagen in joint cartilage). If scientists are able to gain an understanding of the biological, chemical, and genetic factors involved in this remarkable cartilage regeneration, then treatment options for humans might be found.[18]

With these optimistic findings in mind, let's go on to look at cartilage changes in women. Older women seem to incur more cartilage loss than older men, and we'll take a look at reasons why this might be.

Menopausal Women and Cartilage Changes

Even before the onset of knee arthritis, women have been found to have more cartilage volume loss than men. In a study of 102 men and 169 women (ages 50-79 yrs.) with no history of knee pain or arthritis, MRI images of the knees were assessed over a period of approximately two years. The average yearly *declines* in tibial (shin bone) cartilage volume and patellar (kneecap) cartilage volume *were significantly greater in women* than in men. Moreover, in comparison with men, women had an increased risk of tibiofemoral cartilage defects progressing over time.[19] In another study of men and women (ages 50-78 yrs.) with no arthritis symptoms, it was found that compared with young adults (ages 20-30 yrs.), femoral cartilage was thinner in both sexes, which is what one might expect with aging.

What was surprising, though, is that in the older adults there was a *decrease in patellar cartilage thickness in the women, but not in the men.*[20] In addition, in a study looking at men and women over about a decade, *only women had a diminished patellar cartilage volume associated with body mass, especially body fat mass.*[21] Why the greater susceptibility to cartilage loss in women? Remember that the most common characteristic among women with menopausal arthritis, aside from menopause, was obesity. Perhaps the associated proinflammatory cytokines that we talked about in Chapter Two are a causal factor here. However, does loss of estrogen after menopause play a role in this as well?

Estrogen and Cartilage

Research has shown over many studies that there are estrogen receptors in cartilage.[22] It really is not clear, though, whether estrogen loss after menopause is actually playing any kind of key role in cartilage degradation. For example, some animal studies that have used a menopausal model with ovariectomized animals have determined that cartilage breakdown is occurring right after the ovaries are removed. Nevertheless, the cartilage breakdown is short-lived! After 6-9 weeks, the indicators of cartilage breakdown go back to the levels of the animals that had not had their ovaries removed.[23] One possible hypothesis that has been extended for why cartilage breakdown may be temporary is this: Gained fat mass after the ovaries have been removed compensates for lost estrogen from the ovaries by added estrogen produced from the increased fat cells. Compared with animals that did not have their ovaries removed, the ones that did gained weight. This increase in adipose tissue may mean that more estrogen is released from the adipose tissue in these animals. This may offset the lack of estrogen from the ovaries and decrease the indicators of cartilage breakdown.[24] After menopause, estrogen is produced in many areas of the body such as body fat. Body fat is responsible for the bulk of the conversion of androgens to estrogen.[25] So, this seems like it could be a possible reason for a lessening of cartilage breakdown. In the research cases summarized, the specific indicator of cartilage breakdown was elevated CTX-II which is a fragment of type II collagen. It is correlated with joint damage, and it is countered by estrogen.[26]

Does added estrogen after menopause such as in estrogen replacement therapy (ERT) help preserve cartilage, then? Most research studies on women do not really address the effect of ERT on cartilage markers of osteoarthritis. Instead, they look at self-reported symptoms such as knee pain, or they use a clinical diagnosis rather than actual x-ray results. We have summarized much of these findings in Chapter Three. One recent review study, though, did *exclude* self-reported symptoms such as knee pain as well as clinically diagnosed osteoarthritis.[27] They specifically wanted to assess only the structural changes of osteoarthritis. They sought to determine whether estrogen, both what is naturally in a woman's body and what is added in therapy such as ERT, would affect structural changes such as cartilage volume. What they found was that in three randomized controlled trials and in one non-experimental study, there was evidence that estrogen supplementation affects cartilage turnover. Estrogen was associated with CTX-I and II levels that are markers for cartilage breakdown in one study. Moreover, women on estrogen replacement for more than 5 years had greater tibial cartilage than those who had never undergone ERT. Although some studies did not show an effect of estrogen on structural factors related to osteoarthritis, these researchers concluded that estrogen does have an effect upon the health of the joint. Whether estrogen specifically obtained through outside supplementation is beneficial was unclear at this point. This is because the types of hormone therapies differed (e.g., HRT, ERT) as did what was examined (e.g., biomarkers of cartilage breakdown, x-ray images, MRI images) along with a few other factors, as well.[28]

In looking more closely at some of the studies in the above review, some interesting facts emerge. Although estrogen replacement therapy had seemed to affect tibial cartilage positively, this was not found for patella cartilage in which there were no differences between the women who were on ERT and those not on ERT. The researchers speculated that this may be due to different mechanisms or ways that knee osteoarthritis develops in these two different knee locations.[29] Also, in a study examining a variety of medications that prevent bone from being reabsorbed (to include estrogen) a very important finding was noted: There was no association between any of the anti-resorptive medications and changes in knee osteoarthritis on x-ray or reported knee pain. They did find, though, that there was less subchondral bone loss and bone abnormalities with estrogen supplementation as evaluated by MRI. Estrogen was not associated with less severity of knee pain.[30]

Animal models of menopause (those in which the animals' ovaries are surgically removed) have proven to be useful for studying the effects of estrogen and estrogen loss on cartilage in postmenopausal women.[31] These studies allow for better controlled, experimental research. A review of the research with animal models assessing the effects of loss of estrogen and of estrogen treatment on cartilage contained some interesting findings. Eleven out of the 14 studies reviewed showed that there was cartilage damage in sexually mature rats that had been ovariectomized (ovaries removed). However, the effects of estrogen treatment on cartilage resulted in beneficial effects for animals in *only half* of the studies (11 out of 22).[32] From these studies, and those reviewed on postmenopausal women, it seems that nothing definitive really can be said at this point about whether estrogen replacement is protective against onset or worsening of osteoarthritis. Beyond just the methodological and other issues with the overall research, the complexity of other contributing factors has to be considered too. For example, in a large study of knee osteo-arthritis, it was found that as the number of metabolic syndrome risk factors increased, the minimum joint space area *decreased in women* but *not in men.*[33] This study was also looking at structural factors, since joint space narrowing is one of the markers of disease progression in osteoarthritis. I think that this takes us full circle right back to the connection between metabolic syndrome (and leptin resistance) in postmenopausal women, and its association with osteo-arthritis.

Cartilage Degradation on X-Ray and Symptomatic Pain: Far from a Perfect Match

Before going any further, I must bring up an important point relating to cartilage changes, cartilage degradation, and arthritis symptoms. Radiographic findings that diagnose osteoarthritis do not necessarily correspond to self-reported pain with osteoarthritis. This means that you could have breakdown of cartilage on an x-ray but not have any joint pain. Conversely, you could have no breakdown of cartilage on an x-ray and have considerable joint pain. Many different factors can influence whether osteoarthritis (as defined in terms of changes in cartilage and bone on an x-ray) will correspond to reported pain, among them: the number of x-rays taken (e.g., all views of knee compartments vs. isolated views), how pain is defined (e.g., within the last month, for 15 days or more), who is being studied, such as what age group (e.g., ages 40-80 yrs., over age 45 yrs.). Even ethnicity in some cases can be a factor. For example, differences have been found between African American and Caucasian women in terms of the function of pain as a symptom in predicting radiographic osteoarthritis.[34] Factors such as these and others can contribute to the problem of this lack of connection between reported symptoms and x-ray findings. As we shall see in the next chapter, non-joint sources of joint pain (some of which are more common in women than men) are possibly one of the most important reasons for this lack of connection between x-ray evidence of osteoarthritis and reported pain with osteoarthritis. Non-joint sources of pain (i.e., extra-articular sources in the soft tissues surrounding the joint) may be a large source of the pain experienced by women as due to menopausal arthritis.

Ligaments -- The Ties that Bind

Cartilage is critical to joint function because it provides elastic structure and buffering of the bones of the joint against friction as you move. However, without ligaments the inherently unstable knee joint would not be able to function! Ligaments are tough bands of connective tissue containing very strong fibers. The word ligament means "to bind," and, indeed, that is exactly the function of ligaments within the body. Every major joint in our body is sturdily and securely bound together by these tough, fibrous bands. Some joints need more securing than others, though. For example, the knee is not intrinsically stable. In contrast, the elbow is a stable, hinge-type joint. Although the elbow does have ligaments that stabilize it even further, the knee *depends* upon its surrounding ligaments to function. The knee's ligaments are essential in providing it stability. Two ligaments crisscross within the middle of the knee joint itself with two more on either side of the knee joint providing lateral stability. See Figure 7 (presented earlier in the chapter) for the position of these ligaments. Most ligaments are not very "elastic" and they can become stretched out of shape if they have been placed under too much stress. For example, if our muscles are not properly holding up the bones on our body, then the ligaments become overused as a support.[35]

Do Some Female Hormones Cause Joint Laxity?

The effect of estrogen on the anterior cruciate ligament (ACL) has long been a topic in the sports training and sports medicine literature. However, whether hormonal fluctuations influence ACL laxity has remained controversial. Some studies have found that female hormone levels are related to higher joint laxity,[36,37] whereas others have not.[38,39] Do the knee's ligaments change after menopause? Do they in any way contribute to menopausal arthritis? With regard to the hormonal changes at menopause and the effect upon knee ligaments, it is difficult to find any information. The focus within the literature appears to be a gynecological one; the investigations center upon pelvic and urologic issues and related ligaments and their association with estrogen.

Nevertheless, in one animal study, it was found that there were no differences between the non-ovariectomized group and the ovariectomized group in terms of the mechanical or basic compositional properties of their anterior cruciate ligaments. This study also supported the line of thought that knee ligament injury in female athletes is not a result of estrogen's effect on the ligaments.[40]

Another interesting study examined the effects of the hormone resistin, rather than estrogen, on ligaments. This study looked specifically at the ligaments of the trapeziometacarpal joint in perimenopausal women. The trapeziometacarpal joint is the thumb joint that you move when the thumb is pulled away from and back toward the fingers. There is a greater occurrence of arthritis in this joint in women than in men. Since the hormone resistin is known to increase laxity in some ligaments during pregnancy, resistin was suspected as a possible contributive factor in thumb joint laxity. It is thought that if the thumb's attached ligament has too much laxity, then this may predispose one to suffer from osteoarthritis of the thumb joint. Researchers tested for the receptiveness of the ligament tissue to relaxin. They found that there were receptors for this hormone in all of the volar oblique ligaments of the hand (that is, all of the ligaments where the fingers attach to the palm).[41]

Does the hormone relaxin affect other ligaments, such as those within the knee at and after menopause? One "in vitro," laboratory study found that relaxin was found in four out of five female anterior cruciate ligament cells, whereas it was found in only one out of five male anterior cruciate ligament cells.[42] Could some of the knee instability in postmenopausal women going up and down the stairs, for example, be affected by ligaments that have become too lax?

The ACL ligament provides 86% of the restraint upon anterior tibial translation. Anterior tibial translation is basically the pulling of the tibia or shinbone forward that is achieved through quadriceps contraction. The ACL (and the hamstrings) function to try to restrain this pull. Some of the factors that affect whether the ACL is injured are central to the individual's physiology such as joint laxity, the alignment of the lower limbs, and the size of the ligament; others are external to the person's physical makeup such as movement in sports or level of skill.[43] It is baffling why more research on knee laxity in postmenopausal women (and/or in arthritis patients) has not been conducted. It is clear that ligaments and their stability affect movement and certainly could affect the course of arthritis.

Many studies have found gender differences in knee joint laxity. Nevertheless, one study examining all of the various factors that might be involved in causing ACL injuries in males and females found no differences among men and women in terms of knee joint laxity. What they did find, however, was that the strength of the hamstrings and of the quadriceps was different in women and men; and in non-athletes, as opposed to athletes. Men had greater muscle strength than women, and athletes had greater muscle strength than non-athletes. They explained that the reduced muscle strength in women may be a factor leading to increased ACL injuries.[44]

With regard to sports and exercise, there are some findings of particular importance pertaining to cartilage. Mechanical force and loads have been considered essential for the maintenance and regulation of musculoskeletal tissues; they are critical to joint homeostasis. However, if the mechanical loading constitutes an "overload," or conversely, there is too little loading as in disuse, then cartilage destruction occurs. This cartilage destruction can also occur from chronic patterns of joint loading that put excessive load on a joint.[45] This is of particular importance with regard to menopausal arthritis, where due to muscular weakness, abnormal loading on joints can occur. Moderate levels of loading on joints have been shown to be protective of osteoarthritis in both animal and human studies. This is thought to be a result of the moderate mechanical load acting to stimulate synthesis of cartilage cells.[46] In Chapter Seven, I will discuss how this type of loading through exercise not only strengthens muscles and tendons, but also helps promote bone modeling and strong bones. Here we can see that this also extends to cartilage as well!

In fact, research shows that there is a "coupling" that occurs between bone and cartilage, and that if one is affected the other is too. For example, bone marrow lesions are often related to a heightened risk of defects within the cartilage. Moreover, cartilage changes have been associated with remodeling processes in the adjacent bone beneath the cartilage. There may even be a "crosstalk" between bone and cartilage signaling pathways.[47] This vital connection between bone, muscle, tendon, and cartilage is why our exercise program relies on the total functioning unit of muscle-tendon-bone (as described in Chapter Seven). Given this research on cartilage, one might even conceptualize it as a muscle-tendon-cartilage-bone unit! Moreover, this moderate joint loading in exercise has even been associated with a reduction in metalloproteinases (MMPs) in chondrocytes! Recall from Chapter Two that the MMPs are involved in collagen breakdown in cartilage. Joint loading in exercise then could help to maintain cartilage.[48]

Let's go back to ligaments for a moment, however. We've talked a lot about laxity, but what if it's not just ligament laxity that we need to look at. Rather, what if other changes within the ligament may matter with regard to osteoarthritis? At the beginning of this chapter, I had discussed how there is some controversy as to whether the disease process of osteoarthritis is "cartilage-driven" or perhaps driven by other things such as the involvement of the subchondral bone. However, some theorists have even suggested that osteoarthritis might be derived, too, from the involvement of ligaments. These researchers have made the case that the initiation of osteoarthritis might be categorized in terms of whether it is derived from cartilage, bone, ligament, menisci, or synovium involvement.[49]

How could ligaments be a structure where osteoarthritis is initiated? According to Professor Dennis McGonagle of the University of Leeds and colleagues, important changes to ligaments and the areas where they insert into bone can affect the bone and tissues of the joint lining. They noted that in some spontaneous osteoarthritis models, the first changes seen within the knee joint actually occur in the cruciate ligaments, not in the articular cartilage and other joint tissues.[50] Moreover, remember the Heberden's nodes that were commonly found on patients with menopausal arthritis in the classic study by Drs. Cecil and Archer? Well, Professor McGonagle and colleagues noted that in Herberden's nodes, the most marked initial changes are seen in the collateral ligaments.[51] Perhaps then with regard to osteoarthritis, ligaments are more than just ties that bind!

As you can see, unraveling what happens within the disease process of arthritis is an extremely complex scientific endeavor. Although cartilage deterioration is one of the primary characteristics of osteoarthritis, it is not clear whether the process is derived within and driven by cartilage. I have briefly touched upon but a few of the current hypotheses and theories that are circulating within the field of rheumatology at this time.

Of most importance to us in looking at menopausal arthritis are the findings summarized within this chapter that: (1) Even before the onset of knee arthritis, women have been found to have more cartilage volume loss than men; (2) women have been found to have a higher risk than men of tibiofemoral cartilage defects progressing over time; (3) there was a greater decrease in patellar cartilage thickness in older women than in older men; and finally (4) that diminished patellar cartilage volume was associated with body fat mass only in women, not men. Also of importance is the possibility that ligament laxity in women may contribute in some ways to developing problems that could be associated with osteoarthritis. Moreover, in light of the research on ligaments as a possible source of osteoarthritis discussed above, more attention to the actual composition and changes within the ligaments along with cartilage should be of concern.

Finally, since x-ray evidence of cartilage deterioration and self-reported arthritis pain often do not show a connection, this broader perspective on the disease process discussed here may allow us to move beyond cartilage in some important ways. Cartilage is integral to the disease process of osteoarthritis; however, understanding osteoarthritis encompasses more than just cartilage and its breakdown.

Notes for Chapter Five

[1]Warwick, R., & Williams, P. L. (1973). *Gray's anatomy* (35th British ed.). Philadelphia: W. B. Saunders.

[2]Fosang, A. J., & Beier, F. (2011). Emerging frontiers in cartilage and chondrocyte biology. *Best Practice & Research Clinical Rheumatology, 25*(6), 751-766.

[3]Warwick et al. (1973). Op. Cit.

[4]Fosang et al. (2011). Op Cit.

[5]Cormack, D. H. (2001). Essential histology (Medicine series). (2nd ed.). Philadelphia: Lippincott Williams & Wilkins.

[6]Ibid.

[7]Ricklin, P., Rüttimann, A., & Del Buono, M. S. (1971). Meniscus lesions: Practical problems of clinical diagnosis, arthrography and therapy. New York: Grune & Stratton.

[8]Ibid.

[9]Ibid.

[10]Ibid.

[11]Ray, A., & Ray, B. K. (2008). An inflammation-responsive transcription factor in the pathophysiology of osteoarthritis. *Biorheology, 45*(3-4), 399-409.

[12]Cormack et al. (2001). Op. Cit.

[13]Mebarek, S., Hamade, E., Thouverey, C., Bandorowicz-Pikula, J., Pikula, S., Magne, D., & Buchet, R. (2011). Ankylosing spondylitis, late osteoarthritis, vascular calcification, chondrocalcinosis and pseudo gout: Toward a possible drug therapy. *Current Medicinal Chemistry, 18,* 2196-2203.

[14]Bijlsma, J. W. J., Berenbaum, F., & Lafeber, F. P. J. G. (2011). Osteoarthritis: An update with relevance for clinical practice. *Lancet, 377,* 2115-2126.

[15]Ibid.

[16]Buck, R. J., Wyman, B. T., Le Graverand, M. P., Hudelmaier, M., Wirth, W., & Eckstein, F. (2010). Osteoarthritis may not be a one-way-road of cartilage loss -- comparison of spatial patterns of cartilage change between osteoarthritic and healthy knees. *Osteoarthritis and Cartilage, 18*(3), 329-335.

[17]Ibid.

[18]Fitzgerald, J., Rich, C., Burkhardt, D., Allen, J., Herzka, A. S., & Little, C. B. (2008). Evidence for articular cartilage regeneration in MRL/MpJ mice. *Osteoarthritis and Cartilage, 16*(11), 1319-1326.

[19]Hanna F. S., Teichtahl, A. J., Wluka, A. E., Wang, Y. Urquhart, D. M., English, D. R., Giles, G. G., & Cicuttini, F. M. (2009). Women have increased rates of cartilage loss and progression of cartilage defects at the knee than men: a gender study of adults without clinical knee osteoarthritis. *Menopause, 16*(4), 666-670.

[20]Hudelmaier, M. Glaser, C. Hohe, J., Englmeier, K. H., Reiser, M., Putz, R., & Eckstein, F. (2001). Age-related changes in the morphology and deformational behavior of knee joint cartilage. *Arthritis & Rheumatism, 44*(11), 2556-2561.

[21]Teichtahl, A. J., Wang, Y., Wluka, A. E., Szramka, M. , English, D. R., Giles, G G., O'Sullivan, R., & Cicuttini, F. M. (2008). The longitudinal relationship between body composition and patella cartilage in healthy adults. *Obesity, 16*(2), 421-427.

[22]Reginster, J. Y., Kvasz, A., Bruyere, O., & Henrotin, Y. (2003). Is there any rationale for prescribing hormone replacement therapy (HRT) to prevent or to treat osteoarthritis? *Osteoarthritis and Cartilage, 11*(2), 87-91.

[23]Bay-Jensen, A-C., Tabassi, N. C., Sondergaard, L. V., Andersen, T. L., Dagnaes-Hansen, F., Garnero, P., Kassem, M., & Delaissé, J-M. (2009). The response to oestrogen deprivation of the cartlilage collagen degradation marker, CTX-II, is unique compared with other markers of collagen turnover. *Arthritis Research & Therapy, 11*, R9. doi:10.1186/ar2596

[24]Ibid.

[25]Coney, P., Zurawin, R. K., Talavera, F., Gaupp, F.B., & Lucidi, R. S. (2012). Menopause. Retrieved from Medscape Reference - Drugs, Diseases & Procedures http://emedicine.medscape.com/article/264088-overview

[26] Bay-Jensen (2009). Op. Cit.

[27]Tanamas, S. K., Wijethilake, P., Wluka, A. E., Davies-Tuck, M. L., Urquhart, D. M. Wang, Y., & Cicuttini, F. M. (2011). Sex hormones and structural changes in osteoarthritis: A systematic review. *Maturitas, 69*, 141-156. doi: 10.1016/j.maturitas.2011.03.019

[28]Ibid.

[29]Cicuttini, F. M., Wluka, A. E., Wang, Y., Stuckey, S. L., & Davis, S. R. (2003). Effect of estrogen replacement therapy on patella cartilage in healthy women. *Clinical and Experimental Rheumatology, 21*(1), 79-82.

[30]Carbone, L. D., Nevitt, M. C., Wildy, K., Barrow, K. D., Harris, F., Felson, D., Peterfy, C., Visser, M., Harris, T. B., Wang, B. W., & Kritchevsky, S. B., ; Health, Aging and Body Composition Study. (2004). The relationship of antiresorptive drug use to structural findings and symptoms of knee osteoarthritis. *Arthritis and Rheumatism, 50*(11), 3516-3525.

[31]Høegh-Andersen, P., Tankó, L. B., Andersen, T. L., Lundberg, C. V., Mo, J. A., Heegaard, A. M., Delaissé, J. M. & Christgau, S. (2004). Ovariectomized rats as a model of postmenopausal osteoarthritis: Validation and application. *Arthritis Research & Therapy, 6*(2), R169-R180.

[32]Sniekers, Y. H., Weinans, H. Bierma-Zeinstra, S. M., van Leeuwen, J. P., & van Osch, G. J. (2008). Animal models for osteoarthritis: The effect of ovariectomy and estrogen treatment - a systematic approach. *Osteoarthritis and Cartilage, 16*(5), 533-541.

[33]Yoshimura, N., Muraki, S., Oka, H., Kawaguchi, H., Nakamura, K., & Akune, T. (2011). Association of knee osteoarthritis with the accumulation of metabolic risk factors such as overweight, hypertension, dyslipidemia, and impaired glucose tolerance in Japanese men and women: the ROAD study. *Journal of Rheumatology, 38*(5), 921-930.

[34]Bedson, J., & Croft, P. R. (2008). The discordance between clinical and radiographic knee osteoarthritis: A systematic search and summary of the literature. *BMC Musculoskeletal Disorders, 9*(116). doi:10.1186/1471-2474-9-116

[35]Dimon, Jr., T. (2008) Anatomy of the moving body: A basic course in bones, muscles, and joints (2nd ed.). Berkeley, CA: North Atlantic Books.

[36]Heitz, N. A., Eisenman, P. A., Beck, C. L., & Walker, J. A., (1999). Hormonal changes throughout the menstrual cycle and increased anterior cruciate ligament laxity in females. *Journal of Athletic Training, 34*(2), 144-149.

[37]Park, S. K., Stefanyshyn, D. J., Loitz-Ramage, B., Hart, D. A., & Ronsky, J. L. (2009). Changing hormone levels during the menstrual cycle affect knee laxity and stiffness in healthy female subjects. *American Journal of Sports Medicine, 37*(3), 588-598.

[38]Pollard, C. D., Braun, B., & Hamill, J. (2006). Influence of gender, estrogen and exercise on anterior knee laxity. *Clinical Biomechanics, 21*(10), 1060-1066.

[39]Hertel, J., Williams, N. I., Olmsted-Kramer, L. C., Leidy, H. J., & Putukian, M. (2006). Neuromuscular performance and knee laxity do not change across the menstrual cycle in female athletes. *Knee Surgery, Sports Traumatology, Arthroscopy, 14*(9), 817-822.

[40]Wentorf, F. A., Sudoh, K., Moses, C., Arendt, E. A., & Carlson, C. S. (2006). The effects of estrogen on material and mechanical properties of the intra- and extra-articular knee structures. *American Journal of Sports Medicine, 34*(12), 1948-1952.

[41]Lubahn, J., Ivance, D., Konieczko, E., & Cooney, T., (2006). Immunohistochemical detection of relaxin binding to the volar oblique ligament. *Journal of Hand Surgery, 31*(1), 80-84.

[42]Faryniarz, D. A., Bhargava, M., Lajam, C., Attia, E. T., & Hannafin, J. A. (2006). Quantitation of estrogen receptors and relaxin binding in human anterior cruciate ligament fibroblasts. *In Vitro Cellular and Developmental Biology. Animal, 42*(7), 176-181.

[43]Rosene, J. M., & Fogarty, T. D., (1999). Anterior tibial translation in collegiate athletes with normal anterior cruciate ligament integrity. *Journal of Athletic Training, 34*(2), 93-98.

[44]Bowerman, S. J., Smith, D. R., Carlson, M.. & King, G. A. (2006). A comparison of factors influencing ACL injury in male and female athletes and non-athletes. *Physical Therapy in Sport, 7*(3), 144-152.

[45]Sun, H. B. (2010). Mechanical loading, cartilage degradation, and arthritis. *Annals of the New York Academy of Sciences, 1211*, 37-50. doi: 10.1111/j.1749-6632.2010.05808.x

[46]Ibid.

[47]Yokota, H., Leong, D. J., & Sun, H. B. (2011). Mechanical loading: and cartilage maintenance. *Current Osteoporosis Reports, 9*(4), 237-242.

[48]Sun, H. B., Zhao, L., Tanaka, S., & Yokota, H. (2011). Moderate joint loading reduces degenerative actions of matrix metalloproteinases in the articular cartilage of mouse ulnae. *Connective Tissue Research*. Advanced online publication. PMID: 22148954

[49]McGonagle, D., Tan, A. L. , Carey, J., & Benjamin, M. (2010). The anatomical basis for a novel classification of osteoarthritis and allied disorders. *Journal of Anatomy, 216*, 279-291. doi: 10.1111/j.1469-7580.2009.01186.x

[50]Ibid.

[51]Ibid.

Chapter Six

Menopausal Arthritis: Not Just Osteoarthritis Brought on By Menopause!

Beyond the Usual Definition

Menopausal arthritis has generally been considered to be a form of osteoarthritis that may occur as a result of hormonal changes at and after menopause. There is no doubt that osteoarthritis is part of the picture of what is involved in menopausal arthritis. That is why the important new insights into the role of leptin and proinflammatory cytokines in osteoarthritis are invaluable. However, the research that I have reviewed suggests that menopausal arthritis is actually more complex than just a form of osteoarthritis brought on by estrogen decline; it clearly shows that *many more factors* are likely involved in women's experiences of menopausal arthritis.

In Chapter Four, I had mentioned that there are soft tissue disorders such as pes anserine bursitis that can cause knee pain. In this chapter, we will look more closely at pes anserine bursitis. We'll also look at other soft tissue ailments more common in women than men with an eye toward how they can be mistaken for arthritis pain. There are also gender differences in psychological factors that may affect arthritis that I will introduce within this chapter and explore more fully in Chapter Eleven. Could certain psychological factors that are more common in women than men actually result in worsening menopausal arthritis? In addition, the focus in the literature on menopausal arthritis has been upon its association with osteoarthritis. However, the peak onset of rheumatoid arthritis in women occurs at the time of menopause. Is rheumatoid arthritis ever part of what women experience as being "menopausal arthritis?" We will explore whether this may be so within this chapter. First, though, let's look at some factors other than arthritis that might cause knee pain in a woman's life during menopause and thereafter; factors that are *not* directly caused by *any* form of arthritis.

Physical Ailments That Can Cause Arthritis-Like Pain

Osteoarthritis, a disease characterized by degenerative changes within the joints, is often measured by patients' self-reports of pain. It is very important to stress, though, that the *source of pain* in osteoarthritis is unknown; it is simply unclear at this point. The reason is that the hyaline cartilage or joint cartilage has no stimulation by nerves. Other related factors that could cause pain include bone marrow lesions of the bone underneath the cartilage, a thickened joint lining, and abnormal fluid within the joint. Some of the pain may originate from outside of the joint itself in surrounding structures that have pain receptors.[1]

There are usually problems with knee mechanics in osteoarthritis patients, and this may put stress on ligaments and tendon insertions which can cause pain. For example, one study examined pain and disorders outside of the joint itself. These tissue disorders included semimembranosus-TCL bursitis, iliotibial band syndrome, and pes anserine bursitis. This research showed that these types of soft tissue disorders may be the *origin* of the osteoarthritis pain in many cases, *even in patients in which it is thought that the knee joint itself is the source.* The findings showed that prepatellar bursitis and superficial infrapatellar bursitis were commonly found in individuals with radiographic knee osteoarthritis (with or without symptoms). On the other hand, iliotibial band syndrome, semimembranosus-TCL bursitis, and pes anserine bursitis were most common among the patients that did experience symptoms of knee osteoarthritis.[2]

Pes anserine bursitis is of critical importance when considering the causes of menopausal arthritis, and I will discuss it more below. Another important type of bursitis to consider is tibial collateral ligament bursitis that usually causes pain on top of the tibial collateral ligament at the inside of the knee at the joint line.[3] This would be above the area of the pes anserinus. It occurs when the bursa of the semimembranosus tendon is irritated as a result of repetitive or stressful movements of the tendon (e.g., during knee extension, or valgus stress upon the knee). The tendon moves between the tibial collateral ligament and the medial tibial condyle. Researchers from the University of California -- San Francisco, described the tendon as being "scissored" between these two structures. The semimembranosus tibial collateral ligament bursa serves as a cushion to protect the tendon from this shearing force. However, bursitis can occur as a result of either repetitive or chronic stress upon the tendon or an acute trauma.[4]

A third problem which can occur is proximal iliotibial band syndrome. The findings of one study indicated that it may especially be a problem for women. Looking at the incidence of strain at the iliac tubercle, *all cases found were in women.* The iliac tubercle is a bumpy spot or protuberance on the most prominent hip bone, where the iliotibial band inserts. Of the seven cases found within this particular study, four of the women had been athletes and three of the women were overweight.[5]

Clearly, although joint pain in older adults is commonly attributed to osteoarthritis, many other surrounding tissues may be the origins of pain. In one study of older adults and non-joint sources of knee pain such as bursitis, *the majority (71.4%) of the suspected cases occurred in the women, not the men.* Very importantly, this group of women also were more likely to have a chronic, long-standing problem, and *to rate their pain as more severe* than individuals in any other group.[6]

These findings suggest that women's experiences of arthritis may often include some additional painful physical ailments, particularly pes anserine bursitis. Moreover, some of these ailments such as pes anserine bursitis may be mistaken for arthritis. The involvement of nerves which pick up on pain (nociceptors) is of much importance in this type of bursitis. Recall also, as we had talked about in Chapter One, central sensitization can occur where nerves become too stimulated and over-responsive, causing chronic pain. One study investigated the frequency and location of nerve endings in the soft tissue of the knee joint. The pes anserinus was one of the regions of the knee in which *nerve endings were found in the largest quantities.*[7]

Pes Anserine Bursitis: Feels Like Knee Arthritis, But Isn't!

The pes anserine syndrome was first described in 1937 by Dr. Eli Moschcowitz who found that the syndrome (which he called bursitis of sartorius bursa) occurred *almost singularly in women.* His patients complained about pain in the knees upon walking up or down the stairs. Walking on level ground posed no problem and was not associated with any pain. When these patients were examined for knee joint extension as well as flexion, no pain was detected. The joint itself was not sore or tender to the touch. Where he found a tender spot was on the inner tibia (shinbone) exactly where the sartorius, gracilis and semitendinosus muscles conjoin (See Figure 5 in Chapter Four for the location of the pes anserinus). He found his patients typically to have no swelling (or if they did, it was only occasionally). Usually only tenderness was found. Importantly, x-ray examination of the knee joint did not show any arthritis.[8] This could be an important cause of knee pain in menopausal women that is unconnected with radiographic arthritis.

In my case, it definitely was one source of my knee pain (in fact, a very persistent one for quite some time). This problem of separating out arthritis from pes anserine bursitis has been an issue of concern in the medical field. It has been noted that pes anserine bursitis can coexist with osteoarthritis, and that it may actually be the bursitis that is the cause of the knee pain. Caution has been advised in diagnosing osteoarthritis, since mistaking pes anserine bursitis pain for arthritis could lead to invasive treatment. Procedures such as intra-articular injections or joint replacement may be employed with no relief of the pain. It has also been observed that this is a fairly common ailment in middle-aged or older women. In addition, it was found to be particularly a problem in those who are obese, who have persistent but difficult to treat knee pain, or who have been diagnosed with degenerative joint disease. In one study, nearly half of the patients diagnosed with degenerative joint disease had pes anserine bursitis. The position of this bursitis is not the same as in medial knee joint problems such as meniscus injury, nor is it one of the trigger point areas for fibromyalgia. It is uniquely identifiable.[9]

A current review of the literature on pes anserine syndrome indicates that there is not very much understanding of the actual pathology of this disease.[10] If bursitis is confirmed on diagnosis, then corticosteroid injections can be used.[11] However, injection with corticosteroids comes with some very significant risks to include: atrophy or a wasting away of the subcutaneous tissue (the tissue that is just under the skin), skin depigmentation, or a loss of pigment in the skin, and rupture of the tendon.[12] Rupture of the tendon is a very serious risk.

Tendon injury is a debilitating disorder that is particularly problematic if adhesions develop during the healing process. Adhesions are scar tissues made of connective cells that form fibrous bands. When adhesions develop it can severely limit the ability of the tendon to glide once healing is complete.[13] When the muscles contract and relax it is necessary for the tendon to glide easily over tissues. The adhesions form between the tendon and these adjacent tissues. Researchers at the University of Manchester have referred to these adhesions as "a 'hidden disease' with no effective treatment or cure."[14] As such, tendon rupture is something that one would really want to avoid. Moreover, in our program of healing, the muscle-tendon unit is of paramount importance, as we discuss in Chapters Four and Seven. There are ways to heal bursitis naturally, which is how I finally got rid of my pes anserine bursitis (Please see Chapter Nine).

Distressed Nerves and Misaligned Membranes

Another problem that can occur is irritation of the saphenous nerve which is called saphenous neuritis. (Please See Figure 8 for the location of the saphenous nerve.) As you can see in the diagram, the infrapatellar branch of the saphenous nerve curves in toward the middle to lower knee.   It can produce symptoms that mimic other conditions such as osteoarthritis or a medial meniscal tear.[1]

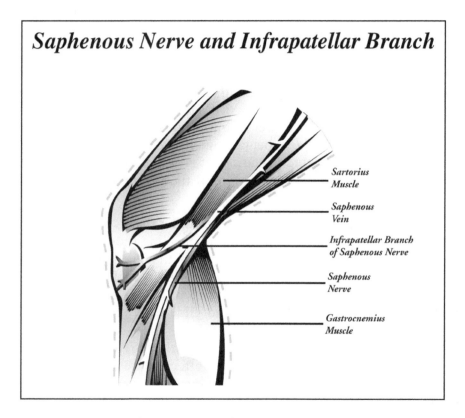

Figure 8 -- Saphenous Nerve and
Infrapatellar Branch

Even the inward fold of the lining of the knee joint capsule can present painful problems not directly related to arthritis. Called "medial plica syndrome," this was highlighted in one study to be a problem especially for women.[16] Synovial plicae consist of membranes which comprise the inward folds of the lining of the knee joint capsule. Commonly found in knees, they are usually without any symptoms or problems. However, if they become irritated they can cause knee pain. In fact, media plica syndrome is a common source of anterior knee pain. It usually manifests as a dull, aching type of pain in the area of the patella on the inner side of the knee (medial patellar area), directly above the joint line. It can also be felt in the area just above the medial patellar area. It is particularly noticeable and bothersome in activities requiring knee flexion and extension (as in climbing the stairs). Other symptoms associated with this syndrome are a "popping," "clicking," or "snapping" in the knee joint and a feeling of tightness in the inside, front of the knee.

The plica is usually very flexible, and it changes its orientation and alters its position with the knee's movements. With inflammation (due to trauma, injury, or strain) the lining of the knee joint swells and the plica may become thickened, and its tissues replaced with fibrous tissue or scar tissue. Medial plica syndrome may lead to mechanical problems with movement and degeneration of the cartilage. It also causes pain due to excessive pressure on areas of the knee abundant with nerve endings.[17] I suspect that I may have had some injuries or inflammation to the medial plica, as this is another area (in addition to the pes anserinus) where I had pain. I discovered the existence of the medial plica when I tried to find out the cause of the "snapping" sound in my knee. I found that orthopedic massage (to be described in Chapter Nine) was particularly helpful to me in repositioning these soft tissues around my knee joint. It was also of much benefit in alleviating my pes anserine bursitis.

From what we've seen here, it is very clear that knee pain that is not visible on x-ray can be caused by other physical problems with the knee. Much of what women experience as "menopausal arthritis" may indeed consist of many of these "non-arthritis" problems. Some of these problems with bursae and nerves may result from dysfunctional use of muscles brought on by muscle mass loss directly following menopause. Recall from Chapter Four that there is a rapid decline in muscle mass and strength directly following menopause.

When X-Rays and Symptoms Don't Match

As mentioned in the previous chapter, radiographic findings that diagnose osteoarthritis have often been found to have little actual correspondence to reported pain.[18] It has even been found that radiographic scores did not correspond well with a person's functioning (such as walking speed and sit-to-stand performance). Osteoarthritis patients with the *same radiographic score* varied considerably in terms of not only pain, but functioning and muscle power.[19] Within the Melbourne Women's Mid-life Health Project, 438 women, aged 45-55 were interviewed each year over eight years. Aches and stiff joints were the most common symptoms and these symptoms increased over time. What was particularly interesting, though, was that aches and stiff joints did not necessarily correspond to radiographic osteoarthritis.[20]

Even women who have similar knee osteoarthritis on x-ray do not necessarily experience the knee pain in the same places. A very interesting study was conducted at the University of Maryland School of Medicine by Dr. Marc Hochberg and colleagues. They found that there are great differences among people in how knee osteoarthritis is experienced, *even if on x-ray their osteoarthritis looks basically the same!* The location of the pain in most patients (85.3%) was usually medial (part of the knee toward the inside part of the body) reported by 33.8% of 68 patients studied, or generalized pain as reported by 51.5% of the patients. These two groups did not differ in demographic or psychosocial variables, *nor did they differ in radiographic characteristics* (such as location of the arthritis or its severity). The ability to function, however, was significantly worse in the generalized pain group. This was particularly the case for activities that involved bending the knee. The question is: Why would this experience of pain differ so greatly, be so heterogeneous in people with osteoarthritis when their joints look so similar on x-ray? The researchers concluded that these findings suggest important differences in the underlying causes of the pain.[21]

So what is happening? How come there is such a wide range of differences in where knee pain is experienced, even when the x-rays show the nature and progression of the knee osteoarthritis as consistent? Moreover, why do some women experience knee pain without radiographic evidence of arthritis? Clearly, the physical soft tissue problems such as bursitis are *prime suspects* in non-radiographic "arthritis" pain. However, might there be other factors not directly physical in nature that may contribute to different *experiences* of this pain?

Bringing Psychological Factors into the Mix

In the Baltimore Longitudinal Study of Aging, Dr. Hochberg and colleagues investigated factors associated with knee pain in participants aged 40 years and over. It was found that women who reported knee pain (without any evidence of radiographic arthritis) had higher anxiety scores than women who did not have knee pain. Self-reported anxiety was unrelated to knee pain in men. These researchers concluded that psychosocial factors may help explain some of the discordance between reported knee pain and knee structural changes indicated in x-rays.[22]

Of course, these findings from the Baltimore Longitudinal Study of Aging do not mean that the pain experienced by women without radiographic evidence of knee osteoarthritis is "all in their heads." The linking of knee pain with anxiety is merely a correlation, an association, *not* a cause and effect relationship in either direction (i.e., knee pain results in anxiety or anxiety results in knee pain). It is possible that the knee pain for women actually *creates* anxiety within their lives. It is also possible that women who are prone to anxiety may experience this emotion in physical manifestations such as arthritis. Perhaps both factors may be at work. However, with pain there must be some kind of *physiological* experience associated with biological processes in the body that cause this pain. If psychological anxiety can result in chemical processes in the body that induce or contribute to knee pain, then what might they be?

One primary physiological response of the body to anxiety is to produce the hormone adrenaline. The effects of adrenaline have an impact upon a multitude of organs in the whole body, and on the important intercellular mediators, the cytokines. For example, it has been found that in rheumatoid arthritis patients, IL-6, cortisol, and epinephrine (adrenaline) were significantly increased in patients who were about to undergo an operation. Once under general anesthesia, the IL-6, cortisol and epinephrine levels significantly declined in comparison with the levels just prior to the anesthesia. They did not find these changes in osteoarthritis patients in this study (however, there were only eight patients with osteoarthritis and twenty-two patients with rheumatoid arthritis which may have influenced these results). They emphasized that mental stress should be reduced in patients with rheumatoid arthritis so that the relationship between the stress-immune and stress-endocrine systems could be altered to control the disease.[23] However, what about osteoarthritis? Wouldn't this form of arthritis, too, be influenced by stress?

Psychological Stress and Inflammation

Psychoneuroimmunology is the study of psychological factors and processes that affect peoples' nervous system and their immune responses. From the first two decades of research, it is now clear that psychological factors *do affect and can alter immune responses.*[24] Researchers in the field of psychoneuroimmunology have explored the effect of psychological factors on some of the cytokines that we have been discussing within this book. For example, research has found that stress may be one of the factors in the initiation and disease progression of cancer. The stress hormone norepinephrine has been found to upregulate proinflammatory cytokines. The term "upregulate" refers to an increase in the cellular response through greater numbers of receptors. Norepinephrine has been found to stimulate progression of melanoma tumor cells by upregulating the proinflammatory cytokines IL-8 and IL-6.[25] However, IL-6 has also been found to be elevated in radiographic knee osteoarthritis.[26] Additionally, it has been associated with synovial inflammation in osteoarthritis patients.[27] The production of the stress hormone norepinephrine, then, would seem like it could have an impact upon cytokines in osteoarthritis, as well.

Psychosocial stressors, such as marital stress, have been associated with a dysregulation of the immune system. In interesting research out of Ohio State University, marital stress has been shown to be associated with the increased production of interleukin-6 (IL-6).

In this research, participants engaged in two different social situations. One situation involved social support and the other one involved marital conflict. In the social support situation, each spouse decided on something that she or he would like to change that was personal (e.g., a problem or individual characteristic, etc.). They were told to expressly avoid discussing any issues that might lead to marital disagreement or conflict. Couples also were asked to tell the "story of their relationship." Conversely, in the marital conflict situation, the couples completed a questionnaire called "The Relationship Problem Inventory." The couples were interviewed about their relationship, and the interviewers determined from this what topics would cause them the most conflict. It was these high-conflict marital topics that they were to then discuss together.

Some of the participants were high in what is called "attachment avoidance." This is a defensive style of relating to others in which a person avoids being close to other people or being intimate with them. The individuals with this attachment avoidance style had an average 11% *increase in* IL-6 during the marital conflict discussion situation in comparison with the social support situation. Individuals lower in attachment avoidance had an average 6% *decrease* in IL-6 production during the marital conflict situation in comparison with the social support situation. These researchers explained that the individuals with an attachment style of avoiding being close to others were more negative in their feelings and behaviors than those without this style. These feelings and behaviors resulted in greater IL-6 production in the body.[28]

Psychological factors influence cytokines and immune function. In addition, they also influence metabolic factors. In a study of women from the Pittsburgh Healthy Women Study, women who were distressed in their marital relationships were significantly more likely to develop metabolic syndrome than those who were satisfied within their marital relationships.[29] Here again, stress may have a large role. Remember that metabolic syndrome greatly increases in women after menopause. As we saw in earlier chapters, metabolic syndrome is connected with a biochemical profile that is associated with osteoarthritis. Researchers have stressed that osteoarthritis and metabolic syndrome have similar inflammatory responses.[30]

Both rheumatoid arthritis and osteoarthritis have been found in some research studies to be associated with metabolic syndrome. In one study of women with early rheumatoid arthritis, there was a greater incidence of metabolic syndrome than in healthy women. Higher systemic inflammation was also associated with metabolic syndrome in women with early rheumatoid arthritis.[31] In a study of osteoarthritis, risk factors for metabolic syndrome (e.g., impaired glucose tolerance, overweight, etc.) were found to be associated with knee osteoarthritis in a large-scale study in Japan, the Research on Osteoarthritis Against Disability (ROAD) study.[32] However, *the metabolic syndrome has been found to be significantly associated with knee osteoarthritis in women, but not in men.*[33] So, as we have seen, women under stress may be more likely to develop metabolic syndrome, metabolic syndrome is more prevalent in post menopause, and metabolic syndrome has been associated with knee osteoarthritis in women (but not men). As such, couldn't there be a complex interaction between stress, metabolic syndrome, and arthritis in women that might be quite characteristic of menopausal arthritis?

Arthritis and Anxiety: A Critical Connection for Women?

As we have just seen, psychological factors can be important in their effects upon the immune system and cytokine production. Although psychological stress as a contributing factor to arthritis has been associated with autoimmune diseases such as rheumatoid arthritis,[34] its role in promoting osteoarthritis has been less researched. Given these general findings from the field of psychoneuroimmunology, it seems clear that psychological stress can promote inflammation and disease.

As we saw earlier, some research suggests that anxiety may play a larger role in inflammation among women. The effects of anxiety on inflammation are dramatically illustrated within the following study: Research examining anxiety and inflammation in middle-aged men and women in Greece (who were chosen randomly from the population) found the following: *Among the 400 middle-aged women* studied (with a mean age of 45 years, plus or minus 12 years), *levels of anxiety were higher* than they were for the men in the study. The group of women with the highest levels of anxiety *had 91% higher C-reactive protein levels and 93% higher interleukin-6 (IL-6) levels.* Moreover, *anxiety was significantly associated with markers of inflammation.* Anxiety was positively correlated with C-reactive protein (CRP) and with interleukin-6 (as well as other inflammatory markers).[35] As you may recall from Chapter Two, these are critical cytokines in the disease process of osteoarthritis! Both IL-6 and CRP have been found to be elevated in radiographic knee osteoarthritis.[36]

In another study that looked at the effects of anxiety and of depression in postmenopausal women with osteoarthritis and rheumatoid arthritis, the effect of anxiety was almost twice the effect of depression in terms of predicting pain. Depression had an effect upon pain only indirectly through decreasing positive feelings and emotions. It was only anxiety that had a direct effect upon arthritis pain.[37]

Going back again to the study cited earlier within this chapter, the Baltimore Longitudinal Study of Aging, women who reported knee pain (without any evidence of arthritis on x-ray) had higher anxiety scores than women who did not have knee pain. There was no association between knee pain and anxiety in men. Moreover, depression was not related to knee pain in either men or women.[38] A picture seems to be starting to emerge with postmenopausal women, anxiety, and arthritis co-occurring in interesting ways.

Anxiety, Childhood Stressors and Adult Onset Arthritis

Let's take a look again at some of the factors involved in the study about marital conflict that we talked about earlier. When we are talking about things like marital conflict, we're referring to interactions that cause stress in a current situation where spouses are engaged in marital dissension. The roots of "attachment avoidance," or the style of relating to others that avoids being close to people, has been theorized to stem from the individual's experiences as an infant and young child.[39] As such, these early life experiences can result in current behaviors (such as in the marital conflict study discussed earlier) that contribute to inflammatory responses in the body. So, what do we know about early stressors and arthritis?

Something that may surprise many is that childhood stressors and adversities are significantly related to adult onset arthritis. In a very large, multi-country study of participants from the World Mental Health Surveys, it was found that 45% of the participants who had experienced two or more stressors or childhood adversities (such as physical or sexual abuse as a child, neglect, family violence, etc.) had developed arthritis by age 65. In contrast, only 35% of those without multiple childhood stressors had developed arthritis. Similarly, those diagnosed with a mood or anxiety disorder prior to the age of 21 had a 60% risk of developing arthritis by age 65. In contrast, those who were not diagnosed with a mood or anxiety disorder prior to the age of 21 had less than a 40% risk of developing arthritis by 65 years of age.[40]

The response to stressors activates the hypothalamic-pituitary-adrenal (HPA) axis and the "fight-or-flight" response. A wearing down of the body can occur if there is excessive activation of this stress response or if it continues when the original stressor is absent.[41] If one continually perceives or feels that one is under threat of being hurt or injured (even in the absence of actual danger), a state of on-going anxiety would essentially result.

In a study which included the prevalence of psychiatric disorders among older adults in the United States, it was found that four times as many women as men suffer from a psychiatric disorder.[42] Moreover, and of specific importance here, women have been found to have a *higher prevalence of anxiety disorders* than men.[43] Recall that in the study cited above, women who reported knee pain (without any evidence of radiographic arthritis) had higher anxiety scores than women who did not have knee pain. There was *no association between knee pain and anxiety in men.* Could a linkage between pain (in this case knee pain) and anxiety, as well as women's greater prevalence of anxiety disorders, be one of the reasons women have a higher prevalence of knee osteoarthritis? We will explore these psychological factors in greater detail in Chapter Eleven, as well as bring into the discussion differences between men and women in the experience of pain. For now, though, keep in mind that the psychological domain is one more dimension that may affect the overall experience of menopausal arthritis.

Rheumatoid Arthritis: Is It Ever Part of the Profile of Menopausal Arthritis?

The peak onset of rheumatoid arthritis in women is menopause.[44] Because of this, one would have to question whether rheumatoid arthritis is ever part of what women experience as menopausal arthritis. We're not talking about rheumatoid arthritis when we are talking about menopausal arthritis, right? Most likely, probably not as a general rule (and certainly not in terms of how menopausal arthritis has been historically defined within the medical literature). However, research seems to indicate that there may be some women who have symptoms that could be differentially attributed to rheumatoid arthritis *or* to hormonal changes at menopause.

Consider this: In a Japanese study, the researchers analyzed in depth, five patient cases with Stage 1 and monocyclic type rheumatoid arthritis. The average age that these women first began experiencing joint symptoms corresponded in time with the onset of menopause (their average age was 51 years). All of the women experienced more than six symptoms characteristic of the menopausal syndrome (e.g., fatigue, myalgia/arthralgia, headache, vasomotor ailments, insomnia, etc.). These researchers concluded that all of the American College of Rheumatology criteria for rheumatoid arthritis (excluding subcutaneous nodules) could be accounted for by a deficit in estrogen associated with the menopausal syndrome. They asserted that this is because estrogen is a regulator of inflammatory cytokines (e.g., IL-1, IL-6, TNF-α), and these are produced in greater quantities as a result of estrogen deficiency. They also cited research that found that IL-6 produces antibodies such as rheumatoid factor. *They concluded that estrogen deficiency consistent with the menopausal syndrome may generate joint symptoms resembling rheumatoid arthritis.*[45] What if rheumatoid arthritis symptoms only begin to appear right at menopause? In light of these researchers' findings, is it possible that arthritis symptoms that co-exist with the menopause could possibly be mistaken for an early stage of rheumatoid arthritis?

Rheumatoid arthritis is considered to be a "female-predominant" disease.[46] Research does seem to suggest that sex hormones exert an effect upon the development and the clinical manifestations of rheumatoid arthritis.[47] Recall back to Chapter Three where we had discussed the influence of estrogen on various diseases. Estrogen has been shown to affect the release of proinflammatory cytokines through its modulating effects upon CD16.[48] Because of this, a close connection with arthritis, indeed, might possibly occur. For example, CD16 expression has been considered as a potential marker of osteoclast precursors (chemicals needed to form osteoclasts) in inflammatory arthritis.[49] Osteoclasts, of course, are the large cells involved in the absorption and elimination of bone; they break bone down. In addition, CD16+ monocytes were found to be significantly increased in rheumatoid arthritis patients in comparison with healthy individuals (control group). Those patients with an increased presence of CD16+ monocytes were considered to have "active disease" due to the increased number of tender and swollen joints, and levels of other factors.[50] If loss of estrogen can cause an increase in these proinflammatory cytokines, then how does one determine whether arthritis symptoms are due to "menopausal arthritis" or to "rheumatoid arthritis" when these symptoms develop right at the menopause?

This is, of course, something that needs careful consideration. It would seem vitally important for women in menopause to consider cautiously and judiciously, along with their physicians, what their symptoms may mean and what may be causing them. This is especially so since according to some in the field of rheumatology, rheumatoid arthritis has been considered to be difficult or challenging to diagnose in its early stages. Researchers from Stanford University School of Medicine have argued that *not only is there a wide range of presentations of the disease, and variations in the course of the disease, but there is no "laboratory gold standard" through which to establish either the presence of rheumatoid arthritis or the absence of it.*[51]

It has been reported that there is a current acceptance that one should begin DMARD (disease-modifying antirheumatic drugs) as soon as possible, even within the first 12 weeks of the disease if it has been determined that the rheumatoid arthritis will go on to become disabling.[52] This makes careful consideration even more important, and particularly so when one considers the studies of gender differences in outcomes using antirheumatic drugs that are described below.

Gender Differences in Rheumatoid Arthritis Disease Progression and Treatment Effects

It is of great concern that some of the pharmaceutical drugs used to treat rheumatoid arthritis may not necessarily be as effective with women as they are with men. In a Swedish study comparing men and women on remission rates and effectiveness of treatment for rheumatoid arthritis, the researchers found that the sex of the patient was a main factor in outcome. There were significantly fewer women than men achieving remission from rheumatoid arthritis, and the course of the disease strikingly worsened in women, although *at the onset of the study there were no certain differences in disease activity.*[53] They did note that the score on the Disease Activity Score 28-joint count (DAS28) and pain scores were higher in women than men at baseline; however, there were no significant differences in terms of morning stiffness or physician assessment of disease activity. Physical performance scores showed no significant gender difference either. They received the same treatments as the men had received (disease-modifying anti-rheumatic drugs or glucocorticoids). Nevertheless, even though all of these factors were the same or similar at the beginning of the study, *women had poorer outcomes.*

Moreover, there were no differences attributable to age (mean age of the participants at the onset of the study was 58 years) or differences in the length of time that they had experienced the disease (average disease duration at the onset of the study was 6.2 months). At the follow-up period, disease activity as assessed by the DAS28 was significantly reduced in both genders; however, women had *significantly less change than men.* With regard to the physician's assessment, women had significantly *increased disease activity* at both 2 years and 5 years and pain was also much greater at both follow-ups compared to the men. The remission rates after two years were 32.1% for women as compared with 48.0% for men; and at five years they were 30.8% for women as compared with 52.4% for men.[54]

The study findings above were reported in 2007. In a more current study out of the University of California, Los Angeles published in 2010, researchers again obtained similar results. Women and men had comparable disease activity at baseline, but, again, treatment responses were worse in women (to DMARDs -- disease-modifying antirheumatic drugs in this case). The women in this study had more progression of the disease, even though they received similar treatments. On the self-reported measures (e.g., pain, fatigue, etc.) women's scores were worse than men's at the beginning of the study and throughout the course of the study. This was despite the fact that they had similar radiographic indications of the disease. What can account for these gender differences? Men had more bone erosion, and women more joint space narrowing, but the researchers viewed their disease activity on x-rays as comparable. What is troubling is that compared with the men's expression of the disease, the *women's expression of the disease progressed and worsened when receiving similar treatment.* Moreover, men were more likely to have their rheumatoid arthritis go into remission.[55] Why would this be? Is it possible that the disease is very different in men and in women, or that men and women respond in different ways to the DMARDs? Hopefully, researchers in the field of rheumatology will find answers to some of these questions soon and more effective drugs might be developed for women.

It is also critically important to point out here that many of the biologics used to treat rheumatoid arthritis can have substantial negative side effects to include liver damage and serious infections, and some side effects that are potentially life threatening (e.g., infections such as tuberculosis, critical damage to blood cells, allergic reactions and convulsions, and cancer).[56]

In light of the fact that women have not been shown to fare as well on the biologics as men in the treatment of rheumatoid arthritis, and with concern over the potential and substantial negative side effects, it seems prudent to be especially cautious in diagnosis. As noted earlier, researchers from Stanford University School of Medicine have referred to the difficulty in diagnosing rheumatoid arthritis in its early stages; they stressed that there is no "laboratory gold standard" to establish its presence or absence.[57]

I must emphasize, however, that these are my personal observations as a researcher and a writer and not medical advice. The information and positions put forth here are in no way to substitute for consultation with your physician or medical health provider. I am providing this information because I believe that based upon my research it is important to be an informed consumer when it comes to health decisions. Rheumatoid arthritis is considered to be a serious disease as reported by the American College of Rheumatology. People's symptoms, as well as their outcomes can greatly differ, and the inflammation may not be limited to joints but may also develop in organs as well.[58]

As a side note to the influence of estrogen on rheumatoid arthritis, one might wonder whether estrogen replacement therapy might help. The effects of postmenopausal hormone therapy on the risk of developing rheumatoid arthritis and on the severity of disease symptoms were studied in the Women's Health Initiative randomized controlled trials. Hormone therapy (estrogen only and estrogen with progestin) did not have a statistically significant effect upon either the risk of onset of rheumatoid arthritis or the severity of symptoms. Non-statistically significant findings were noted, however, that showed a reduced risk for developing rheumatoid arthritis as well as improved joint pain symptoms. Hormone therapy did not improve swelling, though, nor did it stop new joint pains from occurring.[59]

Let's come back to the issue of whether rheumatoid arthritis could ever be part of the profile of menopausal arthritis from another perspective. Menopausal arthritis is usually associated with osteo-arthritis. It is interesting that there are some overlaps between the two diseases of osteoarthritis and rheumatoid arthritis that have recently been found. As discussed in Chapter Two, inflammation is also associated with osteoarthritis, not just rheumatoid arthritis. This is now well-established within the field of rheumatology.[60] It is only over the last decade that this has become so recognized and realized within the more recent medical literature; prior to this, osteoarthritis had been generally thought of as a primarily "non-inflammatory" disease. I am not sure how this line of thought really transpired, though, since "arthritis" literally means "inflammation of the joint."

Perhaps it is because, in contrast to osteoarthritis, rheumatoid arthritis seems to be so strongly characterized by inflammation. Also, the concept of inflammation in arthritis, from an historical perspec-tive, was apparently based upon the number of leukocytes (white blood cells) in the synovial fluid.[61] For example, an important leukocyte protein (L-1) was observed at low concentrations in the synovial (joint lining) fluid of patients with osteoarthritis, as compared with high concentrations in the synovial fluid of patients with rheumatoid arthritis. High concentrations of this leukocyte protein were found in rheumatoid arthritis patients with marked swelling of the joints. These researchers had concluded that this leukocyte protein was a potential biomarker of local and systemic inflammation.[62]

Indeed, this more pronounced inflammation in rheumatoid arthritis (and the particular markers of inflammation used) may have shifted a focus away from inflammation in osteoarthritis. Nevertheless, pioneering research by Dr. Hugo E. Jasin in 1985 demonstrated that immune complexes were present in *both* rheumatoid arthritis and osteoarthritis patients. Extracts from cartilage showed that more than 60% of the rheumatoid arthritis samples contained collagen II antibodies. Moreover, not just the rheumatoid arthritis cartilage samples, but 50% of the osteoarthritis cartilage samples, too, contained collagen II antibodies.[63] In fact, Dr. Jasin emphasized that inflammation was part of the disease process of osteoarthritis, and it could occur along a range from minimal cellular changes to joint lining, to severe synovitis, or inflammation of the joint lining.[64]

Finally, it is now well-recognized that inflammation is not singularly found within rheumatoid arthritis. Indeed, osteoarthritis and rheumatoid arthritis have adipocytokines in common as well. Current research findings show that leptin, adiponectin, and resistin have been found in the joint synovial fluid from individuals with rheumatoid arthritis as well those with osteoarthritis. Research also suggests that leptin is involved in *both* disease processes and that inflammation may be mediated by adiponectin, resistin, or both.[65]

Along with similarities such as the expression of common adipocytokines in both rheumatoid and osteoarthritis, there are more connections between rheumatoid arthritis and osteoarthritis that have not been fully explored as of yet. Osteoarthritis and rheumatoid arthritis have been commonly partitioned off into two very separate diseases. However, new research in proteomics is identifying some overlaps in biomarkers of these diseases.

Researchers at the University of Texas Southwestern Medical Center have written that we are entering the "dawn of a new era" in rheumatology. Through the use of a methodology known as "proteomics" they have identified *several biomarkers of disease common to both osteoarthritis and rheumatoid arthritis.*[66] Proteomics, by the way, is defined as the study of all of the proteins that are contained within a particular cell, tissue or organism. Scientists estimate that there may be between one to ten *million* discrete proteins within the human body. However, in relation to the potential body of proteins, currently only a small number have been identified.[67]

Through systematic analysis, biomarkers of disease can be identified through proteins and patterns of proteins within blood or tissue, for example. These scientists from the University of Texas Southwestern Medical Center conducted a review of the literature and found proteomic overlaps between rheumatoid arthritis and osteoarthritis. As we shall see shortly, though, many of these biomarkers may have very different roles in the two diseases. The researchers from the University of Texas Southwestern Medical Center noted that in both rheumatoid arthritis and osteoarthritis, higher levels of annexin 1 may function to inhibit inflammatory cytokines such as interleukin-1 (IL-1), tumor necrosis factor-alpha (TNF-α), and IL-6. They suggested that it was possible that in both diseases the elevated annexin 1 may represent the body's attempt to restrain or suppress inflammation. Annexin 1 is a protein that may have anti-inflammatory properties.[68]

However, in one study of rheumatoid arthritis patients, annexin 1 did not seem to play its beneficial anti-inflammatory role. Instead, research out of New York University School of Medicine indicated that in these rheumatoid arthritis patients, annexin 1 was secreted by the synovial fluid, and it activated chemical factors that in turn stimulated metalloproteinase 1. As discussed in Chapter Two, metalloproteinases break down cartilage. Thus, in this case, annexin 1 may serve to worsen the destructive process within rheumatoid arthritis.[69]

The researchers at the University of Texas Southwestern Medical Center had also found that in *both* osteoarthritis and rheumatoid arthritis that synovial fibroblasts have a heightened expression of TPI or triosephosphate isomerase (a critical enzyme in energy production).[70] However, in another study it was found that although the presence of TPI is common to both rheumatoid arthritis and osteoarthritis patients, it seems to play a substantial and perhaps unique role in the chronic inflammation of osteoarthritis. Even though the presence of the same protein (enzyme) was detected in both diseases, it may mean different things in terms of the processes of inflammation. It may function as an autoantigen in osteoarthritis patients where anti-TPI autoantibodies were found in 24.1% of the synovial fluid samples. In contrast, less than 6% of the synovial fluid samples from rheumatoid arthritis patients had anti-TPI autoantibodies.[71]

One of the problems with many cytokines and other molecules in arthritis is that they can sometimes have anti-inflammatory, as well as proinflammatory effects (just as we had discussed earlier with regard to interleukin-6). As noted above, this has recently become known with regard to annexin 1, as well. The researchers out of New York University School of Medicine and colleagues had found that annexin 1, previously most known for its important anti-inflammatory effects, now had been shown to also have a proinflammatory role in rheumatoid arthritis. With regard to the biologic therapies for rheumatoid arthritis, these researchers emphasized that a more specific knowledge of how the tissue destruction process is mediated is required for improved therapeutic strategies. They pointed out that there are considerable numbers of rheumatoid arthritis patients that have not shown a positive benefit from the use of biologic therapies. Thus, they stressed that it is important to obtain a clearer grasp of the regulatory effects of the various cytokines and other molecules involved in the disease process to develop better therapeutics to prevent erosion.[72]

All of the ways that proinflammatory and anti-inflammatory cytokines operate within osteoarthritis and rheumatoid arthritis are simply not clear as of yet. However, one thing is clear. Estrogen (and loss of estrogen at menopause) can affect many of the involved cytokines. Nevertheless, the experience of menopausal arthritis, is indeed, much more complex than simply osteoarthritis brought on by estrogen decline. Furthermore, osteoarthritis is far more complex than a simple "wear and tear" disease of aging. There are many factors that need to be considered in understanding menopausal arthritis to include physical problems that might mimic arthritis pain in women, such as pes anserine bursitis. Moreover, we now know that inflammation is involved and that adipocytokines like leptin are associated with osteoarthritis and menopausal arthritis. As a result, we are in a position then to take action to stop inflammation and to correct soft tissue disorders such as bursitis. As we've seen, it is also important to consider differences between women and men in psychological factors such as anxiety. Stressors (and even stressors stemming from childhood) may influence whether women develop osteoarthritis and how they experience it. We will take a look at these psychological factors in much more depth in Chapter Eleven. Finally, some key diagnostic criteria for rheumatoid arthritis might also be accounted for simply by a decline in estrogen at menopause; as such, it would be very important to consider carefully with one's medical doctor any diagnosis of rheumatoid arthritis.

Menopausal arthritis is complex. With this knowledge that more is involved than the process of osteoarthritis alone, and that osteoarthritis (and rheumatoid arthritis too) are more complex than originally thought, we are now in a position to do something about changing the experience of menopausal arthritis. Menopausal arthritis is complex; however, with this knowledge we can begin to heal.

Notes for Chapter Six

[1]Hill, C. L., Gale, D. R., Chaisson, C. E., Skinner, K., Kazis, L., Gale, M. E., & Felson, D. T. (2003). Periarticular lesions detected on magnetic resonance imaging: Prevalence in knees with and without symptoms. *Arthritis & Rheumatism, 48*(10), 2836-2844. doi: 10.1002/art.11254

[2]Ibid.

[3]Kerian, R. K., & Glousman, R. E. (1988). Tibial collateral ligament bursitis. *American Journal of Sports Medicine, 16*(4), 344-346.

[4]Rothstein, C. P., Laorr, A., Helms, C. A., & Tirman, P. F. J. (1996). Semimembranosus-tibial collateral ligament bursitis: MR imaging findings. *American Journal of Roentgenology, 166*(4), 875-877.

[5]Sher, I., Umans, H., Downie, S. A., Tobin, K., Arora, R., & Olson, T. R. (2011). Proximal iliotibial band syndrome: What is it and where is it? *Skeletal Radiology.* Advance online publication. PMID: 21499978

[6]Wood, L. R. J., Peat, G., Thomas, E., & Duncan, R. (2008). The contribution of selected non-articular conditions to knee pain severity and associated disability in older adults. *Osteoarthritis and Cartilage, 16*, 647-653. doi: 10.1016/j.joca.2007.10.007

[7]Biedert, R. M., Stauffer, E., & Friederich, N. F. (1992). Occurrence of free nerve endings in the soft tissue of the knee joint: A histologic investigation. *American Journal of Sports Medicine, 20(*4), 430-433.

[8]Moschcowitz, Eli. (1937). Bursitis of Sartorius bursa: An undescribed malady simulating chronic arthritis. *Journal of the American Medical Association, 109*(17), 1362.

[9]Gnanadesigan, N., & Smith, R. L. (2003). Knee pain: osteoarthritis or anserine bursa? *Journal of the American Medical Directors Association, 4*(3), 164-166.

[10]Helfenstein, Jr., M., &, & Kuromoto, J. (2010). *Anserine syndrome. Revista brasileira de reumatologia, 50*(3), 313-327.

[11]Ibid.

[12]Ibid.

[13]Bluman, E. M., Allen, S. D., & Fadale, P. D. (2006). Tendon repair and regeneration: An overview. In W. R. Walsh (ed.) Repair and regeneration of ligaments, tendons, and joint capsule (Orthopedic biology and medicine). New Jersey: Humana Press.

[14] Taylor, S. H., Al-Youha, S., Van Agtmael, T. V., Lu, Y., Wong, J., McGrouther, D. A., & Kadler, K. E. (2011). Tendon is covered by a basement membrane epithelium that is required for cell retention and prevention of adhesion formation. *PLoS one, 6*(1), e16377. doi: 10.1371/journal.pone.0011337

[15]Morganti, C. M., McFarland, E. G., & Cosgarea, A. J. (2002). Saphenous neuritis: A poorly understood cause of medial knee pain. *Journal of the American Academy of Orthopaedic Surgeons, 10*(2), 130-137.

[16]Blok, A., Weiss, W., Dolata, T., & Szczepaniec, M. (2005). Medial synovial plica. *Ortopedia, Traumatologia, Rehabilitacja, 7*(4), 397-400.

[17]Sznajderman, T., Smorgick, Y., Lindner, D., Beer, Y., & Agar, G. (2009). Medial plica syndrome. *Israel Medical Association Journal, 11*, 54-57.

[18]Bedson, J., & Croft, P. R. (2008). The discordance between clinical and radiographic knee osteoarthritis: A systematic search and summary of the literature. *BMC Musculoskeletal Disorders, 9*,116. doi:10.1186/1471-2474-9-116

[19]Barker, K., Lamb, S. E., Toye, F., Jackson, S., & Barrington, S. (2004). Association between radiographic joint space narrowing, function, pain and muscle power in severe osteoarthritis of the knee. *Clinical Rehabilitation, 18*(7), 793-800.

[20]Szoeke, C.E., Cicuttini, F. M., Guthrie, J. R., & Dennerstein, L. (2008). The relationship of reports of aches and joint pains to the menopausal transition: A longitudinal study. *Climacteric, 11*(1), 55-62.

[21]Creamer, P., Lethbridge-Cejku, M., & Hochberg, M. C. (1998). Where does it hurt? Pain localization in osteoarthritis of the knee. *Osteoarthritis and Cartilage, 6*(5), 318-323.

[22]Creamer, P., Lethbridge-Cejku, M., Costa, P., Tobin, J. D., Herbst, J. H., & Hochberg, M. C. (1999). The relationship of anxiety and depression with self-reported knee pain in the community: Data from the Baltimore Longitudinal Study of Aging. *Arthritis Care and Research, 12*(1), 3-7.

[23]Hirano, D., Nagashima, M., Ogawa, R., & Yoshino, S. (2001). Serum levels of interleukin 6 and stress related substances indicate mental stress condition in patients with rheumatoid arthritis. *Journal of Rheumatology, 28*(3), 490-495.

[24]Coe, C. L., & Laudenslager, M. L. (2007). Psychosocial influences on immunity, including effects on immune maturation and senescence. *Brain, Behavior, and Immunity, 21*(8), 1000-1008. doi: 10.1016/j.bbi.2007.06.015

[25]Yang, E. V., Kim., S. J., Donovan, E. L., Chen, M., Gross, A. C., Webster, M. J. I., Barsky, S. H., & Glaser, R. (2009). Norepinephrine upregulates VEGF, IL-8, and IL-6 expression in human melanoma tumor cell lines: Implications for stress-related enhancement of tumor progression. *Brain, Behavior, and Immunity, 23*(2), 267-275.

[26]Livshits, G., Zhai, G., Hart, D. J., Kato, B. S., Wang, H., Williams, F. M., & Spector, T. D. (2009). Interleukin-6 is a significant predictor of radiographic knee osteoarthritis: The Chingford Study. *Arthritis and Rheumatism, 60*(7), 2037-2045.

[27]Pearle, A. D., Scanzello, C. R., George, S., Mandl, L. A., DiCarlo, E. F., Peterson, M., Sculco,T. P., & Crow, M. K. (2007). Elevated high-sensitivity C-reactive protein levels are associated with local inflammatory findings in patients with osteoarthritis. *Osteoarthritis and Cartilage, 15*(5), 516-523.

[28]Gouin, J-P., Glaser, R., Loving, T. J., Malarkey, W. B., Stowell, J., Houts, C., & Kiecolt-Glaser, J. K. (2009). Attachment avoidance predicts inflammatory responses to marital conflict. *Brain, Behavior, and Immunity, 23*(7), 898-904. doi: 10.1016/j.bbi.2008.09.016

[29]Troxel, W. M., Matthews, K. A., Gallo, L. C., & Kuller, L. H. (2005). Marital quality and occurrence of the metabolic syndrome in women. *Archives of Internal Medicine, 165*(9), 1022-1027.

[30]Katz, J. D., Agrawal, S., & Velasquez, M. (2010). Getting to the heart of the matter: Osteoarthritis takes its place as part of the metabolic syndrome. *Current Opinions in Rheumatology, 22*(5), 512-519.

[31]Dao, H-H., Do, Q-T., & Sakamoto, J. (2010). Increased frequency of metabolic syndrome among Vietnamese women with early rheumatoid arthritis: A cross-sectional study. *Arthritis Research & Therapy, 12*(6), R218. Retrieved from http://arthritis-research.com/content/12/6/R218

[32]Yoshimura, N., Muraki, S., Oka, H., Kawaguchi, H., Nakamura, K., & Akune, T. (2011). Association of knee osteoarthritis with the accumulation of metabolic risk factors such as overweight, hypertension, dyslipidemia, and impaired glucose tolerance in Japanese men and women: the ROAD study. *Journal of Rheumatology, 38*(5), 921-930.

[33]Inoue, R., Ishibashi, Y., Tsuda, E., Yamamoto, Y., Matsuzaka, M., Takahashi, I., Danjo, K., Umeda, T., Nakaji, S., & Toh, S. (2011). Medical problems and risk factors of metabolic syndrome among radiographic knee osteoarthritis patients in the Japanese general population. *Journal of Orthopaedic Science*. Advance online publication. PMID: 21915668

[34]Stojanovich, L., & Marisavljevich, D. (2008). Stress as a trigger of autoimmune disease. *Autoimmunity Reviews, 7*, 209-213.

[35]Pitsavos, C., Panagiotakos, D. B., Papageorgiou, C., Tsetsekou, E., Soldatos, C., & Stefanadis, C. (2006). Anxiety in relation to inflammation and coagulation markers, among healthy adults: The ATTICA Study. *Atherosclerosis, 185*, 320-326.

[36]Livshits et al. (2009). Op. Cit.

[37]Smith, B. W., & Zautra, A. J. (2008). The effects of anxiety and depression on weekly pain in women with arthritis. *Pain, 138*(2), 354-361. doi: 10.1016/j.pain.2008.01.008

[38]Creamer, et al. (1999). Op. Cit.

[39]Bowlby, J. (1982). *Attachment and loss. Vol. 1: Attachment (2nd ed.)*. New York: Basic Books (Original work published 1969).

[40]Von Korff, M., Alonso, J., Ormel, J., Angermeyer, M., Bruffaerts, R., Fleiz, C. de Girolamo, G., Kessler, R. C., Kovess-Masfety, V., Posada-Villa, J., Scott, K. M., & Uda, H. (2009). Childhood psychosocial stressors and adult onset arthritis: Broad spectrum risk factors and allostatic load. *Pain, 143*(1-2), 76-83. doi: 10.1016/j.pain.2009.01.034

[41]McEwen, B. S. (2007). Physiology and neurobiology of stress and adaptation: Central role of the brain. *Physiological Reviews, 87*, 873-904. doi: 10.1152/physrev.00041.2006

[42]Gum, A. M., King-Kallimanis, B., & Kohn, R. (2009). Prevalence of mood, anxiety, and substance-abuse disorders for older Americans in the National Comorbidity Survey-Replication. *American Journal of Geriatric Psychiatry, 17*(9), 769-781.

[43]McLean, C. P., Asnaani, A., Litz, B. T.,& Hofmann, S. G. (2011). Gender differences in anxiety disorders: Prevalence, course of illness, comorbidity and burden of illness. *Journal of Psychiatric Research, 45*, 1027-1035. doi: 10.1016/j.jpsychires.2011.03.006

[44]Islander, U., Jochems, C., Lagerquist, M. K., Forsblad-d'Elia, H., & Carlsten, H. (2011). Estrogens in rheumatoid arthritis; the immune system and bone. *Molecular and Cellular Endocrinology, 335*, 14-29.

[45]Nagamine, R., Maeda, T., Shuto, T., Nakashima, Y., Hirata, G., & Iwamoto, Y. (2001). Menopausal syndrome in female patients with rheumatoid arthritis. *Modern Rheumatology, 11*(3), 230-233. doi: 10.1007/s101650170009

[46]Walitt, B., Pettinger, M., Weinstein, A., Katz, J., Torner, J., Wasko, M. C., Howard, B. V., & Women's Health Initiative Investigators. (2008). Effects of postmenopausal hormone therapy on rheumatoid arthritis: The Women's Health Initiative randomized Controlled Trials. *Arthritis & Rheumatism, 59*(3), 302-310. doi: 10.1002/art.23325.

[47]Ibid.

[48]Ibid.

[49]Chiu,Y. G., Shao, T., Feng, C., Mensah, K. A., Thullen, M., Schwartz, E. M., & Ritchlin, C. T. (2010). CD16 (FcRyIII) as a potential marker of osteoclast precursors in psoriatic arthritis. *Arthritis Research & Therapy, 12*, R14. doi: 10.1186/ar2915.

[50]Kawanaka, N., Yamamura, M., Aita, T., Morita, Y., Okamoto, A., Kawashima, M., Iwahashi, M., Ueno, A., Ohmoto, Y., & Makino, H. (2002). CD14+, CD16+ blood monocytes and joint inflammation in rheumatoid arthritis. *Arthritis & Rheumatism, 46*(10), 2578-2586. doi: 10.1002/art.10545.

[51]Sokolove, J., & Strand, V. (2010). Rheumatoid arthritis classification criteria – It's finally time to move on! *Bulletin for the NYU Hospital for Joint Diseases, 68*(3), 232-238.

[52]Symmons, D. P. M. & Silman, A. J. (2006). What determines the evolution of early undifferentiated arthritis and rheumatoid arthritis? An update from the Norfolk Arthritis Register. *Arthritis Research & Therapy, 8*(4), 214. doi: 10:1186/ar1979

[53]Forslind, K., Hafstr_m, I., Ahlmén, M., & Svensson, B.; for the BARFOT Study Group (2007). Sex: a major predictor of remission in early rheumatoid arthritis? *Annals of the Rheumatic Diseases 66*, 46-52. doi: 10.1136/ard.2006.056937

[54]Ibid.

[55]Jawaheer, D., Maranian, P., Park, G., Lahiff, M., Amjadi, S. S., & Paulus, H. E. (2010). Disease progression and treatment responses in a prospective DMARD-naive seropositive early rheumatoid arthritis cohort: Does gender matter? *Journal of Rheumatology, 37*(12), 2475-2485.

[56]Consumer Reports Health Best Buy Drugs (2010). Evaluating prescription drugs used to treat the symptoms of rheumatoid arthritis: The biologics. Comparing effectiveness, safety, side effects and price. Retrieved from http://www.consumerreports.org/health/resources/pdf/best-buy-drugs/BBD_Rheumatoid_Arthritis.pdf

[57]Sokolove et al. (2010). Op. Cit.

[58]American College of Rheumatology (2012). Rheumatoid arthritis. Retrieved from: http://www.rheumatology.org/practice/clinical

[59]Walitt et al. (2008). Op. Cit.

[60]Gómez, R., Conde, J., Scotece, M., Gómez-Reino, J. J., Lago, F., & Gualillo, O. (2011). What's new in our understanding of the role of adipokines in rheumatic diseases? *Nature Reviews. Rheumatology, 7*(9), 528-536. doi: 10.1038/nrrheum.2011.107

[61]Abramson, S. B., & Attur, M. (2009). Developments in the scientific understanding of osteoarthritis. *Arthritis Research & Therapy, 11*(3), 227. doi: 10.1186/ar2655

[62]Berntzen, H. B., Olmez, U., Fagerhol, M. K., & Munthe, E. (1991). The leukocyte protein L1 in plasma and synovial fluid from patients with rheumatoid arthritis and osteoarthritis. *Scandinavian Journal of Rheumatology, 20*(2), 74-82.

[63]Jasin, H. E. (1985). Autoantibody specificities of immune complexes sequestered in articular cartilage of patients with rheumtoid arthritis and osteoarthritis. *Arthritis and Rheumatism, 28*(4), 241-248.

[64]Jasin, H. E. (1989). Immune mechanisms in osteoarthritis. *Seminars in Arthritis and Rheumatism, 18*(4), 86-90.

[65]Toussirot, E., Streit, G., & Wendling, D. (2007). The contribution of adipose tissue and adipokines to inflammation in joint diseases. *Current Medicinal Chemistry, 14*(10), 1095-1100.

[66]Vanarsa, K., & Mohan, C. (2010). Proteomics in rheumatology: The dawn of a new era. *F1000 Medicine Reports 2*, 87. Published online December 8. doi: 10.3410/M2-87

[67]Alic, M. (2010). Proteomics. In J. L. Longe (Ed.), 3rd ed., *The Gale encyclopedia of cancer* (pp. 1027-1030). Farmington Hills, MI: Gale, Cengage Learning.

[68]Vanarsa et al. (2010). Op. Cit.

[69]Tagoe, C. E., Marjanovic, N., Park, J. Y., Chan, E. S., Abeles, A. M., Attur, M., Abramson, S. B., & Pillinger, M. H. (2008). Annexin-1 mediates TNF-alpha-stimulated matrix metalloproteinase secretion from rheumatoid arthritis synovial fibroblasts. *Journal of Immunology, 181*(4), 2813-2820.

[70]Vanarsa et al. (2010). Op. Cit.

[71]Xiang, Y., Sekine, T., Nakamura, H., Imajoh-Ohmi, S., Fukuda, H., Nishioka, K., & Kato, T. (2004). Proteomic surveillance of autoimmunity in osteoarthritis: Identification of triosephosphate isomerase as an autoantigen in patients with osteoarthritis. *Arthritis & Rheumatism, 50*(5), 1511-1521.

[72]Tagoe et al. (2008). Op. Cit.

Part Two: *The Road to Healing*

Part I: Exercise for Menopausal Arthritis – What Works?

Almost everyone agrees that exercise is important to help prevent and to alleviate arthritis. The American College of Rheumatology recommends exercise to help prevent the symptoms of many kinds of arthritis from possibly worsening. It is emphasized on their website that finding the right balance between different types of exercise such as therapeutic, recreational and competitive (if one is on that level) is vital.[1]

In a very recent, comprehensive review of the research on the benefits of exercise in osteoarthritis (knee and hip), Drs. Kim Bennell and Rana Hinman of the University of Melbourne, Australia, noted that exercise is recommended in all clinical guidelines to help manage osteoarthritis. However, they emphasized that the best exercise for osteoarthritis and the frequency at which it should be performed are unknown. They noted the lack of research-based guidelines for hip osteoarthritis, and emphasized that very little research has been done on the effects of exercise on hip osteoarthritis. Although current international treatment guidelines recommend exercise for those with hip osteoarthritis, this was based primarily upon the opinions of experts in the field, not upon scientific evidence.[2]

The summarized findings of this wide-ranging review were as follows: (1) In one examination of the literature on hip osteoarthritis and exercise trials, there was only a small benefit for pain relief and no benefit with regard to people's perceptions of physical functioning. (2) Another study concluded that there was insufficient evidence to support the idea that exercise therapy by itself (in the short-term) is able to effectively reduce pain, increase physical functioning, and improve the quality of life for people with hip osteoarthritis. (3) Still another study assessing the literature concluded that therapeutic exercise, in particular that which includes supervision and a strength training component, can be an effective intervention in hip osteoarthritis.[3]

Drs. Bennell and Hinman also noted that although aquatic exercise has been recommended for hip osteoarthritis, there is little research in this area in comparison with land-based exercise. The findings of a review on aquatic exercise (combining both hip and knee osteoarthritis patients) found a small to moderate effect on function and on quality of life. There was no significant effect found for aquatic exercise on walking ability or range of motion.[3] Since knee and hip osteoarthritis involve joints with very different functions, it is hard to know whether positive results are equally effective for both types of arthritis. The knee and hip osteoarthritis patients were not analyzed separately within the study.[4]

For women suffering from menopausal arthritis, knee osteoarthritis is the primary joint affected, and fortunately there was a substantial amount of research on knee osteoarthritis. Land-based exercise was found to have a consistent record of improvements in knee pain and physical functioning. In fact, they reported that one meta-analysis of exercise for knee osteoarthritis demonstrated improvement for pain and functioning similar to benefits reported from NSAIDs (non-steroidal anti-inflammatory drugs) with substantially fewer problems from side effects.[5] This is important, as a new study published in the American Journal of Medicine looked at long-term aspirin use with important conclusions regarding dosage. They reported that regular use of aspirin is associated with gastrointestinal bleeding, with the risk more related to dose used than how long one uses the medication. The researchers concluded that the lowest effective dose should be used.[6]

Although acetaminophen has been viewed as not being an NSAID, as it works differently within the body than do the traditional NSAIDs, it too is often used for arthritis symptoms. Importantly, new risks for hospitalization due to gastrointestinal bleeding with acetaminophen have been reported.[7] Moreover, in patients 65 years and older, it was found that using a traditional NSAID along with acetaminophen may increase the risk of gastrointestinal bleeding in comparison with use of either of them singularly.[8]

Topic of Interest #6

Speaking of NSAIDs and Acetaminophen - Some Specific Findings of Importance

Research conducted out of Ball State University has found that acetaminophen (a COX-2 inhibitor) may possibly impair tendon mechanical properties after training.[9] These researchers also stress that there are numerous findings showing that COX-inhibiting drugs may have the ability to alter tendon metabolism within the extracellular matrix. The importance of the extracellular matrix, of course, was discussed in Chapter Two. COX-2 (Cyclooxygenase-2) is an enzyme that increases the rate of production of prostaglandins such as PGE2. PGE2 is associated with inflammation in arthritis. Inhibiting COX-2 can help prevent this inflammation. However, what if there is a downside to this in terms of tendon metabolism? That is essentially what these researchers found.[10] Tendon metabolism is complex and involves the breaking down of some components, and the building up of others. After one exercises, there is both a breaking down of collagen which occurs over a period of a few hours, and there is also protein synthesis that occurs over a period of days.[11]

The researchers at Ball State University looked at the effects of 12 weeks of progressive resistance training (three times weekly) on tendon mechanical properties such as whether there is excessive strain on the tendon. They did not find deformation or strain on the patellar tendon in the control group or in the group that used ibuprofen; these mechanical properties were unchanged in these groups after exercise. In contrast, in the group taking acetaminophen, there was increased patellar deformation and strain. Acetaminophen seemed to be interfering with the ability of the patellar tendon to adapt to resistance training.[12] As these researchers pointed out, many older people are encouraged to improve their health through exercise, but at the same time are taking COX-inhibiting drugs on a daily basis. They noted that the improvements in tendon strength and decreased strain on the tendons that has been found in older adults with exercise in previous research may not occur if the tendon's properties are unfavorably altered.[13]

Quite surprisingly, the same lead researcher from Ball State University along with colleagues, also found that acetaminophen (and ibuprofen) did *not* appear to interfere with muscle mass and strength gains as a result of resistance training. They found that that the over-the-counter doses when used in combination with resistance training, enhanced muscle mass and strength in older adults.[14]

However, please take notice! *The combination of reduced tendon strength and increased muscle strength is not a combination that you want to have!* Athletes in training know that muscles develop faster than tendons when it comes to gaining strength and increasing power. For example, weightlifting competitors are well aware that training for muscle strength is progressive and comes with visible results; however, in order to get to their maximum levels of weightlifting, they must train for tendon strength to match their muscle strength.[15] So, caution is advised when combining resistance training exercise with COX-2 inhibitors (to include acetaminophen).

Strength Training -- Does It Help Older Women with Arthritis?

In the review above that had shown the positive effects for land exercise upon arthritis, gender differences were not explored. The research literature does provide evidence that strength training, for example, can promote muscle growth and strength even in people who are well into their seventies.[16] However, the problem with many of these studies, for our purposes in developing an exercise program for women with menopausal arthritis, is that generally they (1) *do not examine gender differences* in their findings, (2) do not look at *age differences* in older people, and (3) do not look *specifically at women in menopause with osteoarthritis.*

For example, in one such study that did use older osteoarthritis patients as participants, it was found that those in the strength training group did improve in physical functioning (to include time in ascending the stairs and completing chair stands). However, there was *no analysis of gender differences* in these physical performance outcomes.[17] Why is this of particular importance?

Anyone with menopausal arthritis knows that stair climbing activities (to include both ascent and descent) are typically a major problem and are usually accompanied by knee pain. For example, there is one study that has been referred to in the literature as showing that men and women were able to increase in performance in activities such as stair climbing as a result of resistance exercise training; however, this study combines the findings of men and women. There was no breakdown of the training effects upon women and men separately. Rather, the researchers statistically *adjusted for the differential effects of sex.*[18] This uses statistical methods to, in essence, remove gender differences in the data analysis. *This does not provide us with the specific information we need about women*!

Whether women specifically are able to improve in functioning on stair climbing as a result of strength training is *exactly what we need to know.* For example, in one study that actually did analyze their findings by gender, here is what they found: Although stair climbing performance increased by 57% in the strength training group (as compared to a control group without strength training), it was *only the males who made gains in stair climbing performance.* There were no significant differences between men and women in terms of the response in building muscle.[19] So, why wouldn't the similar responsiveness to resistance training in women when compared with the men, translate into heightened performance on the stair climbing task for women?

Several key factors may be of importance here. First of all, older women and men begin strength training with some very distinct biophysiological and physical functioning differences. Importantly, the course of muscle loss is very different for older women and men. Men lose muscle more gradually over time, whereas women show a marked decrease in muscle mass after menopause.[20]

Moreover, there are likely some basic and marked gender differences in physical functioning at the beginning of these training protocols. For example, in a study using the Dynamic Gait Index (a measure of gait, balance, and fall risk), gender differences were most prominent and explicit in stair climbing. The lower score on the Dynamic Gait Index (DGI) among women compared with men was a result of how they functioned in stair climbing. Sixty-five percent of the women chose to hold a handrail, in contrast to 39% of the men.[21] Indeed, in a very large study of gender differences in health outcomes (of individuals aged 65 or over) some very striking differences in stair climbing functioning emerged. Women declined in ability at a much earlier age than did men on this task. Women who were between 65-74 years of age showed the same limitations in stair climbing that were found in men who were between the ages of 75-84 years age! Women also reported greater difficulty with stair climbing more often than men (55.7% for women versus 41.3% for men).[22]

Could gender differences in the prevalence of knee osteoarthritis be partly involved? In an extensive review of the literature, the prevalence of knee osteoarthritis was higher for women than for men regardless of how osteoarthritis was defined (e.g., self-reported, radiographic, symptomatic).[23] We have also seen that it is the knee where menopausal arthritis usually develops first and the place that it affects the most. Also, as noted in Chapter Six, soft tissue problems that are more common in women (such as pes anserine bursitis) may be factors in stair climbing pain.

Sadly, it appears that even total knee replacement is not a gender equalizer with regard to stair climbing performance. Research has found that following total knee replacement, improved ability in stair climbing and other physical functioning was significantly better for men. Men had better functioning scores prior to the operation and after the operation in comparison with women (and this was with the *same diagnosis*). The higher functioning scores were due to better walking and stair climbing scores at both times. After the knee replacement, there were no gender differences in the change in walking function for either sex; however, women had *less improvement than men in their ability to climb the stairs.* These researchers noted that this gender difference in stair climbing post-operation is most likely a continuation of the *same gender effect that was present before the operation.* Moreover, they did not think that this gender effect in function was something that could be remedied by changes in the fit of the prosthetic, or its shape or size.[24] So what *is* this *"gender effect"*?

Could it have something to do with differences in the way muscles respond to physical exercise and physical functioning tasks in men and women? What research seems to show is that women's muscles do not respond to strength training in exactly the same way that men's do. There are simply some important gender differences in how older adults respond to strength training, and these should not be overlooked or ignored.

For example, let's look at a study that actually did examine and analyze for gender differences in strength training effects. The participants were between 65 and 75 years of age and underwent a strength training program consisting of three training sessions per week over a period of approximately nine weeks. In this study, they focused upon knee strength in the dominant leg as an outcome measure of training with the untrained leg serving as a control or comparison. Exercise of the knee extensors was considered to involve "heavy resistance" and "high-volume" exercise. What they found in terms of training effects was that the absolute increase in strength of the trained leg was greater for men than women, but, the *relative change* in strength was similar.[25] However, in this case, the *relative change in strength* that was *similar* in men and women was based upon *1-RM strength.* This is the maximum amount of weight that a person can lift in a *single* repetition.[26]

Here is what was of much importance within the above study: *Isometric strength* (peak force at knee flexion) in the trained knee extensors of men significantly increased in strength, whereas *in women it did not.* Moreover, *isokinetic strength* significantly increased in the trained leg in men, *but in women it did not.*[27] From these findings, it seems that the ability to improve muscle strength and quality is possible for both men and women, but there are *important gender differences.* The lack of a training effect on isometric and isokinetic strength appears to suggest that there may be some limitations in the ability to generate muscle force in more sustained efforts and in terms of muscle endurance among older women.

There are also gender differences that have been found in the activation of the quadriceps muscle group. One study looked at the recruitment efficiency of the quadriceps. Recruitment efficiency is the ability of muscle tension to increase steadily by expanding the active motor units without wasted effort. They found that recruitment efficiency of the quadriceps was different in males and females. At knee angles of 50-70 degrees, all three quadriceps muscles in men showed significantly greater improvement in recruitment efficiency than in women.[28]

This ability to efficiently recruit muscle fibers contributes to the capacity of the muscle to be more resistant to fatigue. The rate at which a muscle fatigues matters in terms of the ability to generate muscle power. The speed of movement determines the velocity of the contraction, and thus, a fatigued muscle will have a diminished speed of contraction; this leads to a reduction in muscle power. With muscle fatigue, muscle power declines.[29]

Gender Differences in Physical Functioning: Searching for the Root Causes

Stair Climbing -- A Tall Order?

Let's take a look at some of the research in biomechanics and related areas that may help us in understanding why there are such marked gender differences in stair climbing performance. In a study conducted out of the Mayo Clinic, it was found that during stair climbing, women had a greater peak knee flexion angle than men. The researchers thought that perhaps this greater peak knee flexion among women is most likely a result of the significant height differences between the men and women within the study. They suggested that the higher prevalence of osteoarthritis in women may, in part, be due to the increased loading on the knee that results from this need for a greater degree of knee flexion.[30] Gender differences in body height (as related to stair climbing activities) have been largely unstudied. This is because it has been generally thought that the standard height of most stair risers is well within the functional range of most people to navigate without problem.

I know that once I began to try to go up and down the stairs properly positioned with weight evenly distributed, I had to change my biomechanics. Prior to doing this, I had basically been "crashing" down the stairs with harsh landings on each step. I found that to avoid this I needed to greatly increase my degree of knee flexion. I am 5'4" in height. As you may recall from the classic study of Drs. Cecil and Archer, the average height of the women with menopausal arthritis was 5'3". Perhaps height and stair climbing problems may be an important link in understanding some of the mechanical causes of menopausal arthritis. The males that I have observed (with heights of 5'8" and above) do not seem to have to use as great a knee flexion angle as I have to use. Interestingly, as I began to use greater knee flexion, it required more "ankle work" to position my feet on the steps. Stair climbing requires both muscle strength and joint flexibility. Not only do your thigh and ankle muscles need to be strong, but you must also have *flexibility* in your knee and ankle joints to function well in stair climbing activities. Now when I descend the steps, I feel the chain of muscles (and strong flexible tendons) that are working to allow me to flex all of my joints in smooth succession upon stair descent.

Deftly Descending Down the Stairs or Dangerously Dropping Down the Stairs: It's All a Matter of Muscle Chains

When it comes to stair activities, perhaps the more difficult and potentially damaging of the two is stair descent. Some study findings show that females may have an increased risk of injury in descending the stairs because of delays in activating muscles and decreased activity of the vastus medialis muscle.[31] The contraction of the vastus medialis muscle upon stair descent is an "eccentric" or lengthening contraction. So, would developing the vastus medialis muscle through eccentric exercise help? Research suggests that one might need to take into account gender differences in muscles exercised eccentrically. In a Danish study of gender differences in step exercise, women sustained more muscle damage to the vastus lateralis muscle during eccentric exercise than men. These researchers concluded that gender-specific step training programs may be needed to avoid this type of muscle damage in women.[32]

Based upon findings such as these, it may be important that precaution is taken not to overexert muscles that are involved in stepping movements in eccentric exercise. Many exercise programs isolate muscles in eccentric and concentric exercises. The exercises within this book are part of the natural movement of whole muscle chains, instead of isolated muscle exercises. You can begin to develop the vastus medialis, along with the entire quadriceps group of muscles in the natural movement of "Exercise 2 -- Point Toe Lift," and "Exercise 3 -- Heel Lift." When you work these muscles and muscle groups together (instead of isolating them), you help contribute to their ability to work as total units. Not only will you develop your vastus medialis muscle, but you will be developing it within natural movement and neuromuscular patterns that may help with stair ascent. Also be keenly aware of the fact that natural, functional movements such as stair climbing, walking, bending, reaching, etc. use *muscle chains, not isolated muscles!*

Step-down activities also require other muscle recruitment, as well. It is commonly thought that this activity requires, among other muscles, strong hip muscles (to include gluteus maximus as a hip extensor). Research shows that men and women differ in the electromyographic (EMG) recruitment of some muscles; that is, they differ in the efficient increase in the number of activated motor units as the strength of a muscle contraction increases.[33] A motor unit consists of a motor nerve cell and the muscle fibers to which it specifically sends impulses causing these muscle fibers to activate. How, specifically, is this related to step-down activities and possible problems in stair descent?

Working Your Gluteus Maximus to the Max: Why the Problem of "Underused Glutes" Is One of Your Knees' Worst Enemies

Researchers in the Program in Physical Therapy at the Mayo Clinic conducted a study examining knee valgus positioning (where the lower legs are angled outwards and the knees are collapsed inwards) and how it relates to hip muscle strength, and hip muscle recruitment. They examined this with the exercise of the single-leg step-down.[34] Knee valgus loading involves a turning in of the knee (such as from excessive rotating inwards of the hip). As I will discuss below, this valgus force can cause many knee problems. The researchers at the Mayo Clinic found that *reduced* knee valgus positioning in women during the single-leg step-down task may have more to do with the *recruitment of the gluteus maximus* than it does with external hip rotation strength, or the ability to rotate and utilize the hip on step down.[35] Much attention has been paid to hip muscle strength with regard to step-down functioning; the finding that the gluteus maximus (primary buttocks muscle) was possibly more central to women in this regard is an eye-opener. Before looking at this critical use of the gluteus maximus, let's briefly look at why reducing knee valgus positioning is so important.

Knee valgus stress has been found to be more prevalent in women than in men. The valgus loading that causes the knee to turn inward can be associated with soft tissue problems as well. For example, it is a cause of semimembranosus tibial collateral ligament bursitis as noted within Chapter Six. This very persistent and painful condition may be a problem for many women with menopausal arthritis. In addition, valgus stress is associated with many knee injuries in sports, as it is thought that increased valgus stress or force may lead to greater anterior cruciate ligament (ACL) loading. As noted earlier in the book, ACL injuries have been found to be more common in women than in men. Indeed, this connection between valgus knee loading and ACL injury is one possible explanation for the gender differences found in noncontact ACL ruptures.[36]

In an exercise program designed for women, then, it is important to build strength in the gluteus maximus and to decrease activities which cause valgus knee loading. The researchers at the Mayo Clinic reported findings from another study that found that knee valgus positioning was reduced in men during a single-leg squat, whereas it increased in women.[37] Because of this importance of the gluteus maximus in female biomechanics connected with knee pain, our exercise program emphasizes increasing gluteus maximus strength. This muscle is exercised, however, along with *all* of the muscles within its muscle chain. The exercises increase strength in the gluteus maximus as it exists as an integral part of the whole kinetic chain of muscles. At the same time, the exercises also incorporate isometric components focusing on the muscle itself. Isometric strength can be increased, but it is important that it be done in increments over time. As we age, our bodies need the chance to develop in a more gradual way than is done in the intense exercise protocols of some of the strength training programs. Because knee valgus positioning has been found to increase in women in the single-leg squat, our program does not include traditionally performed single-leg squat exercises.

It is a common observation in the popular literature among trainers and others involved in sports that women tend to underuse their gluteal muscles, and this results in less body strength and control of movements.[38,39] It is apparent from the Mayo Clinic study above that recruitment of the gluteus maximus may be important in reducing knee valgus positioning. If it is possible to help reduce knee valgus by activating the gluteus maximus, then exercises strengthening this muscle (as part of a kinetic muscle chain) would be very important.

Begin with "Exercise # 4 -- Rear Lift" that puts minimal strain on the joints, but does work the gluteus maximus. This exercise is vital to strengthening the gluteus maximus (and gluteus medius) *with* the hamstrings as they function together in movement. You will take excess strain off of your hamstrings through the activation of your gluteus maximus. This will decrease the likelihood of exercise fatigue and cramping that can result from isolated isotonic exercise of the hamstrings.

"Exercise #4 -- Rear Lift" will allow both muscle groups to be strong and decrease muscle fatigue. Some of the exercises in this book also incorporate contractions that will strengthen your gluteal muscles, even when the primary focus is upon another muscle group. For example, in "Exercise #11 -- Shoulder Turns" (even though the focus is the upper body), when you tuck in your buttocks and hold it tucked you are incorporating an isometric exercise component. This will help to tone and strengthen the gluteus maximus. Start with these exercises first, and you will be in a better position to do the squat exercise in the program ("Exercise #8 -- Body Lowering") when you advance in strength.

What Do You Have in Common with a Male Triathlete? More Than You May Think!

Dr. Christopher Powers of the University of Southern California and Tracey Wagner of Kaiser Permanente, Woodland Hills, California, and colleagues wrote up this very interesting case study of an elite, male triathlete who suffered from exercise-associated muscle cramping of the hamstrings. In his rehabilitation, an intervention to increase gluteus maximus strength was employed. They reasoned that since the hamstrings and the gluteus maximus act as agonists in the loading phase of running, that strengthening the gluteus maximus would lessen the relative amount of work required by the hamstrings. As a result, they predicted that the exercise-associated muscle cramping in the hamstrings would decrease. This is exactly what happened; the results of their electromyographic analysis (EMG) provided support for their hypothesis.[40]

An additional aspect of this case study is very interesting. The triathlete was given a pre- and post-test of the step-down task. Prior to treatment he showed a greater amount of hip internal rotation and adduction. Sound familiar? Just like the women in the Mayo Clinic study above, he was using a knee valgus positioning on step down. He was able to lessen this after he had undergone the strengthening of his *gluteus maximus muscle*.

The researchers involved in the triathlete's case study noted that two of the functions of the hamstrings are to decelerate hip flexion and also decelerate knee extension through eccentric contractions.[41] This is the case with the triathlete's running exercise, but it is also the case with stair descent! Principles that make sense for this male triathlete may also be just as important for a woman with menopausal arthritis (who is *underusing her glutes, and overusing her hamstrings* on stair descent). Both are "over-exercising" their hamstrings, although the reasons for the overworking of the hamstrings are obviously of quite different origin!

The Strongest Glutes in the Gym Will Get You Nowhere Without the Power and Spring of Your Ankles and Feet

Women and men have been found to differ with regard to the stiffness of their ankles, with men having greater musculotendinous stiffness compared with women. With regard to "stiffness" here we are talking about optimal connective tissue stiffness that helps to support the joints. This would suggest of course that there might be ankle joint stability differences between men and women, with men experiencing more stability. Because of this, it has been suggested that exercise interventions for women should involve activities that develop and maintain ankle function as a key component.[42] We have specifically developed "Exercise 15 -- Stepping and Holding Your Ground" to develop strength and flexibility in the ligaments, tendons and muscles of the lower legs, ankles, and feet. As you practice this exercise, you will begin to gain greater control of *how* and *where* you place your feet through the strengthening of muscle-tendon units and muscle chains and the proper and optimal movement of ligaments. As you develop more flexible ankles and control of your ankle movements, stair climbing will be much, much easier.

It is not just the ankles, but also the feet, that are involved in stair climbing; it is important to also focus upon the muscles and tendons that move the feet and the toes. When one goes up the stairs, strong "dorsiflexion" of the metatarsophalangeal joints is required.[43] Dorsiflexion refers to pulling the joints upwards as in standing on tip toes. The metatarsophalangeal joints are the joints that connect the metatarsal bones to the toes (for example, your big toe joint is the first of these joints, and the little toe joint is the fifth). When you go up the stairs, the muscles and tendons surrounding these joints must be strong!

The whole stability of the ankle is helped through the actions of the muscles in and around the foot and ankle.[44] With an emphasis on strengthening the quadriceps that appears in much of the literature on osteoarthritis, the importance of strengthening the foot and ankle muscles is often neglected. Concentrate on "Exercise #15 -- Stepping and Holding Your Ground" to greatly improve the muscles within your foot and around your ankle. When doing this exercise, you will not only tone and strengthen these muscles, but will reinforce and build the muscles all the way up the kinetic muscle chain from your lower leg up to your thighs and buttocks muscles.

Also concentrate on "Exercise 1: Toe Raise," and "Exercise 3: Heel Lift." In Exercise 1 you are strengthening the dorsiflexion of the metatarsophalangeal joints, and in Exercise 3, you are using dorsi-flexion of your foot which flexes the foot upwards decreasing the distance and angle between the upper surface of the foot and the front of the leg. Also practice "Exercise 2 - Point Toe Lift." In Exercise 2, you are using a plantar flexion of your foot which extends the foot and increases the distance and angle between the top surface of the foot and the front leg. As you go through the full set of exercises, you will find that these and many of the other exercises use plantar flexion and dorsiflexion of the feet. You will begin to feel how the muscles that allow for movement of your feet and ankles are vitally connected to the other active muscles of whole kinetic muscle chains.

This is a Book About Menopausal Arthritis and an Exercise Program for Women with Menopausal Arthritis!

As we have seen throughout this book, women and men are different when it comes to arthritis symptoms and different with re-gard to training effects upon muscle and tendon. The exercises within our program incorporate important knowledge from the sports train-ing literature and related areas, as well as fundamental principles of the practice of martial arts. They have been developed by a master within the martial arts, Shihan Herbert Wong (an 8th Degree Black Belt in Okinawan and Japanese Karate). He has practiced in many forms of the Asian martial arts to include Chi Kung, Tai Chi, and Kung Fu health exercises. Shihan Wong is personally dedicated to demystifying the principles behind Asian exercise forms. So, although the exercises rely in important ways upon principles from Asian Chi Kung training, you don't need any knowledge of the martial arts to perform them! You will build not only muscle strength, but also tendon strength and bone strength.

Practitioners of the Asian martial arts such as Tai Chi, Chi Kung, and Karate, etc. are well aware of the importance of tendon strength. In fact, the advanced practitioners and older master teachers are able to utilize more their tendon (rather than muscle) strength which will continue to be effective and strong as the person ages, even if muscle strength begins to diminish. As one ages and as one's muscular strength declines, the martial arts practitioner makes up for this lessening of muscle mass by integration of the muscle-tendon units into a powerful and coordinated body system (such integration results sometimes in *even greater strength and power* than in the practitioner's youth when the reliance was more on muscles alone). Given the research reviewed on the critical limitations in muscle building in older women, this is why this exercise program is so perfectly suited to menopausal women. Moreover, because this exercise program does not use uncomfortable props such as "bands" or require one to get into floor positions for exercise, it is especially suited to menopausal women with arthritis (who may find that these kinds of props and positions put undue strain and pressure on the joints).

An Introduction to the Muscle-Tendon-Bone Unit

Many times exercise programs for arthritis never mention bones! If they do, it's often just in reference to bone deformation that may be occurring with arthritis. Why concentrate on bones, too, in our healing program? Your bones are vital and alive and they are an integral part of the body that is exercised in conjunction with muscles and tendons! That is why, within our exercises, we will be referring continually to the muscle-tendon-bone-unit.

When you exercise your muscles, they pull on the tendons *and* the bones, strengthening them both. This "loading" is integral to the development of these tissues. In fact, research shows that the bone formation marker BAP (bone-specific alkaline phosphatase) may increase as a result of increased bone modeling due to the loading on the bone that occurs during exercise.[45] Bone modeling is the process through which your bone actually changes its size and shape to adapt to the loading that it is undergoing. In this process it also rids itself of damage and keeps itself strong.[46]

Bone cells recognize and react to mechanical stimuli. To be healthy, your bones must remodel and adjust to different types of loading conditions. When the bone undergoes a mechanical stress, bone cells are subject to both breaking down and building up bone tissue in the remodeling process. Fluid is actually transported through the bone. Some researchers have hypothesized that a greater fluid-flow rate allows the bone to receive nutrients more efficiently and to rapidly remove waste. The coordination of the remodeling process seems to take place through this flow of fluid. Moreover, this flow takes place when the bone undergoes mechanical loading or stress.[47] When you think of bone in this way, you can recognize it for what it is: living tissue that senses where it needs to be strong, builds new tissues, discards damaged tissues, and does this all with the movement of a vital flow of fluid that coordinates the remodeling.

Speaking of bone modeling, let's go back to the topic of gender differences. As men age it appears that their bodies naturally compensate for potential losses in bone mass and strength through increases in bone size; *this does not occur in women.* After menopause, women even show a greater inclination toward disconnection of their trabecular network.[48] Trabecular bone is spongy bone, and it is composed of a fine latticework; it has pockets of hollows which make it look like a sponge. It comprises most of the tissue that makes up the bone. In fact, bone tissue has been described as "analogous to a stiff and dense, fluid-filled sponge."[49] (Remember the bone fluid that was described above.)

This spongy bone network consists of "rods" and "plates" connected together. The disconnection of this spongy bone takes place through the plates becoming "rod-like," and losing the substance of the plate. Further, even the rods can become disconnected. The architecture of the bone basically deteriorates and comes apart.[50] For example, although it obviously does not incorporate all of the complexity of the situation, the following analogy does give you a feeling of how this bone can come apart. Imagine for a moment that this spongy bone network consists of wooden toy pieces comprised of sticks that connect to flat pieces, as in the construction toys. The deterioration of the trabecular bone would be similar to disconnecting some of the flat wooden construction toy pieces and replacing them with more sticks, and then taking out some of the sticks. It is, in essence, a changing of the shape and a deconstructing of the parts of the spongy bone network. The good news is that mechanical loading in exercise can help maintain the connections within the latticework of this spongy bone, and this happens through the modeling process.[51] Recall that the bone modeling process allows your bone to actually change its size and shape to adapt to mechanical loading. In light of the gender differences in the disconnection of this spongy bone network, the importance of exercises for women that emphasize the muscle-tendon-and bone unit cannot be overstated. As I emphasized earlier, *gender differences matter*!

We sometimes think only of the transfer of mechanical stress from muscle to bone. The more compliant quality of muscle is superbly adapted to transfer the mechanical stress from muscle to bone. Stress is dissipated not just from muscle to the tendon, but across the entire muscle-tendon-bone unit.[52] However, the force also goes in the opposite direction as well. When you land heavily with your foot (especially on hard surfaces) you are literally sending "shock waves through the body" as it has been described by Professor M. Benjamin and colleagues.[53] When you hit the ground with your foot, the reaction force goes from the ground to bone, from bone to tendon, and from tendon to muscle.

This force achieves some absorption from the Achilles tendon, but considerable stress from bone to tendon leaves the Achilles tendon vulnerable to injury. Professor Benjamin and colleagues were discussing this in terms of forces generated during exercise such as running and jumping. However, when you do not have sufficient muscular strength upon stair descent you land heavily on each step and this intense force from bone to tendon to muscle occurs. As these researchers explained, if there is insufficient strength in the anterior tibialis and soleus muscles, as well as the gastrocnemius, then the foot will not be aligned well when it lands. Because of this lack of control of the foot, the heel bone (calcaneus) will be misaligned changing the insertional angle of the Achilles tendon into the heel bone. This sets the Achilles tendon up for possible injury.[54]

Most strength training exercise books that I have come across have not emphasized the tendons within the muscle-tendon unit. The muscle-tendon unit is a very vital and specialized part of your musculoskeletal anatomy. Within it is the myotendinous junction, an extraordinary region (see Figure 9) where tension generated by muscle

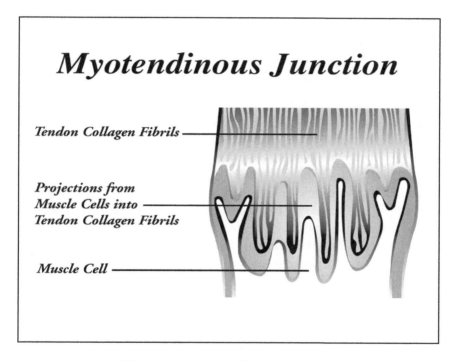

Figure 9 - Myotendinous Junction

is transferred from inside the muscle fiber cells to connective tissue cells outside of the muscle. Finger-like projections of muscle cells insert into the collagen fibrils of the tendon, and the collagen fibrils make their way into the tunnels formed between the muscle projections.[55]

Exercise that promotes both strength and endurance is critical to the health and vitality of the muscle-tendon unit. Weak muscles put more strain on the tendons. Strained tendons have to absorb more load and experience more stress than if they had been supported by a strong muscle. You need *both* strong muscles and strong tendons for the efficient functioning of your joints. Back to the importance of including bones, if you have weak bones in menopause you set yourself up for injuries that can prevent you from being able to put the needed mechanical loading on your tendons. You will not be building tendon *or* bone strength through mechanical loading in exercise if this occurs. It is a vicious cycle! So, strive to keep this vital muscle-tendon-bone unit strong.

Tendons Need Exercise -- But, Not Too Much Exercise

Considering knee osteoarthritis pain, decreased quadriceps tendon thickness has been found to be a risk factor.[56] An unexercised tendon will lose thickness. Nevertheless, it is critical to exercise in such a way that you do not put undue stress upon your tendons. As research suggests, repeated stress or mechanical loading to a tendon may cause fatty and calcified tissues to develop within the tendon. For example, in animal research it was found that repetitive mechanical loading on the tendons (e.g., treadmill running) caused a marked increase in PGE(2) or prostaglandin E2. This messenger molecule, increased through repetitive tendon strain, may ultimately result in promoting tendon degeneration. Under the condition of repetitive tendon strain, PGE(2) appears to have an effect resulting in decreased tendon stem cells (cells that would ordinarily help in the repair of tendon cells). In this case the tendon stem cells not only decreased, but were also *induced to form into fat cells and bone cells.*[57]

Building Tendon Strength in Women

Researchers at the Institute of Sports Medicine, Copenhagen, found that women had less tendon strength than men, and their tendons were less responsive to physical training than were men's tendons. They had looked at the patellar tendon (the tendon surrounding the knee cap), and physical training led to a larger patellar tendon in men, but *not in women*. Men also had greater collagen synthesis after exercise than women. Interestingly, higher levels of estrogen in women led to *less* collagen production. All of this is very critical, because tendon mechanical strength (the ability to endure stress without failure) was weaker in women than in men which could lead to a higher risk of injury.[58]

We have already seen in the chapter on muscles and tendons, that tendons become less flexible, resilient, and strong with aging in both men and women. However, since women may also have less tendon mechanical strength, this must be taken into consideration in planning an appropriate and effective exercise program. You want to increase the health of your tendons, not open them up to injury!

The "Body Lowering" exercise in this book is an invaluable exercise to help develop your tendon strength and the muscle-tendon unit. Beneficial effects of this type of exercise for older women are illustrated in a similar exercise used within a scientific study of low-load resistance training on the tendons of older women. In a study conducted out of the University of Tokyo, middle-aged and elderly women performing a low-load squat exercise (using body weight) significantly increased the elasticity of their tendons; this was in comparison to a control group that did not receive any training intervention but simply continued their daily routines and activities. In this squat exercise, the women began in an upright position lowering themselves to a preferred squat depth (in which the thighs were parallel to the ground) and then in a continuous motion resumed their upright position. The researchers at the University of Tokyo also reported findings within this same study that showed that with advancing age there is a decline in the elasticity of the tendons in the women they had studied. Importantly, their research suggests that the low-load, squat exercise is extremely beneficial in tendon strengthening. [59]

Their squat exercise appears to be quite similar to the squat exercise within this book (although it is unclear whether the back was kept vertically aligned as they lowered into the squat). Our squat exercise does keep the back vertically aligned, and does not use as low of a squat as the one within their research study (based upon their description). There should be less chance of injury, while still developing the strength of the tendons. Within "Exercise 8 -- Body

Lowering," you will also lower your body to a depth that is comfortable for you, and then rise back to the upright position. In this exercise you do hold the pose for about 5 seconds before returning to the upright position. This is an excellent exercise, as tendons are gently stretched and the body is lowered only a few inches; it is not a deep squat. You will feel the stretch upon your tendons, though. What is critical here is to go very slowly, and increase the overall tendon strength in the tendons of both your ankles and your knees. This squat is different from the typical "modified squat" in which the back is not kept in a vertically aligned position. The strength of the "Body Lowering" exercise in this book is that it keeps the upper body in its vertical plane. The lowering into this position activates the upper and lower leg muscles and tendons to strengthen them. However, this will only be true if you keep your upper body in the vertical plane.

Tendon Health and Menopause: A Connection with Overweight and Obesity?

For overweight and obese menopausal women, researchers have found that there is a direct association between body weight and stiffness in the muscle-tendon unit. Again, as noted earlier, stiffness can be used to indicate positive strength or conversely to mean a loss of elasticity and quality. Excessive stiffness can increase the risk of bone injuries and insufficient stiffness can increase the risk of soft tissue injuries.[60] It is excessive stiffness that is being examined within this study. Since obesity is highly associated with menopausal arthritis the following findings are critical. Menopausal women who were of *normal weight* had the same degree of stiffness in the muscle-tendon unit as women who were *not yet menopausal*. However, for each category of greater weight gain (pre-obese, obesity class I, and obesity class II), the muscle-tendon unit stiffness significantly increased. One interpretation provided for why this might occur is that fat may have infiltrated the leg muscle tissue; movement restriction, as well as postural and stability issues of obesity may all work to produce this resulting muscle-tendon stiffness.[61]

Topic of Interest #7

Fat that Infiltrates Muscle May Weaken Physical Functioning

Perhaps one of the most harmful aspects of this infiltration of fat into muscle is that it has been found to unleash harmful pro-inflammatory cytokines right into the muscles themselves! Australian researchers, Dr. Itamar Levinger and colleagues, performed a most interesting study on nineteen patients with knee osteoarthritis and fourteen patients without knee osteoarthritis. Participants in the knee osteoarthritis group were selected to have matched ages and body mass index (BMI) with those in the non-knee osteoarthritis group. The participants underwent both strength measurements and muscle biopsies. It was found that the patients with knee osteoarthritis had *significantly greater levels of inflammatory cytokines* such as Inter-leukin-6 (IL-6), tumor necrosis factor-alpha, and other inflammatory chemicals *within their muscles*! They also had reduced muscle strength compared with the participants without knee osteoarthritis. Higher levels of the gene expression of tumor necrosis factor alpha, for example, *were associated with diminished muscle strength.*[62]

Although one would simply assume that less muscle strength would be associated with poorer physical performance, this, indeed, has been supported in findings of a study at Florida State University. These researchers found that a higher infiltration of fat into muscle tissue was linked to worsened physical performance. They also found that higher fat mass was related to worsened physical performance, and higher muscle mass to improved physical performance. What was especially important was that higher muscle mass, particularly in the lower extremities, was related to enhanced performance. Nevertheless gender mattered. It was not only muscle mass, but fat mass too, that was of significance in women. In women only, it was higher muscle mass and lower body fat that were associated with better physical functioning.[63]

The Key Principles of Our Exercise Program

The most important emphasis of our exercise program is to build strong muscle-tendon-bone units as they exist naturally in full kinetic muscle chains. This is what will optimize your ability to have adequately supported joints, and thus to prevent much of the joint pain associated with menopausal arthritis. There are eight key principles that will enhance your ability to do this.

1. Improving Knee Functioning

In an exercise program for women with menopausal arthritis there must be an emphasis upon the strengthening of the muscles and tendons that surround the knee. Most arthritis exercises focus on specific muscles, such as the quadriceps. However, it is vitally important to strengthen not only other muscles involved in whole muscle chains, but also the tendons too. This is especially so, given the research reviewed above on muscle and tendon strength in women. By strengthening muscles and tendons (within kinetic chains of muscles) you will increase muscle power and physical functioning and decrease stress upon your knee joints.

2. Alleviating Soft Tissue Problems

As you may recall from Chapter Six, several bursitis conditions (such as pes anserine bursitis) are more prevalent in women than in men. An exercise program that promotes rather than hinders the health of the surrounding soft tissues such as the bursae is vital. You do not want to irritate already inflamed tissues. Rather, it is critical to locate the muscles that are not functioning well (either through being shortened or weakened) and to address bursitis and other soft tissue and muscle pain at their root causes. Doing preparatory massage work prior to initiating the exercise program may be beneficial; it can help correct muscle dysfunction and soft tissue displacement that may cause pain and that will not be helped or corrected through exercise alone. In Chapter Nine, I will discuss tissue displacement issues, as well as corrective massage techniques that may be helpful. It can also be advantageous to continue therapeutic massage techniques as you progress along within the exercise program.

3. Making Biomechanics Work for You, Not Against You

There are gender differences in gait patterns and in the bio-mechanics of how some exercises are performed that are relevant to healing from menopausal arthritis. It is commonly thought that both men and women can gain from a universal exercise such as walking. However, walking is a surprising example of a well-regarded activity in which there are gender differences; men and women differ in bio-mechanics that affect performance and the potential to prevent or heal from arthritis.

In a study conducted out of Stanford University and the VA Palo Alto Health Care System, hip joint torque (or twisting force) among healthy older walkers was explored. The researchers analyzed gait patterns and found that the women had greater hip joint moments or torque. The results of their study suggested that walking resulted in greater joint stress for the women as compared with the men. They cautioned that this could point toward greater risk of hip joint deterioration in older women walkers as compared to men. They also cited research that found that older women had less hip cartilage volume than older men (and this was independent of other factors).[64] As you can see, gender and age differences in tissues such as cartilage, as well as some gender-specific biomechanics, may matter greatly as factors in healing outcomes. Recall also the gender differ-ences in knee valgus landing in single leg squats discussed earlier. It is critical to engage in physical exercise activities that do not put excess strain upon your joints. This is one of the reasons why the exercises in this book, focusing upon a diverse range of movements, may be more beneficial for people with arthritis than a general, repetitive exercise activity such as walking.

4. Building Muscle Power

Research is beginning to reveal that impaired muscle power (which is different than "strength") may be a critical factor limiting mobility in older persons.[65] In a very large study of 839 elderly persons (aged 65 years or older), leg muscle power was found to be more associated with many mobility tasks (to include stair climbing) than was leg muscle strength.[66] What is the essential difference be-tween muscle strength and muscle power? Strength is the ability to

exert force, and power is "the ability to exert force quickly."[67]
Maintaining balance in some tasks may be related to the ability to
rapidly generate force when performing a task. For example, if one
performs a task that is time-limited such as crossing the street before
the light changes, or if one needs to maintain balance after one has
been thrown off-balance by something, muscle *power* may be critical.[68]

Physiological factors in aging that may be involved in muscle
power include: changes in muscle fiber composition and quality,
neuromuscular decline in the firing rate of muscle units, and altered
muscle contraction during multi-joint activities.[69] Some of these
problems may not be easily improved. That is why we are empha-
sizing the development of strong tendons and muscle-tendon-units
within our exercises. Your ability to function well is not all based
upon the working of your muscles alone! As you begin to develop
your muscles as components of muscle chains, you will find that
muscle power is increased. Remember, power is a product of muscle
force and speed. As you strengthen your muscles in ways that
incorporate whole chains of muscles, you will increase muscle force.
Moreover, as these chains of muscles begin to work together in a
coordinated and smooth fashion, you will build speed and thus increase power.

5. *Exercising to Improve Physical Functioning*

To improve in everyday physical functioning it is essential to
stay as close to natural (actual natural task) movements as possible. It
has been suggested that strength training with the goal of performing
specific tasks should focus on the movements involved in performing
the actual tasks (not just strengthening of muscles in exercise using
general movements).[70] Indeed, once you have begun to strengthen
your muscles with the exercises in this book, beginning to practice
stair climbing is an excellent way to improve your ability to do stair
climbing. If you want to be good at climbing the stairs, then climb
the stairs! As you may recall from earlier in the book, when I first
began to do this, my muscles were so weak I would wobble as I
ascended the stairs. With practice, I found that I gained strength in
the very muscles that I needed to perform this activity. As these
muscles gained in strength, the kinetic chains of muscles could then

begin to function as a whole. One caveat here, though, is that until these muscles build in strength, you may be both building muscle and still placing strain upon the joints until the muscles are stronger. As such, using the stair climbing as an exercise should occur toward the end of the program when you have already built up strength through the muscle chain exercises.

6. Exercising Using Whole Muscle Chains

The chains of muscles that you are developing involve the working of muscles over multiple joints. Why is multiple joint movement so important? A very unique Japanese study looked at the effects of exercise with single joint movement compared with multiple joint movement. These researchers found that exercise focusing on multiple joints may contribute to a better quality of muscle activity. Moreover, it may improve the stability of the pelvis when standing upon a single leg.[71] This is, of course, important to stair climbing and descent as there is a shifting of weight from one leg to the other during this activity. *All* of our exercises utilize these muscle chains and involve multiple joints working together.

In contrast, many muscle strengthening exercise programs for arthritis use repetitions of what is called "open chain" exercises. A single muscle group and a single joint are usually isolated (e.g., seated knee extension exercises). They are performed with added weights or without weights. Knee extension exercises are often advised for strengthening the quadriceps muscles in those with knee osteoarthritis. In many protocols, weights are added at the ankle. In contrast, closed chain exercises involve the strengthening of multiple muscle groups and involve more than one joint. As explained by Nicole Nichols, ACE-certified personal trainer and AFAA-certified group fitness instructor, the open chain knee extensions stress the knee with the generation of a shear force. This not only stresses the knee, but also the anterior cruciate ligament. Worse yet, adding weights on the "distal" portion of the leg at the ankle increases the risk for injury. Nicole Nichols advises that closed chain exercises provide a safer option for your joints, and this is especially so for the knee. The compressive force that is produced in closed chain exercises such as squats and lunges actually provides a stabilizing effect upon the joint. Working many muscles simultaneously, this type of exercise is closer to the activities of daily living; hence, closed chain exercises can improve your functional ability in physical activities.[72]

7. Addressing Gender Differences in Joint Laxity

Joint laxity is a factor that may put people at higher risk for joint and soft tissue injury. Osteoarthritis has also been frequently found to co-exist with hypermobility of the joints. In a study of rheumatology clinic patients conducted out of the University of Missouri School of Medicine, it was found that *all* of the patients with joint hypermobility *were women*. This was the case, even though only 75% of the patients within the study were women.[73] Concentrate on "Exercise #15 -- Stepping and Holding Your Ground" to increase your attention to developing muscles and tendons to counter joint laxity, and to increase your ability to develop and strengthen these muscles and tendons. This exercise will specifically develop all of the critical muscles and tendons that help to provide stability to the hip, knee, and ankle joints. It also incorporates isometric contraction as you "grip" the ground with your feet. This will help you to strengthen and tone the very muscles that you need in order to walk with a balanced gait. Similarly, in "Exercise #11 -- Shoulder Turns," when you grip the floor with both of your feet, you are also incorporating isometric contractions in your lower legs. So, although the focus in this exercise is primarily upon upper body movement, you are also increasing muscle strength in your lower legs that will help you to strengthen muscles and tendons important to countering joint laxity.

8. Reducing Your Risk of Injury

Differences in health status were explored in a comprehensive review of the literature of strength training and physical functioning in older adults. The authors assessed 121 different trials of strength training with older adults. Overall, the review provided evidence that progressive resistance strength training can improve muscle strength and performance in some activities (such as getting up from a chair and gait speed). For the participants with osteoarthritis, it was found that there was reduced pain.[74]

Nevertheless, when looking at strength training trials in older adults with regard to the occurrence of adverse effects, these same researchers found the following: in 121 trials of progressive strength training in older adults (age 60 years and older), 43 of the trials involved the reporting of adverse events. Thus, *in 35.5% of the progressive strength training trials there were adverse events reported. Most of them were related to musculoskeletal problems (e.g., joint pain, muscle strains).*[75] This is why our program emphasizes gradual progression of strengthening in natural movements using whole chains of muscles slowly to minimize the risk of injury.

In another study of a home-based exercise program for knee pain and knee osteoarthritis, it was found that people in the exercise groups did significantly better than those in the control groups (no exercise conditions) at 6, 12, and 18 months in terms of pain reduction. However, at 24 months, only 48.1% of those assigned to exercise groups had completed the program. The most common physical reasons for not completing the program had to do with problems such as hip or back pain. Also, some reported that the exercise band caused pain around their ankles.[76] *The fact that equipment such as this can cause pain is, by the way, why you will see no exercise bands or other such props within our exercise program. Moreover, getting up and down off of the floor can be painful and difficult for people with arthritis; as such, all of the exercises within this book are done from standing positions with no floor exercises!*

9. *Avoiding Everyday Lifestyle Options That Can Worsen Your Arthritis*

For an exercise program to be of benefit, you must be sure that you are not "undoing" your gains by adopting everyday lifestyle choices and activities that can worsen your joint pain. For example, it is critical to keep an upright posture (not to lean forward when you walk as this puts too much stress upon the knees). Moreover, as we discussed earlier, even some activities such as walking may cause a problem for some older women. Assess how you feel after various activities, and do not just assume that they must be good for you. Also, activities that involve repetitive motion over a long period of time may not be optimal when you have joint pain. The exercises in this book use whole chains of muscles in a natural way. They are also not repetitive in nature; they are varied in the muscle chains that they work.

Topic of Interest #8

How Wearing the Wrong Kind of Shoes Can Worsen Your Arthritis

I had found that sometime right around menopause and there-after, I had begun to twist my ankle (walking in my favorite clogs); I went catapulting to the ground on more than one occasion. It seemed that my ankle would just "give out," or I thought that perhaps I may have tripped on some kind of stone, or pothole, or something. My ankle had never done this before I had entered menopause. I didn't know it at the time, but I was beginning to lose strength in my ankles, particularly in my left ankle. I finally had to give up wearing my favorite footwear, my clogs, which I had loved for their comfort.

When I began to research this book, I found out something rather surprising. Peak medial knee loads (peak knee external adduc-tion moments) were *greatest* in people wearing *clogs* and stability shoes, and they were the least in people sporting flip-flops or going barefoot![77] This is important because increased medial knee joint loads are associated with the severity and progression of osteoarthritis and with pain in osteoarthritis. As the researchers of this study ex-plained, the entire lower extremity is an interrelated unit, both mechanically and functionally. So, alterations in one aspect of this unit, in this case the foot, can have a tremendous impact upon the loading pattern of distant areas such as the knee.[78] Also, with regard to my weak ankle, it was not just the muscles of the lower leg that move the ankle that were weak, but rather problems and imbalances within the *whole flexor muscle sling* that included these muscles! My ankle problem originated far from my ankles. Its initial origin was in my weak hip flexors! Please see again the flexor muscle sling in Figure 1 in Chapter Four.

It is not just clogs (and stability shoes), however, that can be a problem. A new review of the literature on footwear and knee adduc-tion moment was conducted by researchers at the University of Otago in New Zealand and University of Constance, Germany. These re-searchers found that there are several types of shoes that can lead to higher maximum loads on the medial knee joint in healthy individuals as compared with barefoot walking. Within this review, the shoes that were associated with greater medial knee loads included those with higher heels, sneakers, and dress shoes.[79] The importance of greater medial knee loads cannot be overstressed. In fact, one study found that each 1% increase in peak knee adduction moment (over a period of 6 years) was associated with nearly 6.5 times greater risk of the worsening of knee osteoarthritis.[80]

Examining seventeen studies with healthy participants and nineteen studies with participants with medial knee osteoarthritis, the researchers at the University of Otago and colleagues concluded that foot wear with similar knee loadings to barefoot walking may be best for people with medial knee osteoarthritis.[81]

I now walk barefoot at home as often as I can, or I wear shoes that provide similar foot movements (such as some sandals provide). The type of clog that I had been wearing for years was essentially the same one as within the research study above. Mine was the same brand, worn often by healthcare workers, with a stiff sole and heel height of 50 mm; a slip-on with no back support.[82] It was an extremely comfortable shoe. I would have never guessed that it could actually exacerbate and make my arthritis worse.

All of my shoes now have flexible soles. Only with the change to flexible soles could I begin to work and feel all of the muscles of my legs, ankles, and feet. Moreover, by being able to use all of these muscles, I greatly increased my stability in walking and in stair climbing.

10. Supplementing Exercise with Other Therapeutics May Be Needed

A meta-analysis study of people with knee osteoarthritis looked at the effects of strength training alone, exercise therapy alone (which included strength training, range of motion exercises and aerobics), and exercise therapy with passive manual mobilization of the joints. Effect sizes for pain reduction were small for strength training alone and for exercise therapy alone. In contrast, effect sizes were moderate when passive manual mobilization of the joints was added to the exercise therapy.[83]

What is passive manual mobilization of the joints? Usually performed by physical therapists, it is a form of manual therapy. As we saw in Chapter Five, the articular surface of the joints is covered with smooth cartilage that assists in allowing the joints to move freely without having the bones grate against each other. When one performs a knee extension, there is movement at the junction of the tibia and the femur. The femur stays steady, while the tibia moves forward. The tibia is also gliding over the surface of the articular base of the femur. The types of movement between the two joint surfaces, such as that between the femur and tibia, are called "slides" or "glides." The movement between the two surfaces of the bones of the joint has been termed "joint play." In passive manual mobilization, the therapist applies a force to a joint that is not being moved by the person through their own voluntary muscle contraction. The mimicked movement is controlled and powered by the therapist. Mobilizations are usually done slowly; whereas, manipulations are done more quickly such as in a thrust motion. Mobilizations are performed when, due to injury or illness, a person's mobility, and range of motion are impaired.[84]

The joint oscillations or mobilizations by the therapist are done within the available range of motion of the joint (the range that is limited by either pain or tissue resistance). Joint mobilizations are used to restore the proper relationship between the structures of the joint and to reduce pain. It is thought that pain is reduced through an improvement in joint lubrication and through increased circulation in the tissues that surround the joint. This therapeutic technique has also been thought to help muscle tone through its neuromuscular components and to heighten proprioceptive awareness.[85] We will come back to other forms of manual manipulation, as well, in Chapter Nine on "Healing from the Outside."

Finally, when you engage in exercise, be sure that you are providing your body with ample nutrients and all of the assistance it needs to repair itself afterwards. An adequate intake of protein, as well as some carbohydrates, and healthful dietary fat are needed to repair and build your vital muscle-tendon-bone units.

Topic of Interest #9

Launch Your Satellite Cells into Action!

Speaking of repairing muscles after exercise, satellite cells are critical. You may be thinking as I had, what is a satellite cell? Well, these are very specialized muscle cells that for the most part stay inactive and still. They basically hide in the basement (in this case, basement membrane) until they are needed upstairs, so to speak! Did you ever wonder how your body repairs its muscles after a physical workout? These satellite cells come to the rescue of your strained muscles that have been damaged or broken down following intense exercise. They flourish in the area and generate new muscle fibers. Through cell divisions they grow and then begin to unite and merge with the damaged and deconstructed muscle cells.

A study out of Umea University in Sweden has stressed the importance of exercise as one of the most critical things one can do to stem excessive muscle loss that is associated with what is termed sarcopenic obesity. Sarcopenic obesity is a marked reduction in lean body mass and an increase in fat mass. These researchers emphasized that exercise, along with activating the satellite cells and good nutrition, constitute the best things that one can do to help prevent the excessive muscle loss of sarcopenia and to counter sarcopenic obesity.[86] In addition to exercise, are there additional ways to activate your satellite cells? The findings of one new study show that melatonin may be involved in supporting the repair of muscles after injury. In this animal research, melatonin was found to reduce inflammation and to raise the number of satellite cells.[87] Melatonin is a natural chemical compound found within the body, and in mammals it is secreted by the pineal gland. It is secreted when there is darkness such as at night. So, to increase muscle repair it would be important to get adequate sleep at night, with little light introduced into your environment (as with night lights, turning on the bathroom lights, etc.).

Exercise to Counter Menopausal Arthritis -- In Sum

Building muscle strength is one important way to help support your joints. However, *what is most important is strengthening muscles along with tendons and bones, and doing so across whole muscle slings or kinetic muscle chains!* What is critical to understand is the importance of the *unified actions* of your muscles and the continual use of the muscle-tendon-bone unit in exercise and in daily living. A muscle's development depends upon its stimulation and use (e.g., active repetition, load or weight on the muscle, etc.) while tendon development depends less on the stimulation via repetition and more on the stretch, elasticity, and load on the tendon. Keep in mind that mechanical load is important for *bone* too, and that when you work your muscles and tendons, the tendons exert mechanical load on the bone helping to induce modeling, remodeling and stronger bones. Also recall that as discussed in Chapter Five, cartilage synthesis has been shown to be stimulated as a result of moderate mechanical load, so you are promoting healthier cartilage too. When you begin to develop and strengthen your *muscle-tendon-bone units* through our exercises, you should begin to see much improved ability in all of your physical functioning (to include those formidable tasks of stair ascent and descent)! So, let's begin to form strong and supple bodies that can climb stairs with ease!

Notes for Chapter Seven - Part I

[1]Westby, M., (reviewed by the American College of Rheumatology Patient Education Task Force (2009). Exercise and arthritis. American College of Rheumatology. Retrieved from http://www.rheumatology.org/practice/clinical/patients/diseases_and_conditions/exercise.asp

[2]Bennell, K. L., & Hinman, R. S. (2011). A review of the clinical evidence for exercise in osteoarthritis of the hip and knee. *Journal of Science and Medicine in Sport, 14*, 4-9. doi: 10.1016/j.jsams.2010.08.002

[3]Ibid.

[4]Ibid.

[5]Ibid.

[6]Huang, E. S., Strate, L. L., Ho, W. W., Lee, S. S., & Chan, A. T. (2011). Long-term use of aspirin and the risk of gastrointestinal bleeding. *American Journal of Medicine, 124*(5), 426-433.

[7]Zhang, W., Nuki, G., Moskowitz, R. W., Abramson, S., Altman, R. D. Arden, N. K., Bierma-Zeinstra, S., Brandt, K. D., Croft, P., Doherty, M., Dougados, M., Hochberg, M., Hunter, D. J., Kwoh, K., Lohmander, L. S., & Tugwell, P. (2010). OARSI recommendations for the management of hip and knee osteoarthritis: part III: Changes in evidence following systematic cumulative update of research published through January 2009. *Osteoarthritis Cartilage, 18*(4), 476-499.

[8]Rahme, E., Barkun, A., Nedjar, H., Gaugris, S., & Watson, D. (2008). Hospitalizations for upper and lower GI events associated with traditional NSAIDs and acetaminophen among the elderly in Quebec, Canada. *American Journal of Gastroenterology, 103*(4) 872-882.

[9]Carroll, C. C., Dickinson, J. M., LeMoine, J. K., Haus, J.M., Weinheimer, E. M., Hollon, C. J., Aagaard, P., Magnusson, S. P., & Trappe, T. A. (2011). Influence of acetaminophen and ibuprofen on in vivo patellar tendon adaptations to knee extensor resistance exercise in older adults. *Journal of Applied Physiology, 111*, 508-515. doi: 10.1152/japplphysiol.01348.2010

[10]Ibid.

[11]Kjaer, M. (2009). The secrets of matrix mechanical loading. *Scandinavian Journal of Medicine and Science in Sports, 19*(4), 455-456.

[12]Carroll et al. (2011). Op. Cit.

[13]Ibid.

[14]Trappe, T. A., Carroll, C. C., Dickinson, J. M., LeMoine, J. K., Haus, J. M., Sullivan, B. E., Lee, J. D. Jemiolo, B., Weinheimer, E. M., & Hollon, C. J. (2011). Influence of acetaminophen and ibuprofen on skeletal muscle adaptations to

resistance exercise in older adults. *American Journal of Physiology. Regulatory, Integrative and Comparative Physiology, 300*(3), R655-R662.

[15]Robson, D. (2011). Learn how to build great tendon and ligament strength and enhance power and overall. Meridian, ID: Body Building.com, LLC. Retrieved from: http://www.bodybuilding.com/fun/drobson18.htm

[16]Liu, C. J., & Latham, N. K. (2009). Progressive resistance strength training for improving physical function in older adults. *Cochrane Database of Systematic Reviews*, (3), CD002759.

[17]Baker, K. R., Nelson, M. E., Felson, D. T., Layne, J. E., Sarno, R., & Roubenoff, R. (2001). The efficacy of home based progressive strength training in older adults with knee osteoarthritis: A randomized controlled trial. *Journal of Rheumatology, 28*(7), 1655-1665.

[18]Fiatarone, M. A., O'Neill, E. F., Ryan, N. D., Clements, K. M., Solares, G. R., Nelson, M. E., Roberts, S. B., Kehayias, J. J., Lipsitz, L. A., & Evans, W. J. (1994). Exercise training and nutritional supplementation for physical frailty in very elderly people. *New England Journal of Medicine, 330*(25), 1769-1775

[19]McCartney, N., Hicks, A. L., Martin, J., & Webber, C., E. (1995). Long-term resistance training in the elderly: Effects on dynamic strength, exercise capacity, muscle, and bone. *Journal of Gerontology, 50*, B97.

[20]Mangione, , K. K., Miller, A. H., & Naughton, I. V., (2010). Cochrane Review: Improving physical function and performance with progressive resistance strength training in older adults. *Physical Therapy, 90*(12), 1711-1715.

[21]Herman, T., Inbar-Borovsky, N., Brozgoi, M., Giladi, N., & Hausdorff, J. M. (2009). The Dynamic Gait Index in healthy older adults: The role of stair climbing, fear of falling and gender. *Gait & Posture, 29*(2), 237-241. doi: 10.1016/j.gaitpost.2008.08.013

[22]Cameron, K. A., Song, J., Manheim, L M., & Dunlop, D. D. (2010). Gender disparities in health and healthcare use among older adults. *Journal of Women's Health, 19*(9), 1643-1650. doi: 10.1089/jwh.2009.1701

[23]Pereira, D., Peleteiro, B., Araújo, J., Branco, J., Santos, R. A., & Ramos. E. (2011). The effect of osteoarthritis definition on prevalence and incidence estimates: A systematic review. *Osteoarthritis and Cartilage, 19*(11), 1270-1285.

[24]Ritter, M. A., Wing, J. T., Berend, M. E., Davis, K. E., & Meding, J. B. (2008). The clinical effect of gender on outcome of total knee arthroplasty. *Journal of Arthroplasty, 23*(3), 331-336. doi: 10.1016/j.arth.2007.10.031

[25]Tracy, B. L., Ivey, F. M., Hurlbut, D., Martel, G. F., Lemmer, J. T., Siegel, E. L., Metter, E. J., Fozard, J. L., Fleg, J. L., & Hurley, B. F. (1999). Muscle quality. II. Effects of strength training in 65- to 75-yr-old men and women. *Journal of Applied Physiology, 86*(1), 195-201.

[26]Ibid.

[27]Ibid.

[28]Pincivero, D. M., Salfetnikov, Y., Campy, R. M., & Coelho, A. J. (2004). Angle- and gender-specific quadriceps femoris muscle recruitment and knee extensor torque. *Journal of Biomechanics, 37*(11), 1689-1697.

[29]Sargeant, A. J. (2007). Structural and functional determinants of human muscle power. *Experimental Physiology, 92*(2), 323-331. doi: 10.1113/expphysiol.2006.034322

[30]Hughes, C. A., Kaufman, K. R., Morrey, B. F., Morrey, M. A., & An, K. N. (2000, July 19-22). Gender differences in knee kinematics and kinetics during stair climbing and level walking in adults with osteoarthritis of the knee. Paper presented at the *24th Annual Meeting of the American Society of Biomechanics* (University of Illinois at Chicago).

[31]Sung, P. S., & Lee, D. C. (2009). Gender differences in onset timing and activation of the muscles of the dominant knee during stair climbing, *Knee, 16*(5), 375-380.

[32]Fredsted, A., Clausen, T., & Overgaard, K. (2008). Effects of step exercise on muscle damage and muscle Ca2+ content in men and women. *Journal of Strength Conditioning Research, 22*(4), 1136-1146.

[33]Pincivero et al. Op. Cit.

[34]Hollman, J. H., Ginos, B. E., Kozuchowski, J., Vaugh, A. S., Krause, D. A., & Youdas, J. W. (2009). Relationships between knee valgus, hip-muscle strength, and hip-muscle recruitment during a single-limb step-down. *Journal of Sport Rehabilitation, 18*, 104-117.

[35]Ibid.

[36]Russell, K. A., Palmieri, R. M., Zinder, S. M., & Ingersoll, C. D. (2006). Sex differences in valgus knee angle during a single-leg drop jump. *Journal of Athletic Training, 41*(2), 166-171.

[37]Hollman et al. (2009). Op. Cit.

[38]Verstegen, M., & Williams, P. (2009). *Core performance women: Burn fat and build lean muscle.* New York: Avery.

[39]Riley, L. (2008, January 18). With ACL tears, prevention is the key: Athletes must relearn how to use muscles. *Hartford Courant.* Retrieved from http://articles.courant.com/2008-01-18/features/0801180375_1_acl-tears-female-athletes-rebecca-lobo

[40]Wagner, T., Behnia, N., Ancheta, W-K. L., Shen, R., Farrokhi, S., & Powers, C. M. (2010). Strengthening and neuromuscular reeducation of the gluteus maximus in a triathlete with exercise-associated cramping of the hamstrings. *Journal of Orthopaedic and Sports Physical Therapy, 40*(2), 112-119.

[41]Ibid.

[42]Sung, P. S., Baek, J-Y., & Kim, Y. H. (2010). Reliability of the intelligent stretching device for ankle stiffness measurements in healthy individuals. *Foot, 20,* 126-132. doi: 10.1016/j.foot.2010.09.005

[43]Calais-Germain, B. (2007). Anatomy of movement (Rev. ed.). Seattle: Eastland Press.

[44]Ibid.

[45]Shen, C-L., Williams, J. S., Chyu, M-C., Paige, R. L., Stephens, A. L., Chauncey, K. B., Prabhu, F. R., Ferris, L. T., & Yeh, J. K. (2007). Comparison of the effects of tai chi and resistance training on bone metabolism in the elderly: A feasibility study. *American Journal of Chinese Medicine, 35*(3), 369-381.

[46]Seeman, E. (2009). Bone modeling and remodeling. *Critical Reviews in Eukaryotic Gene Expression, 19*(3), 219-233.

[47]Kernen, E., de Rooij, N., Huyghe, J., Smit, Th., van Duyl, W., Tanase, D., & French, P. J. (2005). Microelectrodes for measuring streaming potential in bone. *Sensors, 2005 IEEE.* doi: 10.1109/ICSENS.2005.1597823

[48]Mosekilde, L. (2000). Age-related changes in bone mass, structure, and strength--effects of loading. *Zeitschrift für Rheumatologie, 59*(Suppl. 1), 1-9.

[49]Knothe Tate, M. L. (2003). "Whither flows the fluid in bone?" An osteocyte's perspective. *Journal of Biomechanics, 36,* 1409-1424. doi: 10.1016/S0021-9290(03)00123-4

[50]Wehrli, F. W., Ladinsky, G. A., Jones, C., Benito, M., Magland, J., Vasilic, B., Popescu, A. M., Zemel, B., Cucchiara, A. J., Wright, A. C., Song, H. K., Saha, P. K., Peachey, H., & Snyder, P. J. (2008). In vivo magnetic resonance detects rapid remodeling changes in the topology of the trabecular bone network after menopause and the protective effect of estradiol. *Journal of Bone and Mineral Research, 23*(5), 730-740. doi: 10.1359/JBMR.080108

[51]Mosekilde (2000). Op. Cit.

[52]Benjamin, M., Toumi, H., Ralphs, J. R., Bydder, G., Best, T. M., & Milz, S. (2006). Where tendons and ligaments meet bone: Attachment sites ('entheses') in relation to exercise and/or mechanical load. *Journal of Anatomy, 208,* 471-490.

[53]Ibid.

[54]Ibid

[55]Józsa, L. G., & Kannus, P. (1997). Human tendons: Anatomy, physiology, and pathology. Champaign, IL: Human Kinetics

[56]Mermerci, B. B., Garip, Y., Uysal, R. S., Do_ruel, H., Karabulut, E., Ozoran, K., & Bodur, H. (2011). Clinical and ultrasound findings related to pain in patients with knee osteoarthritis. *Clinical Rheumatology, 30*(8), 1055-1062.

[57]Zhang, J., & Wang, J. H. (2010). Production of PGE(2) increases in tendons subjected to repetitive mechanical loading and induces differentiation of tendon stem cells into non-tenocytes. *Journal of Orthopaedic Research, 28*(2), 198-203.

[58]Magnusson, S. P., Hansen, M., Langberg H., Miller, B., Haraldsson, B., Westh, E. K., Koskinen, S., Aagaard, P., & Kjaer, M. (2007). The adaptability of tendon to loading differs in men and women. *International Journal of Experimental Pathology, 88*(4), 237-240.

[59]Kubo, K., Kanehisa, H., Miyatani, M., Tachi, M., & Fukunaga, T. (2003). Effect of low-load resistance training on the tendon properties in middle-aged and elderly women. *Acta Physiologica Scandinavica, 178*, 25-32.

[60]Faria, A. , Abrantes, G. R., Brás, R., & Moreira H. (2009). Triceps-surae musculotendinous stiffness: relative differences between obese and non-obese postmenopausal women. *Clinical Biomechanics, 24*(10), 866-871.

[61]Ibid.

[62]Levinger, I, Levinger, P., Trenerry, M. K., Feller, J. A., Bartlett, J. R, Bergman, N., McKenna, M. J., & Cameron-Smith, D. (2011). Increased inflammatory cytokine expression in the vastus lateralis of patients with knee osteoarthritis. *Arthritis and Rheumatism, 63*(5), 1343-1348. doi: 10.1002/art.30287

[63]Shin, H., Panton, L. B., Dutton, G. R., & Ilich, J. Z. (2011). Relationship of physical performance with body composition and bone mineral density in individuals over 60 years of age: A systematic review. *Journal of Aging Research.* Advance Online Publication. PMID: 21318048

[64]Boyer, K. A., Beaupre, G. S., & Andriacchi, T. P. (2008). Gender differences exist in the hip joint moments of healthy older walkers. *Journal of Biomechanics, 41*(16), 3360-3365.

[65]Herman, S., Kiely, D. K., Leveille, S., O'Neill, E., Cyberey, S., & Bean, J. F. (2005). Upper and lower limb muscle power relationships in mobility-limited older adults. *Journals of Gerontology (Series A - Biological Sciences and Medical Sciences) 60A*(4), 476-480

[66]Bean, J. F., Leveille, S. G., Kiely, D. K., Bandinelli, S., Guralnik, J. M., & Ferrucci, L. (2003). A comparison of leg power and leg strength within the InCHIANTI Study: Which influences mobility more? *Journals of Gerontology (Series A - Biological Sciences and Medical Sciences), 58A*(8), 728-733.

[67]Bean, J. F., Kiely, D. K., Herman, S., Leveille, S. G., Mizer, K., Frontera, W. R., & Fielding, R. A. (2002). The relationship between leg power and physical performance in mobility-limited older people. *Journal of the American Geriatrics Society, 50*(3), 461-467.

[68]Bean et al. (2003). Op. Cit.

[69]Ibid.

[70]Taunton, J. E., Martin, A. D., Rhodes, E. C., Wolski, L. A., Donelly, M., & Elliot, J. (1997). Exercise for the older woman: Choosing the right prescription. *British Journal of Sports Medicine, 31*, 5-10.

[71]Imada, K., & Katoh, H. (2010). Exercise focused on multiarticular movement to improve muscle activity during gait and single-leg standing for participants with hip osteoarthritis by using electromyogram and three-dimensional motion analysis. *Journal of Physical Therapy Science, 22*, 425-428.

[72]Nichols, N. (2008). Fitness defined: Open and closed chain exercises. Retrieved from http://www.dailyspark.com/blogs_author_view_all.asp?author=126539 (SparkPeople).

[73]Bridges, A. J., Smith, E., & Reid, J. (1992). Joint hypermobility in adults referred to rheumatology clinics. *Annals of the Rheumatic Diseases, 51*, 793-796.

[74]Liu et al. (2009). Op. Cit.

[75]Liu, C. J., & Latham, N. (2010). Adverse events reported in progressive resistance strength training trials in older adults: 2 sides of a coin. *Archives of Physical Medicine and Rehabilitation, 91*(9), 1471-1473.

[76]Thomas, K. S., Muir, K. R., Doherty, M., Jones, A. C., O'Reilly, S. C., & Bassey, E. J.; on behalf of the Community Osteoarthritis Research Group (2002). Home based exercise programme for knee pain and knee osteoarthritis: randomized controlled trial. *British Medical Journal, 325*, 752.

[77]Shakoor, N., Sengupta, M., Foucher, K. C., Wimmer, M. A., Fogg, L. F., & Block, J. A. (2010). The effects of common footwear on joint loading in osteoarthritis of the knee. *Arthritis Care & Research, 62*(7), 917-923. doi: 10.1012/acr.20165

[78]Ibid.

[79]Radzimski, A. O., Mundermann, A., & Sole, G. (2011). Effect of footwear on the external knee adduction moment - A systematic review. *Knee*. Advance Online Publication. doi: 10.1016/j.knee.2011.05.013.

[80]Maly, M. R. (2008). Abnormal and cumulative loading in knee osteoarthritis. *Current Opinion in Rheumatology, 20*(5), 547-552.

[81]Radzimski et al. (2011). Op. Cit.

[82]Shakoor et al. (2010). Op. Cit.

[83]Jansen, M. J., Viechtbauer, W., Lenssen, A. F., Hendriks, E. J.M., & de Bie, R. A. (2011). Strength training alone, exercise therapy alone, and exercise therapy with passive manual mobilization each reduce pain and disability in people with knee osteoarthritis: A systematic review. *Journal of Physiotherapy, 57*, 11-20.

[84]Rossi, M. D. (2002). Joint mobilization and manipulation. In K. Krapp (Ed.), *The Gale encyclopedia of nursing and allied health.* (Vol. 3), (pp. 1342-1344). Farmington Hills, MI: Gale Cengage Learning.

[85]Dutton, M. (2004). Orthopaedic examination, evaluation, and intervention. New York: McGraw-Hill.

[86]Thornell, L. E. (2011). Sarcopenic obesity: Satellite cells in the aging muscle. *Current Opinion in Clinical Nutrition and Metabolic Care, 14*(1), 22-27.

[87]Stratos, I., Richter, N., Rotter, R., Li, Z., Zechner, D., Mittimeier, T., & Vollmar, B. (2011). Melatonin restores muscle regeneration and enhances muscle function after crush injury in rats. *Journal of Pineal Research.* Advance online publication. doi: 10.1111/j.1600-079X.2011.00919.x

Chapter Seven

Part II: The Exercises

■

Before beginning the exercise program, be sure to consult with your medical doctor or physician as to whether the exercises are appropriate for you. Start out slowly, and never overstress or overwork your body. Do not do any exercise if it causes pain. There is a difference between the discomfort of exercising an underused muscle and the pain that may be caused by straining or overtaxing a muscle or tendon; the latter may result in muscle tears, or tendon and ligament injuries. These exercises should be done in comfortable, flexible shoes, or barefoot if comfortable for you on a soft carpet or rug (be sure that the rug is in a fixed position and will not slide around).

Exercise #1: Toe Raise

Place your hands on the door frame to steady yourself.

Stand with your feet just a little less than shoulder-width apart and concentrate on using your calf muscles to raise your heels slowly from the ground until you are on tiptoe. Muscles in the whole kinetic chain will be activated.

Once done, slowly descend until your feet come to rest on the ground. Repeat this exercise for another repetition (start with three repetitions, and slowly increase the number of repetitions).

As you perform the Toe Raise Exercise, focus your attention on strengthening your calf muscles and Achilles' tendons, and on the flexing of the ankles and toes. This exercise will affect the muscle-tendon-bone units of the entire leg with emphasis on the lower leg, feet, and toes.

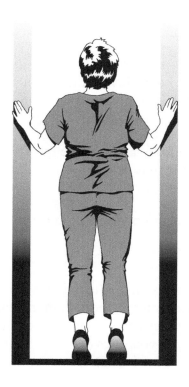

Exercise Tips and Check Points
for Exercise #1: Toe Raise

Be sure to stand upright in a relaxed posture.

Place your hands on the door frame lightly for balance, and do not push or pull on the door frame.

As you raise your body slowly, think of it moving straight upwards as a total unit.

As you lower your body slowly, think of it moving straight downwards as a total unit to the floor.

Be aware of the muscle-tendon-bone units of both of your whole legs (and the kinetic muscle chains).

Be aware of and focus on your calf muscles and Achilles tendons getting stronger.

Be aware of and focus on the flexing of your ankles and toes. This exercise is extremely important in increasing dorsiflexion strength of the muscles and tendons that connect your foot (metatarsal bones) to your toes (e.g., the big toe joint being the first and largest of these joints).

Repeat this exercise several times; however, be sure you do not overdo the repetitions. Begin with about three until you feel yourself getting stronger.

Exercise #2: Point Toe Lift

Place your hands on the door frame to steady yourself.

Stand with your feet about shoulder-width apart, and slightly shift your weight to one leg for support. For the other leg, use your buttocks (gluteus) and back muscles, and slowly lift your leg (with your toe pointed in the direction of the lift) to a comfortable height.

Once done, slowly bring your leg back to floor position, and repeat this for another repetition (start with three repetitions and slowly increase the number of repetitions). Repeat with each leg.

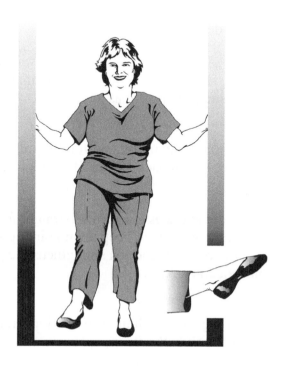

As you perform the Point Toe Lift Exercise, focus your attention on the strengthening of your upper thigh muscles, in particular the muscle in the front and back parts of your thigh along with those of the hip. This exercise will work the muscle-tendon-bone units (and kinetic muscle chains) pertaining to the entire leg with emphasis on the upper leg, groin, hip, and buttocks components.

Exercise Tips and Check Points
for Exercise #2: Point Toe Lift

Be sure to stand upright in a relaxed posture.

Place your hands on the door frame lightly for balance, and do not push or pull on the door frame.

As you lift your leg slowly, keep your leg straight and relax, and think of it moving straight upward as a total unit.

Try to keep your entire body upright as you lift your leg (and try not to bend forward or lean back as you lift and lower your leg).

Be sure that your foot and toes are pointed straight forward (see insert above) using your ankle to keep them pointing straight forward. This foot and ankle motion strengthens the plantar flexion of your foot and ankles.

As you lower your leg slowly, think of it moving straight downward as a total unit to the floor.

Lift and lower your leg up and down with emphasis on the muscle groups of the upper leg, groin, hip, and buttocks.

Lift your leg to a comfortable height. As you continue to practice this exercise, over time you may gradually be able to lift your leg higher.

Be aware of the muscle-tendon-bone units of both your supporting leg and your lifting leg. Also, think of the kinetic chains of muscles all working together.

Be aware of and focus on your upper thigh muscles, in particular the muscles in the front and back parts of your thigh along with those of the hip. Also notice that you are working the muscles along the shinbone.

Be aware of and focus on the lifting and lowering of your leg *slowly*; *do not swing your leg up and down – deliberately lift and lower it slowly* using your muscle groups.

Repeat this exercise several times; however, be sure you do not overdo the repetitions. Begin with about three until you feel yourself becoming stronger.

Exercise #3: Heel Lift

Place your hands on the door frame to steady yourself.

Stand with your feet about shoulder-width apart, and extend one leg slightly forward resting the foot on the heel of your extended leg. Bend your ankle and curl your toes back toward yourself (which will tighten the muscles in the front of your leg – see insert below). This locks in the ankle for the rest of the lift.

Shift your weight slightly to your supporting leg. Use your buttocks (gluteus maximus), back muscles, and front thigh muscles (quadriceps) and slowly lift your leg (with your heel extended and your toes curled toward yourself. Focus on lifting your leg from the heel to a comfortable height.

Once done, slowly bring your leg back to floor position with foot resting on your heel, and repeat this for another repetition (start with three repetitions and slowly increase the number of repetitions). Repeat on the opposite leg.

As you perform the Heel Lift Exercise, focus your attention on the stretching of your back thigh muscles, in particular the muscles in the back parts of your thigh along with the tendon unit behind the knee.

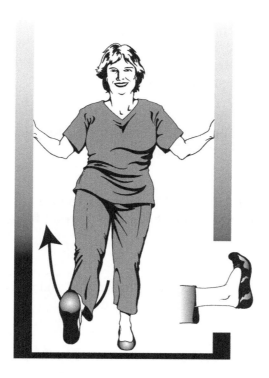

This exercise will affect the muscle-tendon-bone units of the entire leg with emphasis on the upper leg (in particular the hamstrings), hip, groin, and buttocks.

Incidentally, by flexing your ankles and curling the toes back, you will contract the front thigh and lower leg muscle groups and therefore allow for a fuller stretch in the back parts of your leg. You will also be developing the dorsiflexion strength of your ankles and foot.

Exercise Tips and Check Points
for Exercise #3: Heel Lift

Be sure to stand upright in a relaxed posture.

Place your hands on the door frame lightly for balance, and do not push or pull on the door frame.

Try to keep your entire body upright as you lift your leg (and try not to bend forward or lean backward as you lift and lower your leg).

As you lift your leg, keep your leg straight and relax, and think of it moving straight upward as a total unit.

Be sure that your foot and toes are curled back toward yourself (see insert above) using your ankle (and surrounding muscles) to keep them curled toward yourself.

As you lower your leg, think of it moving straight downward as a total unit to the floor coming to a rest on your heel.

Lift your leg from the heel (with your toes curled toward yourself) to a comfortable height. As you continue to practice this exercise, over time you may gradually be lifting your leg higher.

Lift and lower your leg up and down with emphasis on the muscle groups of the upper leg, groin, hip, and buttocks.

Be aware of the muscle-tendon-bone units of both your supporting leg *and* your lifting leg. Also, feel the kinetic chains of muscles working together.

Focus on flexing your ankles and curling the toes back, so that you will contract the front thigh and lower leg muscle groups (and therefore allow for a fuller stretch in the back parts of your leg).

Be aware of and focus on your back thigh muscles (your hamstrings) along with those of the hip.

Be aware and focus on the lifting and lowering of your leg; *do not swing your leg up and down – deliberately lift and lower it* using your muscle groups.

Repeat this exercise several times; however, be sure that you do not overdo the repetitions. Begin with about three until you feel yourself becoming stronger. Repeat with the other leg.

Exercise #4: Rear Lift

Place your hands on the door frame to steady yourself.

Stand with your feet just a little less than shoulder-width apart, and shift your weight to one supporting leg. For the other leg, use your buttocks (gluteus), front-upper leg, and back muscles, and slowly lift your leg to the rear (focusing on lifting the leg from the heel) to a comfortable height. Be sure that when you lift your leg from the heel that your toes are curled toward yourself. Keep the toe pointed toward the ground so that you do not swing the foot sideways.

Once done, slowly bring your leg back to floor position, and repeat the entire sequence again (start with three repetitions and slowly increase the number of repetitions).

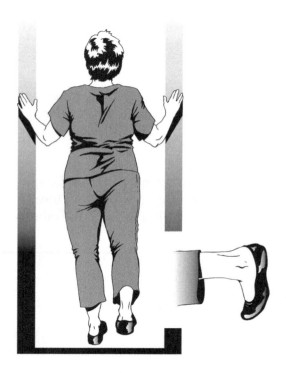

As you perform the Rear Lift Exercise, focus your attention on the strong activation of your buttocks (gluteus) muscles and the stretching of your back thigh (hamstrings) muscles along with the muscle-tendon unit behind the knee.

This exercise will affect the muscle-tendon-bone units of the entire leg with emphasis on the upper back, buttocks, hip, groin, thighs and lower legs.

Incidentally, by curling the toes back toward yourself, you will contract the front thigh and lower leg muscle groups and therefore allow for a fuller stretch in the back parts of your leg.

Exercise Tips and Check Points

for Exercise #4: Rear Lift

Be sure to stand upright in a relaxed posture.

Place your hands on the door frame lightly for balance, and do not push or pull on the door frame

Try to keep your entire body upright as you lift your leg (and try not to bend forward or lean back as you lift and lower your leg).

As you lift your leg to the rear, keep your leg straight and relax, and think of it moving straight upward as a total unit. The natural tendency is for the foot to shift outwards. Instead, keep your foot vertically aligned to the floor. This will allow you to fully use and work your buttocks muscle and its muscle chain.

Be sure that your foot and toes are curled back toward yourself (see insert above) using your ankle and surrounding muscles to keep them curled toward yourself.

As you lower your leg, think of it moving straight downward as a total unit to the floor.

Lift your leg from the heel (with your toes curled toward yourself) to a comfortable height. As you continue to practice this this exercise, over time you may gradually be lifting your leg higher.

Lift and lower your leg up and down with emphasis on the muscle groups of the upper back, buttocks, hip, upper leg, and groin.

Be aware of the muscle-tendon-bone units of *both* your supporting leg and your lifting leg. Also, feel the kinetic chains of muscles working together.

Focus on flexing your ankles and curling the toes toward yourself, so that you will contract the front thigh and lower leg muscle groups (and therefore allow for a fuller stretch in the back parts of your leg).

Be aware of and focus on your back thigh muscles, in particular the muscles in the back parts of your thigh along with those of the hip and buttocks.

Be aware of and focus on the lifting and lowering of your leg; *do not swing your leg up and down – deliberately lift and lower it* using your muscle groups.

Repeat this exercise several times; however, be sure that you do not overdo the repetitions. Begin with about three until you feel yourself becoming stronger. Repeat with the other leg.

Exercise #5: Sideways Lift – Toes Pointed Toward the Lift

Face one side of the frame, and place your two hands on one side of the door frame to steady yourself.

Stand with your feet about shoulder-width apart with your shoulders facing the door frame and your feet pointed in the direction of the door frame.

Slightly shift your weight to one leg, and for the other leg, turn one foot so that it is pointing away from the door frame. For the leg with the foot pointed away from the door frame, use your back, buttocks, hip and upper leg muscles to slowly lift your leg (with your toe pointed in the direction of the lift) to a comfortable height. You will be activating your hip and inner thigh muscles and muscles involving hip rotation.

Once done, slowly bring your leg back to floor position, and repeat this for another whole sequence (start with three repetitions and slowly increase the number of repetitions). Repeat with the other leg.

As you perform the Sideways Lift – Toes Pointed Exercise, focus your attention on the strengthening of your upper thigh muscles, in particular the muscles in the inner and outer parts of your thigh along with those of the groin and hip.

This exercise will affect the muscle-tendon-bone units (and kinetic muscle chains) pertaining to the entire leg with emphasis on the inner and outer thigh, hip, groin, and buttocks components.

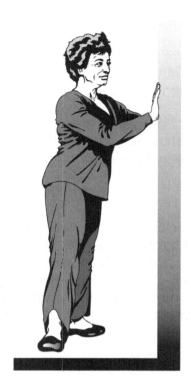

Incidentally, by pointing your toes, you will contract the front thigh and lower leg calf muscle groups and therefore allow for a fuller stretch in the inner and outer thigh parts of your leg.

Exercise Tips and Check Points

for Exercise #5: Sideways Lift – Toes Pointed Toward the Lift

Be sure to stand upright in a relaxed posture.

Place both of your hands on one side of the door frame lightly for balance, and do not push or pull on the door frame.

Try to keep your entire body upright as you lift your leg (and try not to bend sideways or lean back as you lift and lower your leg).

As you lift your leg slowly, keep your leg straight and relax, and think of it moving straight upwards as a total unit.

Be sure that your foot and toes are pointed in the direction of your lift using your ankle to keep them pointed toward your lift.

As you lower your leg slowly, think of it moving straight downward as a total unit to the floor coming to a rest on the ground.

Lift your leg from the top part of the foot (with your toes pointed in the direction of the lift) slowly coming to a comfortable height. As you continue to practice this exercise, over time you may gradually be lifting your leg higher.

Lift and lower your leg up and down with emphasis on the muscle groups of the upper leg, groin, hip, and buttocks.

Be aware of the muscle-tendon-bone units of *both* your supporting leg and your lifting leg.

Focus on flexing your ankles downward and pointing your toes, so that you will contract the front thigh and lower leg calf muscle groups (and therefore allow for a fuller stretch in the inner and outer thigh parts of your leg).

Be aware of and focus on your inner and outer thigh muscles, in particular the muscles in the side and back parts of your thigh and the side of your hip along with those of the groin.

Be aware of and focus on the lifting and lowering of your leg; *do not swing your leg up and down – deliberately lift and lower it* using your muscle groups.

Repeat this exercise several times slowly; however, be sure that you do not overdo the repetitions. Begin with about three until you feel yourself becoming stronger. Repeat with the other leg.

Exercise #6: Sideways Lift – Toes Pointed Toward the Frame

Face one side of the door frame, and place your two hands on one side of the door frame to steady yourself.

Stand with your feet about shoulder-width apart with your shoulders facing the door frame and your feet pointed in the direction of the door frame.

Slightly shift your weight to one leg, and with the other leg, turn one foot at the ankle so that the foot stays pointed at the door frame. To raise the leg use your back, hip, side leg and buttocks muscles to slowly lift your leg (from the heel with your toe pointed in the direction of the door frame) to a comfortable height.

Once done, slowly bring your leg back to floor position, and repeat this whole sequence again (start with three repetitions and slowly increase the number of repetitions). Repeat with the other leg.

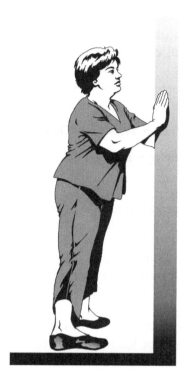

As you perform the Sideways Lift – Toes Pointed Toward the Frame Exercise, focus your attention on the strengthening of your upper thigh, hip and side leg muscles, in particular the muscles in the inner and outer parts of your thigh along with those of the groin and hip. Focus on activating the muscles at the side of your hip and your buttock muscles.

This exercise will affect the muscle-tendon-bone units of the entire leg (and kinetic muscle chains involved in leg movement) with emphasis on stretching the inner thigh, groin, and buttocks components, along with building strong hip muscles.

Incidentally, by pointing your toes toward the door frame, you will contract the front thigh and lower leg calf muscle groups and therefore allow for a fuller stretch in the inner thigh and groin areas.

Exercise Tips and Check Points

for Exercise #6: Sideways Lift – Toes Pointed Toward the Frame

Be sure to stand upright in a relaxed posture.

Place both of your hands on one side of the door frame lightly for balance, and do not push or pull on the door frame.

Try to keep your entire body upright as you lift your leg (and try not to bend sideways or lean back as you lift and lower your leg).

As you lift your leg, keep your leg straight and relax, and think of it moving straight upward as a total unit.

Be sure that your foot and toes are pointed in the direction of the door frame using your ankle (and surrounding muscles) to keep them pointed toward the frame.

As you lower your leg, think of it moving straight downward as a total unit to the floor coming to a rest on the ground.

Lift your leg from the heel of the foot (with your toes pointed in the direction of the frame) to a comfortable height. As you continue to practice this exercise, over time you may gradually be lifting your leg higher.

Lift and lower your leg up and down with emphasis on the muscle groups of the inner thigh, groin, hip, and buttocks.

Be aware of the muscle-tendon-bone units of *both* your supporting leg and your lifting leg.

Be aware of and focus on your inner and outer thigh muscles and groin. Also focus on the muscles at the side of your body to include your hip and side of your thigh.

Be aware of and focus on the lifting and lowering of your leg; *do not swing your leg up and down – deliberately lift and lower it* using your muscle groups.

Repeat this exercise several times; however, be sure that you do not overdo the repetitions. Begin with about three until you feel yourself stronger. Repeat with the other leg.

Exercise #7: Back Leg Push

Place your hands on the door frame to steady yourself.

Stand in a lunge position with one leg in front and the back leg straight (with foot pointed forward and not to the side) and ready to push with your back leg. For the front leg, bend at the knee so that it is over the toes.

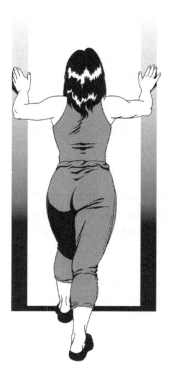

Slowly push yourself forward using the back leg's buttock and leg muscles as you steady yourself with resistance from both arms against the door frame for a count of three. This exercise is very different from a traditional one-leg lunge (or one-leg push), in which the knee is often stressed. By resting your hands on the door frame, you take pressure off of the knee and emphasize strengthening of the hamstrings and the buttocks. You are also working the muscles and tendons around your ankles, as well.

Once done, bring the other leg forward to the same lunge position, and repeat this whole sequence again (start with three repetitions for each leg in the back position, and slowly increase the number of repetitions).

As you perform the Back Leg Push Exercise, focus your attention on the strengthening of your buttocks, upper thighs, calf muscles and Achilles tendons for the back leg, and on the front thigh and calf muscles of the front leg. This exercise will affect the muscle-tendon-bone units of the entire leg (and kinetic muscle chains involved in leg movement) with emphasis on the upper leg, calf, and buttocks components. It is also excellent for strengthening the Achilles tendons.

Exercise Tips and Check Points
for Exercise #7: Back Leg Push

Be sure to stand upright in a relaxed lunge posture.

Place your hands on the door frame lightly for balance, and use the door frame for resistance when you are pushing with your legs.

As you push with your back leg, think of your entire body moving forward as a total unit.

Keep your upper body upright as you push forward; do not lean forward or backward.

Be aware of the muscle-tendon-bone units of both of your entire legs.

Be aware of and focus on your buttocks, upper leg, calf muscles and Achilles tendons getting stronger, as well as the muscle-tendon units that you are working.

Be aware of and focus on the flexing of your ankles and feet as you push forward.

Repeat this exercise several times; however, be sure that you do not overdo the repetitions. Begin with about three until you feel yourself getting stronger. Repeat with the other leg.

Exercise #8: Body Lowering

Stand with your feet about shoulder-width apart, and raise your arms to shoulder height with your palms downward.

With both feet flat on the floor and your posture remaining upright, slowly lower yourself about three to four inches; *however, only go down as many inches as is comfortable for you.* At first, you may not be able to go down this far, but can work toward it as a practice goal to achieve over time. Use your buttocks and leg muscles, and hold the pose for about five seconds.

Be sure that you stay relaxed and maintain an upright posture.

Once done, slowly bring yourself up to the standing position, bringing your arms to your side. Do the above sequences for another repetition (start with three repetitions, and slowly increase the number of repetitions).

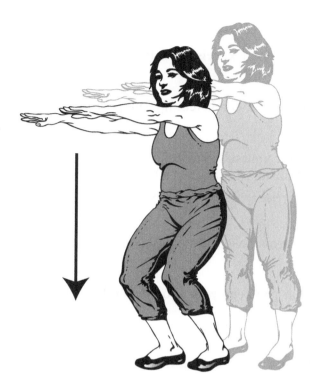

As you perform the Body Lowering Exercise, focus your attention on the strengthening of your front thighs, lower leg and calf muscles, and Achilles tendons. This exercise will strengthen the muscle-tendon-bone units of both of your entire legs. It will also develop the muscles and tendons that surround and support your knee and ankle joints.

Exercise Tips and Check Points
for Exercise #8: Body Lowering

Be sure to stand in a relaxed, upright posture.

As you lower yourself, stay relaxed and be sure that you maintain an upright posture (imagine a string attached to the top of your head, and you are lowered by the string).

Keep your arms raised and parallel to the floor.

Be sure that you keep your shoulders relaxed and down (not popped up or raised).

Keep your upper body upright as you lower yourself; do not lean forward or backward.

Be aware of the muscle-tendon-bone units of both of your entire legs.

Be aware of and focus on your front thigh muscles, calf muscles and Achilles' tendons getting stronger.

Be aware of and focus on the stability of your ankles and feet as you lower yourself.

Repeat this exercise several times; however, be sure that you do not overdo the repetitions. Begin with about three until you feel yourself becoming stronger.

Exercise #9: Shoulders Down

Stand with your feet about shoulder-width apart, and move your arms (at the shoulders) away from your legs to the side so that your palms are about 6 inches from your legs with your palms facing your legs.

With both feet flat on the floor and your posture remaining upright, inhale as you slowly pull down on both shoulders (using the muscles in your upper back), and exhale as you let the feeling of the forces extend out of your fingertips.   Hold this pose for about five seconds. *Do not use the top of your shoulders to pull down.* Rather, *use your upper back muscles* which are the largest muscles in your back.

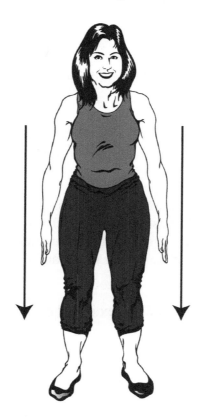

Be sure that you stay relaxed and maintain an upright posture.

Once done, slowly relax your shoulders in the standing position (breathing comfortably), and bringing your arms comfortably to your side. Repeat the above sequences for another repetition (start with three repetitions, and slowly increase the number of repetitions).

As you perform the Shoulders Down Exercise, focus your attention on the strengthening of your shoulders, arms, upper chest, and upper and middle back (particularly the upper back muscles). This exercise will affect the muscle-tendon-and-bone units of the entire chest and shoulder/arm areas with emphasis on the shoulder, upper and middle back, and upper and lower arm components.

Exercise Tips and Check Points
for Exercise #9: Shoulders Down

Be sure to stand in a relaxed, upright posture.

As you lower your shoulders, stay relaxed and be sure that you maintain an upright posture. As you activate your upper back muscles, imagine that your shoulders are being pulled down from under your arms and from your upper and middle back.

Keep your arms lowered and extended out to your side about six inches from your legs.

Be sure that you keep your shoulders relaxed and down (not popped up or raised).

Keep your upper body upright as you lower your shoulders; do not lean forward or backward.

Be aware of the muscle-tendon-bone-units of your entire upper body. Feel the kinetic muscle chains working to keep your entire shoulder/chest area held together as a whole unit.

Be aware of and focus on your shoulder, upper arm, upper and middle back, and lower arm muscles and tendons getting stronger.

Be aware of and focus on the lowering of your shoulders as you feel yourself more centered and stronger in your entire body from the top of your head to the soles of your feet. This exercise helps you to feel the integrity of your whole body. As you extend a feeling of force downwards from your fingertips (using the power of your upper back muscles) the connection between your upper and lower body is reinforced. This feeling of body integrity will help you in keeping your balance as you perform tasks such as ascending and descending the stairs.

Repeat this exercise several times; however, be sure that you do not overdo the repetitions. Begin with about three until you feel yourself becoming stronger.

Exercise #10: Circle Hips

Stand with your feet about shoulder-width apart, and place your palms to each side of your legs (slightly below your hips) with your palms touching your legs.

Both feet should be flat on the floor, and keep your posture upright and relax. Your legs should be relaxed and straight (do not bend at the knee).

Using your hand at the upper thigh to push one side of your hip, and then the other, rotate your hips in a clockwise fashion for five rotations. The circles that you are making with your hips should not be wide circles, but rather, they should be more egg-shaped or "elliptical" (as if the egg's top and bottom were on each side of your hips).

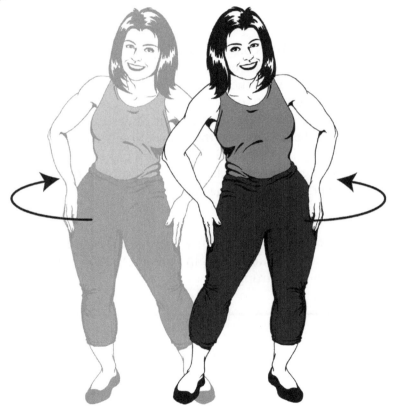

Once done, keep your hands on your legs, take a deep breath and relax while standing upright. Now repeat the above sequence of five rotations going in a counter-clockwise fashion.

Start with two sequences of five rotations clockwise and two sequences of five rotations counterclockwise; slowly increase the number of repetitions of these sequences.

As you perform the Circle Hips Exercise, focus your attention on the stretching of your inner and outer thigh muscles, in particular the muscles in the groin area (such as gracilis and sartorius). Focus also on your activated hip muscles and muscles at your waist. Also notice that the muscle-tendon units of the lower legs, ankles, and feet are being strengthened, as well. In these rotations, feel the support of your ankles in lending stability to your movements.

This exercise will strengthen the muscle-tendon-bone units of the entire leg (and kinetic muscle chains involved in leg movement) with emphasis on the inner and outer thigh, hip, groin, waist, buttocks, and lower leg components. Notice especially how you are activating the muscle chains at the side of your hips as you do the rotations.

Incidentally, by circling from your hips, you will strengthen your thigh and lower leg muscle groups and therefore allow for fuller flexibility in your ankles and feet in your movements.

Exercise Tips and Check Points
for Exercise #10: Circle Hips

Be sure to stand upright in a relaxed posture and with your legs relaxed and straight (but not stiff).

Place the palms to each side of your legs (slightly below your hips) with your palms touching your legs. Use your palms to slightly push your legs in the "elliptical" directions of your rotations.

Try to keep your entire body relaxed and upright as you circle your hips (and try not to bend forward or lean back as you rotate your hips).

As you rotate your hips, think of your body moving as a total unit with the top of your head and soles of your feet relatively stable.

Use your palm at your upper thigh to push one side of your hip, and then the other to accentuate the rotation of your hips in a clockwise (and then in a counter-clockwise) fashion.

Be sure that the circles that you are making with your hips are not "round" circles, but rather, they should be more egg-shaped or "elliptical" (as if the egg's top and bottom were on each side of your hips).

Focus your awareness on the stretching of your inner and outer thigh muscles, in particular the muscles in the groin areas. Two of these muscles (sartorius and gracilis) have tendons that end in the pes anserinus. Ensuring that these muscles are healthy and strong should help to avoid problems such as pes anserine bursitis.

Focus also on your activated hip muscles. These hip flexor muscles may take time to strengthen. These are critical muscles that are needed for you to lift your knees and assist you in performing tasks such as stair climbing.

Be aware of the muscle-tendon-bone units of *both* of your supporting legs, and feel the support of your ankles in lending stability to your movements.

Notice that you are activating the muscle chains at each side of your hips as you do the rotations.

Be aware of and focus on the muscle-tendon-bone units of both of your entire legs (along with the kinetic muscle chains used for leg movement) with emphasis on the inner and outer thigh, hip, groin, waist, buttocks, and lower leg components.

Begin doing this exercise with two sequences of five clockwise rotations and two sequences of five counter-clockwise rotations; however, be sure not to overdo the repetitions until you feel yourself becoming stronger.

Exercise #11: Shoulder Turns

Stand with your feet about shoulder-width apart, and bring your bent arms with palms down to a shoulder height position.

With both feet flat on the floor and your posture remaining upright, slightly lower your body and tuck in your buttocks, and hold it tucked in this isometric stance. Grip the floor with both of your feet by pushing your heels in without actually moving them, and lower your body slightly.

Be sure that you stay relaxed and maintain your upright posture, with your knees slightly bent. Be sure to grip the floor with your feet so that your legs are not moving, only your waist and hips. **V e r y Important**: *Do not move your knees*; this could strain your knees.

You should not be moving your legs and knees; rather, the movement should all be centered in your upper body (while maintaining the isometric contractions in your lower body).

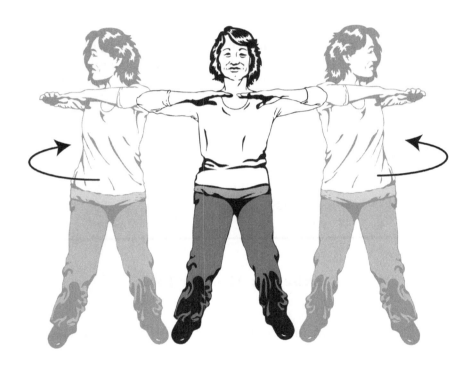

Turn your shoulders to one side, then slowly bring yourself back to the beginning position, then do the same movement to the opposite side. Do three full sequences of shoulder turns (left and right), and slowly increase the number of repetitions.

As you perform the Shoulder Turns Exercise, focus your attention on the strengthening of your waist and hip muscle chains. From the slightly lowered position (with your feet pulled in*) you will be strengthening your front thighs, lower leg and calf muscles, and

Achilles tendons of both legs. This exercise will affect the muscle-tendon-and-bone units of your waist and hips and the two legs with emphasis on the upper leg and lower leg components.

*Your heels should be *pulled in without moving them,* as if you were attempting to click your heels without actually having them move. Be sure to maintain this isometric pull in your heels throughout the full sequence of the exercise.

Exercise Tips and Check Points
for Exercise #11: Shoulder Turns

Be sure to stand upright in a relaxed posture.

As you tuck your buttocks in and slightly lower yourself, be sure to maintain an upright posture (imagine a string attached to the top of your head, and you are lowered by the string as you tuck your buttocks in).

Grip the floor with both of your feet by bringing your heels in (as decribed above, and lower your body slightly). By gripping the floor with both of your feet, you should immobilize the movement of your legs as you turn from side-to-side. This allows you to fully exercise the kinetic muscle chains of your upper torso (and to prevent straining your knees).

Keep your arms raised with your palms parallel to the ground.

Keep your upper body upright as you turn side-to-side; do not lean forward or backward.

As you turn from side-to-side, think of your body moving as a total unit with the top of your head and soles of your feet relatively stable.

Focus your awareness on the strengthening of your waist and hip muscles via the isometric tension and the exercising of the muscles in the groin and waist areas along with the muscle-tendon units of the upper legs and buttocks.

Be aware of the muscle-tendon-bone units of both of your supporting legs in these isometric positions, and feel the support of your ankles in lending stability to your upper-body movements.

Notice that you are activating the muscle chains at your waist, shoulders, and upper and lower back as you turn from side-to-side.

Each side of your hips, upper and lower legs, feet and buttocks are activated in the isometric contractions that you are maintaining throughout the sequence.

Repeat this exercise several times to each side, but be sure you do not overdo the repetitions. Do three in each direction until you feel yourself becoming stronger.

Exercise #12: Shoulder Pulling

Stand with your feet about shoulder-width apart, and grasp with both of your hands your own forearms in front of your chest.

With both feet flat on the floor and your posture remaining upright, slowly pull your own arm in one direction until the elbow of the pulled arm is in front of your chest (providing moderate resistance with your non-pulling arm).

Be sure that you stay relaxed and maintain an upright posture.

Repeat the above sequence for another repetition in the opposite direction (providing moderate resistance with your non-pulling arm).

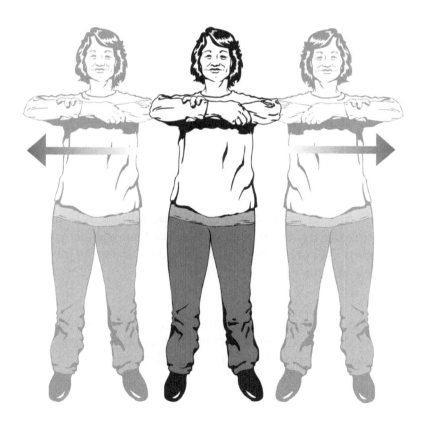

Start with three repetitions (of side to side), and slowly increase the number of repetitions.

As you perform the Shoulder Pulling Exercise, focus your attention on the strengthening of your shoulders and upper arm and lower arm muscles. This exercise will affect the muscle-tendon-bone units of the entire arms and shoulders with emphasis on the upper arm and shoulder components along with the upper back muscles on each side.

Exercise Tips and Check Points
for Exercise #12: Shoulder Pulling

Be sure to stand upright in a relaxed posture and with your legs relaxed and straight (but not stiff).

Grasp with both of your hands your own forearms in front of your chest; try to grasp your forearms as close to your own wrists as possible.

Keep your arms raised and parallel to the floor.

Try to keep your entire body relaxed and upright as you pull on each arm (and try not to bend forward or lean back as you pull on your arm). Be sure to have your shoulders and arms move, and do not move at your waist.

Be sure to pull your own arm in one direction slowly until the elbow of the pulled arm is in front of your chest (providing moderate resistance with your non-pulling arm).

Remember to give yourself resistance against the pulling arm.

As you pull your arms from one side to the other, think of your shoulders, arms and body as moving as a total unit with the top of your head and soles of your feet relatively stable.

Focus your awareness on the stretching and strengthening of your shoulders, arms, upper back and muscles under your arm. Pay

particular attention to the muscle-tendon units of the shoulders and upper arms.

Be sure to feel the support of your waist and legs as you do this exercise.

Notice that you are activating the muscle chains at your shoulders, arms, and upper back as you pull each arm from one side to the other.

Repeat this exercise several times to each side, but be sure you do not overdo the repetitions. Begin with about three until you feel yourself becoming stronger.

Exercise #13: Shoulder Pushing

Stand with your feet about shoulder-width apart, and place one palm against the other with the forearms in front of your chest.

With both feet flat on the floor and your posture remaining upright, put your palms together in front of your chest with your arms still parallel to the ground. Slowly push with one of your palms until the pushing arm's elbow is in front of your chest (providing moderate resistance with your non-pushing arm).

Be sure that you stay relaxed and maintain an upright posture and that you keep your shoulders down (not raised up).

Repeat the above sequences for another repetition in the opposite direction (providing moderate resistance with your non-pushing arm).

Start with three repetitions (side to side), and slowly increase the number of repetitions.

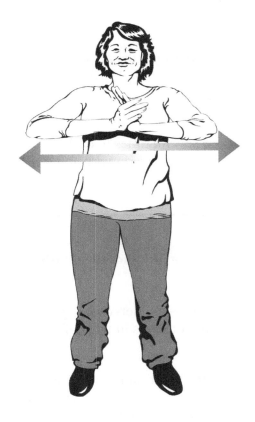

As you perform the Shoulder Pushing Exercise, focus your attention on the strengthening of your shoulders, chest, and upper and lower arm muscles. This exercise will strengthen the muscle-tendon-bone units of the entire arms and shoulders with emphasis on the upper arm and shoulder components along with the muscles on each side of the chest.

Exercise Tips and Check Points

for Exercise #13: Shoulder Pushing

Be sure to stand upright in a relaxed posture and with your legs relaxed and straight (but not stiff).

Push with the palms of your hands with your own forearms in front of your chest.

Keep your arms raised and parallel to the floor, and be sure to keep your *shoulders down* (not raised up) when you move from side-to-side.

Try to keep your entire body relaxed and upright as you push on each arm (and try not to bend forward or lean back as you push on your arm). Be sure to have your shoulders and arms move, and not your waist.

Be sure to push your own arm in one direction slowly until the elbow of the pushing arm is in front of your chest.

Remember to give yourself resistance against the pushing arm.

As you push your arms from one side to the other, think of your chest, shoulders, and arms moving as a total unit with the top of your head and soles of your feet relatively stable.

Focus your awareness on the stretching and strengthening of your shoulder, arm, and chest muscles, in particular the muscle-tendon units of the shoulders and upper arms.

Be sure to feel the support of your waist and legs as you do this exercise.

Notice that you are activating the muscle chains at your shoulders, arms, and chest, as you push your arms from one side to the other.

Repeat this exercise several times to each side, and be sure that you do not overdo the repetitions. Begin with about three until you feel yourself becoming stronger.

Exercise #14: Shoulder Pushing (Variation)

Stand shoulder-width apart in the door frame.

Let your arms hang down, and place the palms of each hand against the door frame so that you can push against it using the muscles of your chest, shoulders, arms, and palms.

Stand with both feet flat on the floor, and be sure to keep your posture remaining upright.

Slowly push using both palms against the door frame for a count of five. Once done, relax your arms to your side.

Repeat this entire sequence again (start with three repetitions, and slowly increase the number of repetitions).

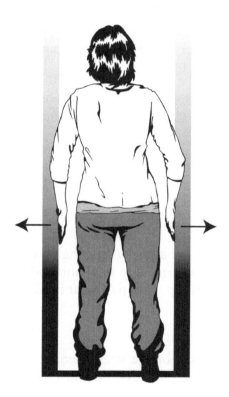

As you perform the Shoulder Pushing Variation Exercise, focus your attention on the strengthening of your shoulder, chest, and upper and lower arm muscles. This exercise will strengthen the muscle-tendon-bone units of the entire arm and shoulder area with emphasis on the upper arm and shoulder components along with the muscles on each side of the chest.

Exercise Tips and Check Points
for Exercise #14: Shoulder Pushing (Variation)

Be sure to stand upright in a relaxed posture and with your legs relaxed and straight (but not stiff) inside the door frame.

Be sure to let your arms hang down, and place the palms of each hand against the door frame so that you can push against it.

Use the door frame for resistance when you are pushing with the muscles of your chest, shoulders, arms, and palms.

Try to keep your entire body relaxed and upright as you push with both arms (and try not to bend forward or lean back as you push with your arms).

As you push with your arms against the door frame, think of your chest, shoulders, and arms as a total unit and connected with your body as a whole. Keep the top of your head and soles of your feet relatively stable.

Focus your awareness on the strengthening of your shoulder, arm, and chest muscles, in particular the muscle-tendon-bone units of the shoulders and upper arms.

Be sure to feel the support of your waist and legs as you do this exercise.

Notice that you are activating the muscle chains at your shoulders, arms, and chest, as you push your arms against the door frame.

Repeat this exercise several times; however, be sure that you do not overdo the repetitions. Begin with about three until you feel yourself becoming stronger.

Exercise #15: Stepping and Holding Your Ground

Stand with your feet about shoulder-width apart, and step forward with your left leg so that the heel "holds" the ground (See Segment A of the Illustration for "Stepping and Holding Your Ground that follows). This "hold" position is a steady "gripping" of the ground with your heel. *You are pulling the heel backwards although you do not actually move or reposition your heel during the pulling action.* When you do this, begin to move your left foot forward shifting the weight off of the right leg without taking it off the ground, and pull your body forward by placing the toes of your left foot down.

 You will transfer your weight to your entire foot after putting your toes down, and then pivoting the toes forward to begin the "holding or grabbing" of the ground (See Segment B of the Illustration). "Grip" the ground with your entire left foot as if you were pulling yourself forward with the left foot. Be sure that the toes of the stepping foot are pointing straight ahead.

This heel-toe movement is very important, and it is very important to keep the toes of the front foot pointed straight ahead at the conclusion of the heel-toe step.

You then simultaneously (1) "grab" the ground with your left toes and entire left foot and pull into the center of your body and (2) "grab" the ground with your right toes and entire right foot and pull into the center of your body, and hold this for a count of five.   In this movement, you are "Holding Your Ground" (See Segment B of the

Illustration - the arrows indicate the direction that you should be "pulling" with each foot *without actually moving the feet*).

Because this "gripping" of the ground is a key component of this exercise, it would actually be optimal to do this exercise in your bare feet on a soft carpet or rug (that is in a fixed position and will not slide around).   In this way, the muscles, tendons and joints within your foot can be tightened or contracted without the physical restrictions of a shoe.

In doing this exercise, you will increase the tone and strength of the muscles surrounding your knees and ankles. It will also strengthen the muscles in your feet. This exercise will help foster stability and counter joint laxity.

Be sure that you stay relaxed and maintain an upright posture.

Once done, you then relax and pivot your left foot at the heel moving your left toes outward two inches (See Segment C of the Illustration as follows).   This puts you into position to then step forward with your right foot.

You step forward with your right leg so that the right heel "holds" the ground (See Segment D of the Illustration for "Stepping and Holding Your Ground that follows). This "hold" position is a steady "gripping" of the ground with your heel. *You are pulling the heel backwards although you do not actually move or reposition your heel during the pulling action.* When you do this, begin to move your right foot forward shifting the weight off of the left leg without taking it off the ground, and pull your body forward by placing the toes of your right foot down (See Segment E of the Illustration as follows).

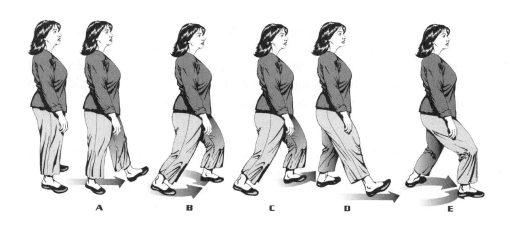

Remember, pull yourself forward with your entire right foot.

This heel-toe movement is very important, and it is very important to keep the toe of the front foot pointed straight ahead at the conclusion of the heel-toe step.

You then simultaneously (1) "grab" the ground with your right toes and entire right foot and pull into the center of your body and (2) "grab" the ground with your left toes and entire left foot and pull into the center of your body, and hold this for a count of five. In this movement, you are "Holding Your Ground" (See Segment E of the Illustration). *Remember, the arrows show the direction of the "pulling" inward; your feet remain* **stable** *and "holding ground."*

You then relax, pivot your right foot at the heel moving your right toes outward 2 inches and begin the sequence again with the left leg.

As you perform the Stepping and Holding Your Ground Exercise, focus your attention on the strengthening of your upper leg (especially the inner thigh), lower leg, calf muscles, Achilles tendons of both legs, and muscles in your ankles and feet. This exercise will strengthen the muscle-tendon-bone units of the hip and entire leg with emphasis on the lower leg components, ankles, and feet.

This very important exercise will increase the tone and strength of the muscles that surround your knees and ankles. "Stepping and Holding Your Ground" will help foster stability and help counter joint laxity by increasing the stability of your knee and ankle movements.

Exercise Tips and Check Points
for Exercise #15: Stepping and Holding Your Ground

Be sure to stand in a relaxed, upright posture.

If you are doing this exercise on a rug surface, be sure that the rug is fixed and will not slide around as you step on it.

As you do this exercise, stay relaxed and be sure that you maintain an upright posture (imagine a string attached to the top of your head, and that you are moving your entire body forward as the string keeps your entire body upright in a vertical plane).

Keep your arms lowered and relaxed hanging comfortably at the sides of your legs.

Be sure that you keep your shoulders relaxed and down (not popped up or raised).

Keep your entire body upright as you move forward and do not lean forward or backward (nor let your head bob up and down).

Be aware of the muscle-tendon-bone units of your entire body moving. Feel the entire muscle chains working to keep your entire body held together and moving dynamically.

Practice the heel-toe movement as this is very important; remember to keep the toes of the front foot pointed straight ahead at the conclusion of the heel-toe step.

Be sure that when you step forward that you land with the heel first and "grab" the ground with your heel (pulling backwards without moving the heel) then pull your body forward.

After putting your foot down and pivoting forward with your foot, remember to "grab" the ground with your entire foot and pull yourself forward.

Remember to simultaneously (1) "grab" the ground with your front toes and entire front foot and pull into the center of your body and (2) "grab" the ground with your rear toes and entire rear foot and pull into the center of your body, and hold this for a count of five.

Imagine in doing this exercise that instead of your feet "Holding the Ground," you put your hands on the ground and try to "squeeze up" a large piece of the ground in your hands. This is the feeling that you should have with your feet as you are "Holding the Ground."

Focus your attention on the strengthening of your upper leg (especially the inner thigh), lower leg and calf muscles, Achilles tendons of both legs, and muscles in your ankles and feet.

Repeat this exercise several times; however, be sure that you do not overdo the repetitions. Begin with about three until you feel yourself becoming stronger.

Exercise #16: Back Leg Stretch

Stand with your feet slightly wider than shoulder-width apart (See Segment A of the Illustration on the following page). With both feet flat on the floor and your posture remaining upright, jut your chin upwards and out as far as it will go by bending your neck back (See Segment B of the Illustration).

You then slowly bend at the waist forward while grabbing both legs with your arms at the back of your legs and aim your jutted chin (keeping your neck bent back) to an envisioned spot about four feet in front of your feet on the floor (See Segment C of the Illustration below) and hold for a count of five.

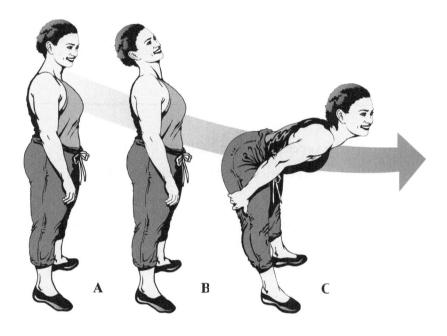

Return to your upright standing position, and be sure that you stay relaxed and maintain an upright posture.

Repeat the above sequences for another repetition. Start with three repetitions, and slowly increase the number of repetitions.

In this exercise, *it is very important that you have jutted your chin upward and out, keeping your neck pulled back.* You then lower yourself by *aiming with your chin.* **Important**: *This keeps the back muscles from being strained and works the legs.*

As you perform the Back Leg Stretch Exercise, focus your attention on the strengthening of your back thigh (hamstrings), knee tendons, calf muscles, and Achilles tendons of both legs. This exercise will strengthen the muscle-tendon-bone units of the entire leg with emphasis on the upper and lower leg components of the back of the leg.

Exercise Tips and Check Points
for Exercise #16: Back Leg Stretch

Be sure to stand in a relaxed, upright posture when you start this exercise.

Begin the exercise by jutting your chin upwards and out as far as it will go by bending your neck back.

Remember to slowly bend at the waist forward while grabbing both legs with your arms at the back of your legs and aim your jutted chin (keeping your neck bent back) to an envisioned spot about four feet in front of your feet on the floor.

As you bend forward, stay relaxed and be sure that your neck is bent backwards with your chin jutted forward.

Be sure to bend forward *slowly*, and hold for a count of five.

Focus your attention on the stretching and strengthening of your back thigh (hamstrings), back knee tendons, calf muscles, and Achilles tendons.

Be aware of the muscle-tendon-bone units of both of your entire legs.

Be aware of and focus on the stretching and stabilizing forces at the back knee tendons and your Achilles tendons as you bend forward slowly. Feel the strong stretch in your hamstrings (*but do not stretch too far if at first it is uncomfortable*).

Repeat this exercise several times; however, be sure that you do not overdo the repetitions. Begin with about three until you feel yourself becoming stronger.

This is an excellent exercise for helping you to stretch your hamstrings and decrease some of the feeling of "stiffness" in the hamstrings.

Chapter Eight

Tips for Weight Loss During Menopause

and After

■

You can make great progress in healing menopausal arthritis without losing any considerable weight (even if you are overweight or in a beginning level of obesity). I was within five pounds of the same weight when I began my program and when I had healed from my menopausal arthritis (between 180 - 185 lbs.).

However, you may want to enhance through weight loss the healing that you have already experienced. In doing so, you may even find that you need fewer supplements to maintain being free of pain and inflammation. Or, perhaps for you weight loss is indicated. In either case, research provides some important pointers for weight loss during menopause.

Oftentimes, women in menopause try to employ the same popular diets that have been touted to help people in general (of all ages) to lose weight. The only problem is that in menopause our bodies are *much different* from when we were younger! In fact, they are markedly different from when we were in premenopause. You may find in menopause that you have a greater appetite than before, at the same time that you may have begun to exercise less and burn fewer calories. There is even a noted difference in energy expenditure during *sleep* with less energy expenditure in postmenopausal women in comparison to premenopausal women![1] Nevertheless, research shows that you *can* lose weight, and I will summarize some of the studies in which menopausal women have successfully accomplished weight loss.

I have focused on what has been found to work optimally for menopausal or postmenopausal women who are overweight or obese, as well as for those who may also have metabolic syndrome or insulin resistance (so common in women who have menopausal arthritis). Provided below are my weight loss tips based upon the results of my research.

The Fundamental Seven: Key Tips for Weight Loss in Menopause

#1 -- Don't Be a Weight-Cycler

In terms of dieting, a "weight-cycler" has been defined as someone who has gone on a diet and lost weight (more than 22 lbs., for example) and then has regained it. You could be a low, moderate, or frequent cycler. Some researchers have defined a frequent cycler as dieting in this way four or more times. In a study of overweight, and obese postmenopausal women, researchers from the University of Montreal found that moderate cyclers (those dieting in this way two to three times) had lower adiponectin levels than non-cyclers. Adiponectin, as noted earlier in the book, is usually lower in women who are suffering from metabolic syndrome. Also, recall from the research noted in Chapter Two, that the balance between adiponectin and leptin may be critical in whether one suffers from knee arthritis; there was less pain with a higher adiponectin/leptin ratio. Frequent cyclers had less ability to resist bingeing, and they had a lower sense of body esteem. This was completely independent from their body mass; that is, the lower sense of body esteem was not dependent upon how fat they were. All in all, frequent cyclers had a higher body mass and percent body fat, larger waist circumference, and a lower resting metabolic rate than women who did not do weight-cycling.[2]

Weight cycling not only carries the metabolic and psychological drawbacks noted above, but it also has been hypothesized that changes in adipose tissue that result from cycling may actually create an environment where there is a deficient amount of oxygen available to the tissues. Adipose or fat tissue that does not have adequate oxygen is the type of fat that secretes leptin! Leptin stimulates macrophages to accumulate in the fat tissue and the macrophages release the proinflammatory cytokines that were talked about earlier in this book. So, according to scientists at the University of Houston, it is possible that weight cycling could produce changes in inflammation that are far worse than just sustained weight gain.[3] Weight cycling is not *only* bad for your ability to become and stay lean, but it *also* fosters the inflammatory environment that contributes to menopausal arthritis.

#2 -- Be Patient

"Patience is a virtue," as the old proverbial saying goes. It could not be truer with regard to weight loss in perimenopause or menopause (especially if you are overweight or obese). For example, a study of young adult women and perimenopausal women found that while both groups of women were able to lose weight, the ability was much more pronounced in the younger women. Although both groups of women did lose weight on the same diet, it took more time for perimenopausal women to lose weight. The researchers thought that this might be due to hormonal or metabolic effects with the younger women burning more calories than the perimenopausal women.[4]

Do not succumb to the temptation to lose weight too fast! It can do you more harm than good in terms of your physical health. For example, in a study of obese postmenopausal women who lost weight at different rates, those who lost weight at a high rate (greater than 1.6 lbs. per week) lost significantly more lean body mass than those who lost weight at a low rate (less than 1.6 lbs. per week). Amazingly, there was no difference between the groups in the loss of fat mass! The faster weight loss rate did not reap greater body composition benefits; these women lost no more fat in the long run, and unfortunately lost more lean body mass.[5] So, losing weight more slowly is a healthier way to go under most circumstances.

#3 -- Reduce Stress (and That Means Dieting Stress, Too)!

Did you know that a preoccupation with weight and restricting the food one consumes is actually linked to weight gain? That's right. As unfair as it may sound, if you are a person who is concerned with dietary restraint, you are more likely to be experiencing stress, higher cortisol levels, and weight gain. This is what was found in studies of community samples.[6] In fact, psychological stress can lead to stress hormones such as cortisol initiating an inflammatory process that ultimately leads to weight gain. The reason is that stress, inflammation, and fat accumulation go hand-in-hand. The pathways from the brain that are active in signals from fat cells are the same as those that are active in responses to psychological stress.[7]

In an example of how dietary restraint (the effort exerted by women to limit food to manage weight) is linked to higher stress levels, researchers measured urinary cortisol excretion in postmenopausal women with varying levels of dietary restraint. Cortisol, as noted above, is a hormone released in response to stress. The women with high or low dietary restraint did not differ in terms of their "perceived stress," (nor did they differ on other important factors such as BMI, energy intake, exercise levels, etc.). Nevertheless, the women with high dietary restraint had higher cortisol excretions which would suggest that *dietary restraint* was possibly a *source* of stress.[8]

Researchers at the University of California, San Francisco, conducted research to find out if telomere length (a biomarker or indicator of aging) is related to dietary restraint (the preoccupation with weight and food intake). They did a study with two groups of women, one premenopausal and one postmenopausal, and they found that shorter telomeres (indicating greater aging) were associated with dietary restriction in *both* the pre- and postmenopausal groups. Telomere shortening is associated with morbidity and mortality, the likelihood of disease and death. So, perceived dietary restriction (not actual caloric restriction) may set one up for premature aging![9]

4 -- Maintain a Sense of Well-Being

It will, no doubt, be easier to lose weight if you maintain a sense of well-being. It appears that it may not be whether you are on a diet or not that seems to lead to feelings of impaired well-being, but rather whether you feel that you are susceptible to hunger and not able to control your cravings. In a study of 101 postmenopausal women, it was not whether women were dieting or not dieting that mattered – there were no significant differences between dieters and non-dieters in terms of psychological well-being. What *mattered* was whether the women felt that they could *not* control their cravings (termed "disinhibition"). Women with the greatest perceived "disinhibition," had lower scores on psychological well-being, and this was the case regardless of their actual weight.[10]

Topic of Interest #10

Milkshakes, Anyone? -- Mindset Over Matter

Dr. Kelly Brownell and colleagues at Yale University performed a study where they told participants that they would be taste-testing two different milkshakes on two occasions. They were informed that the goal of this research was to determine whether the milkshakes tasted similar to each other, and to take notice of the reaction their bodies had to the different dietary components of each shake (e.g., high fat vs. low fat; high sugar vs. low sugar, etc.).[11] One shake was "Indulgence - Decadence You Deserve - French Vanilla" and the other shake was "Sensi-Shake Guilt-Free Satisfaction - 0% fat, 0 added sugar, 140 Calories - French Vanilla." The researchers had also measured the hormone, ghrelin (the gut hormone that increases as a signal for hunger) in the participants after they had consumed the shakes. Ghrelin decreased (indicating that their hunger decreased) after the participants consumed the "Indulgence" shake, which would make perfect sense. In contrast, ghrelin remained level, and didn't change after consuming the "Sensi-Shake." This makes perfect sense also, as one might still have an appetite left over with the low calorie shake.   Only one catch: The researchers had concealed from the participants the true nature of the experiment. They had hidden from them this very critical thing -- the content of both shakes was *identical*, only the labeling on the container was different!

The researchers had not told the participants the real thing that they were trying to find out. What they really had wanted to know was whether actual physiological satisfaction of hunger (as measured by the level of ghrelin) was affected by a person's *mindset* when eating a food. The participants' mindset was what mattered here! If they believed that they were consuming a rich, indulgent milkshake, their appetite declined; they were satisfied. However, if they believed that they were eating a sensible, calorie-restricted shake, their appetite (as measured by ghrelin level) stayed relatively "flat." The way that ghrelin responded in the body was similar to the situation of people actually consuming food with different amounts of calories.[12] However, the ghrelin response here was not caused by the calorie content or nutrient value of the shakes -- *they were the same!* Your mindset when you consume a food matters greatly.

#5 -- *Avoid Weight Regain!*

As you can see from the research on weight cycling, successful maintenance of weight loss over the long run is limited for a large number of women. The problem is that once you have achieved the reduced weight state, you have also set into motion some biological mechanisms and processes that promote the regaining of the weight. In fact, researchers out of Columbia University have referred to obesity as "a disease in which the human body actively opposes the 'cure' over long periods of time. . ."[13] So, one thing that research shows you can do to counteract this problem is to exercise during the weight reduction period. Don't just exercise after the weight reduction period is over. Researchers at Wake Forest University and the State University of New York at Buffalo found that overweight/obese postmenopausal women with the highest decline in physical activity *during* weight loss had the *greatest* weight regain following the weight loss period. Weight regain was *not* associated with the amount of physical activity reported *following the weight loss period*, rather, it *was* associated with the physical activity *during the weight loss period.*[14] This has enormous importance, as I suspect that there are a great number of women who might decide to lose the weight first, and then exercise after weight loss. This might especially be the case if they have chosen a hypocaloric diet or one low in energy intake. A hypocaloric diet has research evidence supporting its use among postmenopausal women. It has been found that a hypocaloric diet combined with varying intensities of exercise is effective in producing weight and fat reduction in postmenopausal women, as well as better insulin sensitivity, glycemic control, and cardio-respiratory health.[15]

Nevertheless, it would be important to consult with your healthcare provider to determine the optimal calories and types of food to consume when you will also be exercising during weight loss (or before going on any diet or exercise regime for that matter). Remember, though, that the *primary goal of the exercises within my healing program for menopausal arthritis is to build strong muscle-tendon-bone units.* You need *sufficient energy intake* (in calories) and *very good nutrition within a balanced diet* to accomplish this.

6 - Use Vitamins, Supplements, and Specific Foods to Assist and Fortify Your Body

One of the most beneficial things that you can do when trying to lose weight is to fortify your body with some specific vitamins and supplements that can both help you to lose weight, and to keep you healthy in the process.

---Try the Synergistic Combo: Genistein, Quercetin, and Resveratrol (along with Vitamin D)

In animal research out of the University of Georgia using ovariectomized lab animals as a model for the menopausal state, it was found that the combined supplementation of vitamin D with genistein, quercetin, and resveratrol had synergistic effects. Genistein (an isoflavone derived from soybeans and other plant sources), quercetin (a flavonoid derived from many fruits, vegetables and other plants sources) and resveratrol (a natural phenol derived from red grape skins and other fruits) when combined with vitamin D, reduced bone loss and weight gain.[16]

---Maintain Calcium Levels During Weight Loss

Menopausal women may have a disrupted ability to efficiently absorb dietary calcium, and they may also consume less of this nutrient.[17] Dr. Sue A. Shapses and colleagues have cautioned that in overweight postmenopausal women, calcium level needs may be elevated during weight loss. In a study of overweight postmenopausal women they found that weight restriction (that included maintaining participants' usual exercise patterns) significantly reduced these women's total amount of calcium absorbed in comparison with the group that maintained their weight. In addition, in the weight loss group that took a high calcium supplement, greater rate of weight loss was associated with suppression of calcium absorption. Nevertheless, the women in the high calcium group did absorb sufficient amounts. For those in the normal calcium supplement group, weight loss resulted in an inadequate level of calcium. The high calcium supplement was needed in order to obtain adequate amounts of calcium. Not sustaining adequate levels of calcium during weight loss, thus, could result in increased bone turnover and loss.[18]

Speaking of maintaining calcium levels to prevent bone loss during weight reduction, there are other matters pertaining to bone mass during weight loss that must be mentioned. It is critical to be aware of the fact that *weight loss leads to decreased bone mass even when one exercises.* Weight loss has been found to be associated with a decrease in bone mineral density (BMD) in both premenopausal and postmenopausal women. This is so, even with a physical activity such as walking added to the program for weight loss. In a unique study (with participants from the Women's Healthy Lifestyle Project) women aged 44-50 years were followed over a period of approximately six years. The effects of weight control on bone mineral density were examined. Premenopausal women lost BMD if they were in the group that experienced weight loss, but they gained BMD if they were in the group that experienced weight gain. Weight loss was related to a greater loss of BMD in the hip in both premenopausal and postmenopausal women who had weight loss percentages of 3% or more. In fact, even in the postmenopausal group who took hormone therapy, if they lost more than 3% of their body weight, they had greater hip BMD loss than those who had gained weight.[19]

In a study out of Washington University School of Medicine that examined the effect of weight loss and exercise on bone metabolism and mass in obese older adults, decreases in hip bone mineral density also occurred. In fact, the researchers concluded that weight loss, even when it is accompanied by exercise, still led to reduced hip bone mineral density in obese older adults. Moreover, in this study the exercise component was quite extensive and varied to include resistance exercises using weight-lifting machines as well as endurance exercises. Participants exercised at moderate intensity that was progressively increased to 80-90% of peak heart rate. Nevertheless, bone mineral density at the hip was lost.[20]

---Beyond Helping to Maintain Bone Mass: Calcium's Fat-Fighting and Muscle-Preserving Effects

In a study of postmenopausal women who filled out a dietary questionnaire of food intake, there was a significant correlation between lower percent body fat and calcium intake, and lower abdominal fat mass and calcium intake (from both dairy and supplements combined). Higher calcium intake was linked to a lower percentage of body fat, and higher dairy intake was linked to lower fat mass.[21] In addition, in a study with ovariectomized laboratory animals as a model for the menopausal state, it was found that fructus ligustri lucidi (a Chinese herb) might reduce calcium loss and help in the body's utilization of vitamin D to improve calcium levels.[22] This herb has the appearance of little, dried red berries and is often found in healing Chinese soups.

Calcium and vitamin D, as well as natural dairy products, appear from the research to be nutritional allies in preserving bone and facilitating muscle preservation and healthy muscle composition. Ensuring that these are part of your menopausal weight loss plan would be very important. If you do take your calcium in supplement form, be sure it also includes the appropriate amount of magnesium, too.

Topic of Interest #11

A Major Concern About Current Popular Drugs Used to Prevent and Treat Osteoporosis

In a very recent article published within the Journal of the American Medical Association in 2011, it was found that use of bisphosphonate (e.g., Fosamax, Boniva, Reclast, etc.) was associated with fractures of the femur shaft or thigh bone. With more than five years of usage, the drug was found to protect against typical fractures such as fracture at the intertrochanteric region or femoral neck (the very top of the thigh bone or in the neck area where it attaches to the pelvis). However, use of the drug for more than five years was found to increase the risk of fracture below this area, *within the thigh bone itself* (the subtrochanteric or femoral shaft area). *The fractures did not occur due to trauma, motor vehicle collisions, or falls from a height.*[23] *Rather, these fractures occurred with minimal trauma.*

In a report of the Working Group of the European Society on Clinical and Economic Aspects of Osteoporosis and Osteoarthritis and the International Osteoporosis Foundation, this type of fracture was described in detail. Most disturbingly, these fractures occurred as a result of minimal or even no trauma. Prior to these fractures, women commonly experienced pain indicating that a disease process or abnormal condition was present. This type of hip fracture usually results from multiple episodes of high energy trauma such as might occur in sports activities. It can also occur due to low energy injuries that occur as a result of bone that is osteoporotic.[24] So, why would a drug that is supposed to build up bone have the result of being associated with a fracture that (in cases with minimal or no trauma such as these) would occur in those with poor bone structure?

Apparently a whole host of things may be happening, all of which (in my opinion) are bad news for anyone who wants to have healthy bone. Perhaps, there are some cases in which the use of this type of drug might make sense medically; again, this is my observation based upon research, not medical advice. Nevertheless, research points toward significantly suppressed bone formation, with diminished or even absent osteoblasts on the bone surface (and osteoclasts were found to be diminished in number, as well).[25,26] Normal bone remodeling needs both osteoblasts (which make bone) and osteoclasts (which break down bone, or resorb it) in order to work properly. The reduction of osteoblasts is troubling, but so too is the reduction in osteoclasts because they work together in the bone remodeling process.

In a study of alendronate (a bisphosphonate drug commonly used as an inhibitor of bone resorption and widely used to treat osteoporosis), severe suppression of bone turnover was found. The bone formation rate among the group taking this drug was almost 100 times lower than in postmenopausal, healthy women who served as controls. Moreover, these researchers noted that studies show that in women also taking estrogen along with this drug, the suppression of bone turnover was *intensified.* Fracture healing while on alendronate seemed to be impaired among the patients studied who had severe suppression of bone turnover. Even after discontinuing alendronate, fracture healing was not obtained even at 8-12 months later in four of these nine patients. The researchers concluded that severe suppression of bone turnover can occur in patients with long term treatment with alendronate, and that when it is accompanied by the use of estrogen (or glucocorticoids) that this severe suppression of bone turnover can occur even earlier.[27] As glucocorticoids are used in the treatment of rheumatoid arthritis and other diseases, (and some women do use estrogen replacement during menopause) this is important for women to know.

---Boosting Folate Levels May Help Prevent Increases in Body Fat

In postmenopausal women, lower levels of serum folate have been associated with adiposity, or the quality or condition of being fat. Among postmenopausal women, overweight women were found to have a 12% lower folate level, and obese women a 22% lower folate level compared with normal weight women. Increases in central and peripheral fat, body mass index, and percent body fat all were found to be significantly related to lower serum folate levels.[28] Folate and folic acid are both forms of the same B vitamin, with folic acid the synthetic form. You can increase the folate in your diet by including green leafy vegetables such as spinach, turnip greens, romaine lettuce, and vegetables such as asparagus and broccoli. Beef liver is a very good meat source of folate, and fruit sources include cantaloupe, papaya, and bananas. Taking it in supplement form as folic acid is another way of increasing folate. If you take it in supplement form, be sure that you are taking it in a complete, balanced B-Complex supplement.

---Two Foods That Might Be Allies in Weight Loss: Soy and Seaweed

Soy (Isoflavones):

Research seems to show that soy may be an important food and supplement to add to your diet to lose weight in menopause. For example, in a Spanish study, 87 healthy, obese postmenopausal women were assigned to either a diet plus exercise group, or diet plus exercise group with the addition of taking a soy isoflavones supplement. At the end of 6 months, leptin and TNF-alpha had declined in both groups. However, only in the group with the added soy supplement did *adiponectin* increase.[29] This is extremely important since, as noted earlier, low adiponectin levels are associated with the metabolic syndrome. Moreover, in a study of 116 postmenopausal women assigned to a Mediterranean diet and exercise, or alternatively to a Mediterranean diet and exercise along with taking a soy isoflavones supplement, the latter group reduced insulin resistance (in women who had insulin resistance at the beginning of the study).[30]

Although there is some controversy over whether some aspects of soy consumption (such as a possible thyroid-depressing mechanism) might be problematic or harmful, it has long been consumed as a dietary staple in China, Japan, and Korea as well as other Asian countries. It originated in China and has been used as a food staple for thousands of years. There are differences, however, between the soy food products consumed in Asia and the soy food products consumed in the United States. In Asia, soy foods are often in fermented form. Microorganisms convert the soybeans to miso, soy paste, and tempeh. In fact, soy sauce is often a product of long fermentation.

In the United States, foods that contain soybeans have become quite popular; however, they are made very differently and the vast majority of soy products are not fermented. Textured soy protein, for example, commonly used in foods as a substitute for meat goes through an extrusion process. This takes out the protein (soy protein isolate) which serves as the primary food product, but eliminates the complex carbohydrates and lipids as well as the isoflavones.[31] The above research study seems to point toward a possible positive effect of isoflavones in soy in managing the metabolic syndrome. Thus, it is important to consume soy products that contain isoflavones. It would seem to be most beneficial to preserve the products in their natural forms for the greatest health benefit as in the forms used in Asian countries. More research is certainly needed, but soy may be worthy of consideration as an important addition to a diet for weight loss.

Seaweed:

In a study of postmenopausal women and their consumption of seaweed and soy products, seaweed supplementation had a small, but significant effect in increasing thyroid stimulating hormone (TSH). Moreover, it was found that soy supplementation did not affect thyroid function measures.[32] These are important findings, as soy has been shown in some reports or accounts to have goitrogenic effects which could lead to hypothyroidism. A well-functioning thyroid gland is important in being able to lose weight. Perhaps in the Japanese diet the seaweed counters any goitrogenic effects of the soy.

In a further study conducted by Dr. Jane Teas and colleagues out of the University of South Carolina Cancer Center, it was found that seaweed might have potential in decreasing some aspects of the metabolic syndrome. For example, it was found that for both men and women (mean age of 47 years) with at least one symptom of the metabolic syndrome, seaweed supplementation (at the higher dose within this study) helped to bring blood pressure down in participants who had high-normal blood pressure at the start of the study. Moreover, in women only, it decreased waist circumference. With increasing amounts of seaweed, increases in waist size reduction occurred. The optimal amount of seaweed supplementation in this study corresponded to the typical amount consumed by most Japanese people.[33]

Topic of Interest #12

Should You Refrain from the Foods That You Crave?

I am sure many of us have heard the maxim that we should stay away from the foods that we crave; they are in essence an addiction, and eating even a small amount of them will make us crave more. There is solid science behind this caution. Reviews of research data and analyses out of Princeton University and Yale University have led researchers to conclude that people may respond to certain foods with possible physiological processes similar to neural responses in drugs of abuse that reinforce addiction to these foods.[34,35] Foods high in fat, salt, and sugar are often preferred by people. Research indicates that these foods seem to have a potential for abuse akin to addictive drugs.[36]

If you crave protein, could it have a similar effect? Well, if you crave protein and refrain from eating it, you probably won't go out of control eating chicken after your protein restriction ends. However, if you crave carbs, then after carbohydrate restriction you just might have a need to consume more croissants than usual (and crave carbs more). This is, indeed, essentially what was found in a study conducted out of the University of Toronto. Carbohydrate restriction initiated a "rebound" effect after dieting; that is, people seemed to try to make up the carbohydrates that they had missed. Protein restriction did not lead to a "rebound" effect. Even though the protein restriction did cause more cravings for protein, protein consumption was not increased (in comparison to people who had not restricted protein).[37]

Moreover, as reported in the Journal of the American Dietetic Association, a review of the literature on food restriction found that it may have some unanticipated negative consequences. Self-imposed restriction of food can result in eating binges, preoccupation with food and eating, unhappiness, increased emotionality, and an inability to concentrate fully on things.[38]

It seems that it would be important to determine whether you are really "addicted" to a particular food or whether it is a food that you can "crave" but without the addictive component. If it does constitute a true food addiction that is unhealthful in nature, then eliminating it would be important. However, restricting a desired food could cause the negative mental and emotional consequences described above. If the desired food is not actually craved as part of a food addiction pattern, then the negative emotional and cognitive effects would be consequences of food restriction that one would want to avoid.

#7 - Foster Exercise Self-Efficacy

Attitudes toward exercise when one gets older seem to be highly associated with whether you are an exerciser or not. For example, Dr. Martha Storandt and colleague at Washington University in St. Louis conducted a study of over 100 women from a community sample (not from a structured exercise program). They explored whether these women found exercise both enjoyable and beneficial in their lives. They also looked at whether women felt self-efficacy in exercise, which is whether they believed that they could perform the exercise adequately or well. They found that younger women, not surprisingly, had more positive attitudes toward exercise than older women. What was interesting, however, was that the older women consisted of two groups – exercisers who had a positive attitude toward exercise, and non-exercisers who had a negative attitude toward exercise. However, a woman's age was even more associated with self-efficacy than whether she was an exerciser or non-exerciser. The only exception to this was for the exercise activity of walking.[39]

Although walking has been found to help reduce metabolic syndrome profiles in postmenopausal women,[40] it has unfortunately also been found to considerably increase their fracture rates. In a very recent study published in the Journal of Bone and Mineral Research, it was found that postmenopausal women (aged 50 years and over) who walk more than 3 hours per week were found to have a 51% increased risk of fracture; or if they had walked for 6 episodes of walking, they had a 56% increased risk of fracture. This was in comparison with women who did no walking. Older men were not spared either; those who walked more than 3 hours per week also had an increased fracture risk compared with those who did no walking. Interestingly, the *total physical activity* in which women engaged (moderate to vigorous in nature) amounting to 2.5 hours per week (or more) was *not* associated with increased fracture risk.[41] The majority of the fractures were low-trauma (resulting from a fall from standing height or less). The researchers speculated that the increased risk with greater walking time and frequency of walking episodes was likely due to the increased risk of slipping or falling while walking outdoors. They suggested that for individuals at high risk for fractures, that individually designed programs to foster muscle balance and function, as well as strength and power, would be important to implement. Among women, a previous history of fracture and cardiovascular disease, a lower body weight and BMI, and poorer physical functioning were associated with greater incidence of low trauma fractures. Menopausal arthritis, as we have seen is associated with a higher body weight and BMI; in addition, balance problems are of concern due to the rapid muscle strength and power deline that women experience following menopause. The exercises within our program are designed to help increase muscle and tendon strength and power, and thus provide better balance and stability in movement.

Moreover, as noted in Chapter Seven, women have been found to have greater hip joint moments (hip joint loads) in walking which results in greater joint stress for women as compared with men. This could potentially result in a greater risk of hip joint deterioration in older women walkers as compared to older men. So, caution is advised in overdoing walking. Although perhaps a very good exercise in most circumstances for the general population, the research discussed above does provide some areas of concern for older women.

Dr. Storandt and colleague framed their perspectives in terms of the noted psychologist Albert Bandura's theory of self-efficacy, that is, whether a person believes and expects that she or he would be able to succeed at doing a particular task or activity (in this case, exercise). Part of the problem is that many of the older women may have felt that they did not have the capability to engage in exercise. The researchers noted that some of this may be a realistic assessment of their ability, but that it could also be a result of a lack of experience with exercise, as well as buying into negative stereotypes about aging.[42]

The importance of one's perception of self-efficacy in behaviors that promote health was addressed within the last decade by Albert Bandura. He emphasized that the level or "quality" of health that one experiences is greatly affected by "lifestyle habits." He noted that one can have a significant impact upon personal health, longevity, and well-being by managing health habits. Stressing that it is important to be aware of this and to control and regulate one's health behaviors, Bandura emphasized, "Self-management is good medicine."[43]

Self-efficacy in health and exercise behaviors does matter in terms of one's outcomes. More specifically, though, what exactly is "self-efficacy?" According to Dr. Albert Bandura, it is one's perception, belief, or expectation that one will be able to succeed at accomplishing a task, performing a behavior, or coping effectively with a situation.[44] This is critical to any person trying to accomplish change in his or her health status, as well as in other domains. So, with many of the underpinnings of Albert Bandura's theory in mind (as well as learning tools from cognitive psychology), here are some suggestions for improving your exercise self-efficacy:

---**Start with activities that you enjoy and that are *easy for you to perform*.** By beginning with an activity in which you know you can achieve success, you will begin to *build* exercise self-efficacy. Begin slowly, with the exercise program in this book. As you become physically stronger, your belief in your ability to perform an exercise will become stronger as well. Get an instructional dance or other exercise video or CD and start to learn the new dance steps or exercise movements. As your moves get *closer* in form to the performers' moves, then you will *increase* your sense of exercise self-efficacy. Always start out slowly, and never go beyond your point of comfort.

   ---Don't just perform one type of exercise. Now that you have gained competence in one form of exercise, add to your exercise repertoire. Perhaps you have gained skill in dancing, for example, as a form of aerobic exercise. Your belief of self-efficacy in exercise *should increase* if you find that you can perform and become competent in an *additional* type of exercise as well. Swimming can be an enjoyable activity for people with arthritis as one is buoyant in the water, and there is minimized stress on the joints. However, be sure not to slip on any wet pool pavement, though – you do not want an injury to hamper your forward movement or seriously impair your health. Gaining and using new skills in another activity (such as swimming) may exercise additional muscle groups or different chains of muscles while increasing your exercise self-efficacy.

   ---Exercise alone at home if you are prone to social anxiety in performing exercise tasks. If having other people watching you is anxiety-producing or you are fearful of negative comments and evaluation from others, then exercise alone at first. This is an important point, because the strong emotions that arise from the fear of people's appraisals can influence your self-efficacy for the exercise task. Negative feelings and emotions usually hamper people's performance. So, provide a comfortable, non-stressful environment for yourself as you learn new tasks.

   ---Build a social support network to maximize your self-efficacy in exercise. People with more social support are more likely to increase self-efficacy beliefs. Some studies have helped to point toward possible factors of importance to women in terms of social support. For example, one study indicated that women receive less social support than men with regard to physical exercise.[45] This is important, because in addition to self-efficacy for physical activity, social support has also been found to be associated with physical activity in women. Interestingly, for men in this study it was self-efficacy for physical activity along with environmental factors (i.e., the availability of recreational facilities), instead of social support that was most associated with physical activity.[46] In a different study of older adults, it was found that self-efficacy and social support have a synergistic effect. Both can be very important to exercise outcomes in older adults. People high in self-efficacy were less likely to be active if they had low social support. Likewise, people with social support were less likely to be active if they had low self-efficacy.[47] So, as you gain in self-efficacy, be sure to include a social support network to reinforce your involvement in exercise.

   ---**Seek out role models for the tasks or behaviors that you want to learn**. You will be more likely to believe that you can be effective at a task (for example, a complex dance step) if you watch other women your age with similar body challenges accurately and efficiently performing it well. The importance of observing active people was positively associated with regular strength training in older Japanese adults in one recent study conducted out of Waseda University.[48] Moreover, if you participate in watching and performing the behaviors of the model, the effect will be even stronger.

   ---**A Coach or Trainer can be helpful for encouraging and persuading one to believe that one can be successful; nevertheless, expectations of self-efficacy that stem from *your own actualized achievements* are *more powerful*.** The reason for this is that you *directly experienced* the performing of the skills successfully. Your mind keeps a record of it, ready to reinforce your expectations that you will succeed again.

   ---**Realize that as you gain skills in one aerobic exercise (and even better in two, or more) that you are actively building your self-efficacy base for future success.** Take an active part in building this strong personal base; when you accomplish a task, congratulate yourself. Experience and feel the success. As you attain new skills or achieve at tasks, be sure to commend your own efforts on the way to your ultimate goals. Instead of waiting for all of your muscles to be strong before you allow yourself to feel success, recognize small gains. Take notice and appreciate your achievements with each muscle strengthened or brought into balance (for example a very weak calf muscle or a tight hamstring muscle). Recognition of these smaller successes will help you to increase your exercise self-efficacy and to achieve more difficult tasks or exercise goals.

---Notice and appreciate that the increased self-efficacy you feel as a result of mastering exercise may be transferring to other areas of your life as well! The fact that you could increase your self-efficacy with the exercises might be generalized to other tasks, too. That is, since you were successful at mastering increasingly difficult exercises and gaining new physical skills, you might extend this faith in your ability to succeed on these tasks to other tasks. This is especially the case if they are, in important ways, related to the self-efficacy gains through exercise (such as dieting to lose weight, for example). The nice thing about fostering your sense of self-efficacy is that as it rises, you will be less vulnerable to negative appraisals from occasional failed attempts at a task.

Succeeding at Weight Loss During Menopause

Succeeding at weight loss during menopause is no easy task. Some of the most important suggestions that I gained from research findings were to approach weight loss conservatively, and to always emphasize nutrition in conjunction with weight loss and exercise. You do not want to lose bone mass and bone mineral density, nor do you want to lose muscle mass. Moreover, with regard to weight loss, it is better to not have a "diet mentality." Being moderate about what you consume (while eating in a style and way that brings happiness and satisfaction to you) should help to keep you off the weight cycling roller coaster.

Is Weight Loss Really Necessary to Tackle Menopausal Arthritis?

Keep in mind that *a major healing plan goal is to reduce the proinflammatory cytokines in your body*, and that you can greatly reduce them through foods, supplements, and herbs. Higher levels of leptin are associated with increased production of cytokines as discussed in Chapter Two. Weight loss has been shown to be associated with reduced plasma levels of leptin in obese people.[49] However, curcumin, an active component of the spice turmeric, has been shown to help reduce leptin levels. Moreover, there are many other herbs, supplements, and foods that decrease cytokine levels. I will be discussing these important supports in Chapter Ten. You will likely be able to alleviate your menopausal arthritis symptoms with minimal, or perhaps even no weight loss (of course, depending upon your initial weight and overall health).

The beneficial effects of reducing leptin and proinflammatory cytokines through foods, supplements, and herbs are especially effective in combination with the other modes of reducing arthritis in this program (i.e., when accompanied by the strengthening of muscles and tendons, and healing of any soft tissue problems). From my own experience and the research I have reviewed, if you are overweight or in a beginning level of obesity you can still be successful in stemming menopausal arthritis without any substantial weight loss. If you strengthen your muscle-tendon-bone units and have an adequate intake of anti-inflammatory herbs, foods, and supplements (along with some of the external healing therapies), then you should be able to find your menopausal arthritis greatly alleviated or even, in essence, eliminated.

Nevertheless, if you are obese, research points toward weight loss interventions as effective in reducing osteoarthritis symptoms.[50,51] Weight loss does reduce leptin levels, and higher leptin levels are associated with the release of proinflammatory cytokines. However, longitudinal data would be important to determine whether the effects of initial weight loss interventions on arthritis symptoms hold over time. If you are considering weight loss as a strategy to help improve your arthritis symptoms, it must be stressed that it should be done without sacrificing your overall health and strength.

Consult your medical doctor on how to proceed, and of course consult your physician or doctor before undertaking *any* kind of weight loss program even if you think that you are in good health. Weight loss in menopause may help to alleviate arthritis symptoms, but if not done cautiously and well, it may bring you more pain than progress. Personally, I chose to heal from my menopausal arthritis first prior to undergoing any major weight loss attempts. Now that I no longer have menopausal arthritis, I plan to use these weight loss tips more fully. From the vital base of a strong, healthy body, I am now in a more advantageous position to begin weight reduction!

Notes for Chapter Eight

[1]Lovejoy, J. C., Champagne, C. M., de Jonge, L., Xie, H., & Smith, S. R. (2008). Increased visceral fat and decreased energy expenditure during the menopausal transition. *International Journal of Obesity (Lond).*, *32*(6), 949-958.

[2]Strychar, I., Lavoie, M. E., Messier, L., Karelis, A. D., Doucet, E,. Prud'homme, D., Fountaine, J., & Rabasa-Lhoret, R. (2009). Anthropometric, metabolic, psychosocial, and dietary characteristics of overweight/obese postmenopausal women with a history of weight cycling: a MONET (Montreal Ottawa New Emerging Team) study. *Journal of the American Dietetic Association, 109*(4), 718-724.

[3]Strohacker, K., & McFarlin, B. K. (2010). Influence of obesity, physical activity, and weight cycling on chronic inflammation. *Frontiers in Bioscience (Elite Ed.)*, *1,2*, 98-104.

[4]Nestares, T., de la Higuera López-Frías, M., Diaz-Castro, J., Campos, M. S., & López-Frías, M. (2009). Evaluating the effectiveness of a weight-loss program for perimenopausal women. *International Journal for Vitamin and Nutrition Research, 79*(4), 212-217.

[5]Arguin, H., Bouchard, D. R., Labonté, M. Carpentier, A., Ardilouze, J. L. , Dionne, I. J. & Brochu, M. (2008). Correlation between the rate of weight loss and changes in body composition in obese postmenopausal women after 5 weeks: a pilot study. *Applied Physiology, Nutrition and Metabolism, 33*(2), 347-355.

[6]Kiefer, A., Lin, J., Blackburn, E., & Epel, E. (2008). Dietary restraint and telomere length in pre- and postmenopausal women. *Psychosomatic Medicine, 70*(8), 845-849.

[7]Black, P. H. (2006). The inflammatory consequences of psychological stress: Relationship to insulin resistance, obesity, artherosclerosis and diabetes mellitus, type II. *Medical Hypotheses, 67*(4), 879-891.

[8]Rideout, C. A., Linden, W., & Barr, S. I. (2006). High cognitive dietary restraint is associated with increased cortisol excretion in postmenopausal women. *Journal of Gerontology, Series A: Biological Sciences, 61*(6), 628-633.

[9]Kiefer et al. (2008). Op. Cit.

[10]Provencher, V., Bégin, C., Piché, M. E., Bergeron, J., Corneau, L., Weisnagel, S. J., Nadeau, A., & Lemieux, S. (2007). Disinhibition, as assessed by the Three-Factor Eating Questionnaire, is inversely related to psychological well-being in post-menopausal women. *International Journal of Obesity, 31*(2), 315-320.

[11]Crum, A. J., Corbin, W. R., Brownell, K. D., & Salovey, P. (2011). Mind over milkshakes: Mindsets, not just nutrients, determine ghrelin response. *Health Psychology, 30*(4), 424-429.

[12]Ibid.

[13]Rosenbaum, M. & Leibel, R. L. (2010). Adaptive thermogenesis in humans. *International Journal of Obesity (London), 34*(Sppl 1), S47-S55.

[14]Wang, X., Lyles, M. F., You, T., Berry, M. J., Rejeski, J., & Nicklas, B. J. (2008). Weight regain is related to decreases in physical activity during weight loss. *Medicine and Science in Sports and Exercise, 40*(10), 1781-1788.

[15]Al-Zadjali, M., Keller, C., Larkey, L. K., & Albertini, L.; Center for Healthy Outcomes in Aging. (2010). Evaluation of intervention research in weight reduction in post menopausal women. *Geriatric Nursing, 31*(6), 419-434.

[16]Lai, C. Y., Yang, J. Y., Rayalam, S., Della-Fera, M. A., Ambati, S., Lewis, R. D., Hamrick, M. W., Hartzell, D. L., & Baile, C. A. (2011). Preventing bone loss and weight gain with combinations of vitamin D and phytochemicals. *Journal of Medicinal Food.* Advance online publication. PMID: 21663481

[17]Shapses, S. A., & Riedt, C. S. (2006). Bone, body weight, and weight reduction: What are the concerns? *Journal of Nutrition, 136*(6), 1453-1456.

[18]Cifuentes, M., Riedt, C. S., Brolin, R. E., Field, M. P. , Sherrell, R. M., & Shapses, S. A. (2004). Weight loss and calcium intake influence calcium absorption in overweight postmenopausal women. *American Journal of Clinical Nutrition, 80*(1), 123-130.

[19]Park, H. A., Lee , J. S., Kuller, L. H., & Cauley, J. A. (2007). Effects of weight control during the menopausal transition on bone mineral density. *Journal of Clinical Endocrinology & Metabolism, 92*(10), 3809-3815. doi: 10.1210/jc.2007.1040

[20]Villareal, D. T., Shah, K., Banks, M. R., Sinacore, D. R., & Klein, S. (2008). Effect of weight loss and exercise therapy on bone metabolism and mass in obese older adults: A one-year randomized controlled trial. *Journal of Clinical Endocrinology and Metabolism, 93*(6), 2181-2187. doi: 10.1210/jc.2007-1473

[21]Heiss, C. J., Shaw, S. E., & Carothers, L. (2008). Association of calcium intake and adiposity in postmenopausal women. *Journal of the American College of Nutrition, 27*(2), 260-266.

[22]Zhang, Y., Dong, X. L., Leung, P. C., Che, C. T., & Wong, M. S. (2008). Fructus ligustri lucidi extract improves calcium balance and modulates the calciotropic hormone level and vitamin D-dependent gene expression in aged ovariectomized rats. *Menopause, 15*(3), 558-565.

[23]Park-Wyllie, L. Y., Mamdani, M. M., Juurlink. D. N., Hawker, G. A., Gunraj, N. Austin, P. C., Whelan, D. B., Weiler, P. J., & Laupacis, A. (2011). Bisphosphate use and the risk of subtrochanteric or femoral shaft fractures in older women. *Journal of the American Medical Association, 305*(8), 783-789.

[24]Rizzoli, R., _kesson, K., Bouxsein, M., Kanis, J. A., Napoli, N., Papapoulos, S., Reginster, J.-Y., & Cooper, C. (2011). Subtrochanteric fractures after long-term treatment with bisphosphonates: A European Society on Clinical and Economic Aspects of Osteoporosis and Osteoarthritis, and International Osteoporosis Foundation Working Group Report. *Osteoporosis International, 22*, 373-390. doi: 10.1007/s00198-010-1453-5

[25]Ibid.

[26]Odvina, C. V., Zerwekh, J. E., Rao, S., Maalouf, N., Gottschalk, F.A., & Pak, C. Y. C. (2005). Severely suppressed bone turnover: A potential complication of alendronate therapy. *Journal of Clinical Endocrinology & Metabolism, 90*(3), 1294-1301.

[27]Ibid.

[28]Mahabir, S., Ettinger, S., Johnson, L., Baer, D. J., Clevidence, B. A., Hartman, T. J., & Taylor, P. R. (2008). Measures of adiposity and body fat distribution in relation to serum folate levels in postmenopausal women in a feeding study. *European Journal of Clinical Nutrition, 62*(5), 644-650.

[29]Llaneza, P., González, C., Fernandez-Iñarrea,J., Alonso, A., Diaz, F., Arnott, I., & Ferrer-Barriendos, J. (2011). Soy isoflavones, diet and physical exercise modify serum cytokines in healthy obese postmenopausal women. *Phytomedicine, 18*(4), 245-250.

[30]Llaneza, P., Gonzalez, C., Fernandez-Iñarrea, J., Alonso, A., Diaz-Fernandez, M. J., Arnott, I., & Ferrer-Barriendos, J. (2010). Soy isoflavones, Mediterranean diet, and physical exercise in postmenopausal women with insulin resistance. *Menopause, 17*(2), 372-378.

[31]Barnes, S. (2010). The biochemistry, chemistry and physiology of the isoflavones in soybeans and their food products. *Lymphatic Research and Biology, 8*(1), 89-98. doi: 10.1089/lrb.2009.0030

[32]Teas, J., Braverman, L. E., Kurzer, M. S., Pino, S., Hurley, T.G., & Hebert, J. R. (2007). Seaweed and soy: companion foods in Asian cuisine and their effects on thyroid function in American women. *Journal of Medicinal Food, 10*(1), 90-100.

[33]Teas, J., Baldeón, M. E., Chiriboga, D. E., Davis, J. R., Sarriés, A. J., & Braverman, L. E. (2009). Could dietary seaweed reverse the metabolic syndrome? *Asia Pacific Journal of Clinical Nutrition, 18*(2), 145-154.

[34]Avena, N. M., Rada, P., & Hoebel, B. G. (2009). Sugar and fat bingeing have notable differences in addictive-like behavior. *Journal of Nutrition, 139*(3), 623-628.

[35]Gearhardt, A. N., Grilo, C. M., DiLeone, R. J., Brownell, K. D., & Potenza, M. N. (2011). Can food be addictive? Public health and policy implications. *Addiction, 106*(7), 1208-1212. doi: 10.1111/j.1360-0443.2010.03301.x

[36]Davis, C., Curtis, C., Levitan, R. D., Carter, J. C., Kaplan, A. S., & Kennedy, J. L. (2011). Evidence that "food addiction" is a valid phenotype of obesity. *Appetite, 57*(3), 711-717. doi: 10.1016/appet.2011.08.017

[37]Coelho, J. S., Polivy, J., & Herman, C. P. (2006). Selective carbohydrate or protein restriction: Effects on subsequent food intake and cravings. *Appetite, 47,* 352-360.

[38]Polivy, J. (1996). Psychological consequences of food restriction. *Journal of the American Dietetic Association, 96*(6), 589-592.

[39]Wilcox, S., & Storandt, M. (1996). Relations among age, exercise, and psychological variables in a community sample of women. *Health Psychology, 15*(2), 111-113.

[40]Roussel, M., Garnier, S., Lemoine, S., Gaubert, I., Charbonnier, L., Auneau, G., & Mauriège, P. (2009). Influence of a walking program on the metabolic risk profile of obese postmenopausal women. *Menopause, 16*(3), 566-575.

[41]Nikander, R., Gagnon, C., Dunstan, D. W., Magliano, D. J., Ebeling, P. R., Lu, Z. X., Zimmet, P. Z., Shaw, J. E., & Daly, R. M. (2011). Frequent walking, but not total physical activity, is associated with increased fracture incidence: A 5-year follow-up of an Australian population-based prospective study (AusDiab). *Journal of Bone and Mineral Research, 26*(7), 1638-1647. doi: 10.1002/jbmr.363

[42]Wilcox et al. (1996). Op. Cit.

[43]Bandura, A. (2004). Health promotion by social cognitive means. *Health Education & Behavior, 31*(2), 143-164. doi:10.1177/1090198104263660

[44]Bandura, A. (1977). Self-efficacy: Toward a unifying theory of behavioral change. *Psychological Review, 84*(2), 191-215.

[45]Hankonen, N., Absetz, P., Ghisletta, P., Renner, B., & Uutela, A. (2010). Gender differences in social cognitive determinants of exercise adoption. *Psychology and Health, 25*(1), 55-69.

[46]Phongsavan, P., McLean, G., & Bauman, A. (2007). Gender differences in influences of perceived environmental and psychosocial correlates on recommended level of physical activity among New Zealanders. *Psychology of Sport and Exercise, 8*(6), 939-950.

[47]Warner, L. M., Ziegelmann, J. P., Schuz, B., Wurm, S., & Schwarzer, R. (2011). Synergistic effect of social support and self-efficacy on physical exercise in older adults. *Journal of Aging and Physical Activity, 19*(3), 249-261.

[48]Harada, K., Oka, K., Shibata, A., Ishil, K., Nakamura,Y., Inoue, S., & Shimomitsu, T. (2011). Strength-training behavior and perceived environment among Japanese older adults. *Journal of Aging and Physical Activity, 19*(3), 262-272.

[49]Maffei, M., Halaas, J., Ravussin, E., Pratley, R. E., Zhang, Y., Fei, H., Kim, S., Lallone, R., Ranganathan, S., Kern, P. A., & Friedman, J. M. (1995). Leptin levels in human and rodent: Measurement of plasma leptin and *ob* RNA in obese and weight-reduced subjects. *Nature Medicine, 1(*11), 1155-1161.

[50]Gudbergsen, H., Boesen, M., Christensen, R., Astrup, A., & Bliddal, H. (2011). Radiographs and low field MRI (0.2T) as predictors of efficacy in a weight loss trial in obese women with knee osteoarthritis. *BMC Musculoskeletal Disorders, 12*, 56. Advance Online Publication. doi: 10.1186/1471-2474-12-56

[51]Riecke, B. F., Christensen, R., Christensen, P., Leeds, A. R., Boesen, M., Lohmander, L. S., Astrup, A., & Bliddal, H. (2010). Comparing two low-energy diets for the treatment of knee osteoarthritis symptoms in obese patients: A pragmatic randomized trial. *Osteoarthritis and Cartilage, 18*(6), 746-754.

Chapter Nine

Healing from the "Outside" – External

Treatments and Applications

■

For many of us, it may be hard to obtain complete relief from our menopausal arthritis solely through what we eat or the supplements that we take. Muscle strengthening and/or weight loss may not seem to be providing full relief, either. What is happening for many women is that there can be some problems less amenable to healing through supplements, exercise, and weight loss alone. These problems include injuries and displacement of soft tissues. There may also be some concentrated areas around the joint where pro-inflammatory cytokines and related chemicals may build up and become "trapped." This can occur within the tissues surrounding the joint and even within the muscle (as noted earlier). If this is the case, help may be needed from the "outside" in conjunction with the other healing measures taken. These external healing practices would include the application of healing oils, creams, and natural substances such as mud packs. They would also include manipulation of the muscles and joints through orthopedic massage and other techniques.

The foods, supplements, and herbs that we will be discussing in Chapter Ten have anti-inflammatory effects working directly upon the expression of cytokines within your body. External applications and treatments can help facilitate this process. They can help increase circulation and bring toxins to the surface, for example. This can facilitate the ability of the body's immune system to eliminate irritants and antigens which may be causing arthritis symptoms.

The Use of External Remedies in Ayurvedic and Traditional Chinese Medicine

The use of topicals and external treatments in healing arthritis is age-old, and traditions from Ayurveda to Traditional Chinese Medicine (dating back to 2,000 - 4,000 BC) have and continue to employ these practices. For example, in Ayurveda there are many medicated oils that are used to help provide external nourishment and to promote healing of the joints. The primary focus in Ayurveda, however, is on correcting low Agni (the energy that creates the digestive fire) in order to cure arthritis. In this healing tradition, arthritis is believed to be caused by improper digestion of foods that allows toxins (Ama) to accumulate within the colon and be transported into the joints. As a complementary practice, oils such as Mahanarayan Oil are massaged into the skin over the joint to decrease stiffness, stop pain, clear out toxins, and ease muscle fatigue. Sweating therapies are also used in Ayurveda in which steam, infused with herbs such as angelica or eucalyptus leaves, add to the potency of the treatment. Ayurveda also employs hot baths in mineral salts (such as Epsom salt) to soothe and help draw toxins out of the joints.[1]

In addition to Ayurveda, one can see this focus on both external and internal healing within Chinese Traditional Medicine as well. External interventions such as acupuncture and Chinese medical massage have traditionally been used to treat arthritis and other chronic diseases. These external remedies are often used in conjunction with herbal remedies, especially if there is any weakness of organs such as with the spleen or kidneys. However, chronic problems that involve body organs or the bowels would often be best corrected with herbal medicine. The cause of arthritis is viewed as arising out of energy imbalances within the body.

In Traditional Chinese Medicine the cause of arthritis is believed to result from "bi zheng" which means "impediment condition." The impediment is essentially seen as a blockage or an obstruction. Any "bi" or impediment condition is accompanied by pain. In Traditional Chinese Medicine, the proper functioning of the tendons and ligaments is the role of the liver. Chronic arthritis is viewed as a disorder that takes hold of the tendons and ligaments that encompass the joints. If the liver does not function properly, the blood may become deficient leading to stiff and dry sinews. In addition, the kidneys are believed to be insufficient in chronic arthritis conditions. They are in charge of proper functioning of the bones and bone marrow; this is why the kidneys are so important to the joint problems of arthritis within Traditional Chinese Medicine.[2]

Are There Empirical Links Between Traditional Healing Systems and Modern Medicine?

As noted above, in the healing tradition of Ayurveda, arthritis is caused by waste products or gases (toxins) absorbed by the colon that end up in the bones and the joints; these toxins are called "Ama." When the colon is not working properly, the toxins are moved into the joints.[3] This concept of "toxins" becoming localized within the joints as a cause of arthritis is not something that one will likely find in a search of the current medical literature. However, there is an ever-increasing knowledge with regard to the nature of proinflammatory cytokines in the processes of *both* rheumatoid arthritis *and* osteoarthritis, and these may be involved in promoting what could be considered to be "toxins."

For example, in osteoarthritis, inflammatory components have been detected in the synovial fluid to include proinflammatory cytokines (that we have discussed earlier) and immunoglobulins.[4] The research literature also shows that a *highly toxic*, free radical called peroxynitrite can be formed by nitric oxide released from synoviocytes (cells which form the membrane lining the joint) and chondrocytes (cartilage cells). Tumor necrosis factor is one of the cytokines that helps form toxic free radicals such as peroxynitrite. Toxic molecules such as peroxynitrite cause oxidative stress or a build-up of too many unwanted products of oxidation (the exposure to oxygen). The oxidative stress is a major cause of cell damage. When peroxynitrite is produced in areas of the body that are undergoing inflammation (in an acid condition) it creates the OH˙ radical (hydroxyl radical).[5] Of all of the highly reactive atoms and molecules that combine with oxygen in this way, OH˙ is the most highly toxic. A powerfully destructive, but short-lived free radical, it need only travel an extremely short distance before it does immense damage to another molecule. In fact, it is estimated that half of all the free radical damage in the human body (and in the body of any organism that uses oxygen to live) is a result of the action of highly toxic OH˙. Preventing macromolecular damage by OH˙ is vital, since these macromolecules (i.e., large, critical molecules such as lipids, proteins, and DNA) are essential to physical functioning.[6]

The damage to these macromolecules causes explicit dysfunction resulting from what is, in essence, a "mutilation" of these macromolecules by highly toxic radicals such as OH˙. Free radical damage is associated with oxidative damage; this has been likened to "rust" within the body tissues. The damage to macromolecules is of extreme importance; it goes beyond the analogy of oxidative damage as a kind of "rust," to something akin to the damaging disfigurement of these molecules.[7] The aggressive reactive oxygen species (ROS), such as OH˙, do not just cause oxidative damage which increases the vulnerability to enzymes that break down cartilage; rather, they also break up DNA and lipid structures, and fragment parts of the matrix. In addition, they cause oxidative damage that heightens the vulnerability of cartilage cells to proteases (enzymes that cause breakdown of proteins).[8] We had discussed earlier in Chapter Two how vital this cartilage matrix is to cellular growth and regeneration. When you see how destructive these effects are from highly toxic radicals such as OH˙, it is extremely clear why "antioxidants" are so critically important to include within your diet to heal. In fact, there is evidence within the literature that a low antioxidant status in rheumatoid arthritis patients is associated with disease activity and inflammation, as well as a higher risk of developing the disease.[9]

With regard to the highly toxic peroxynitrite, melatonin is able to directly neutralize it (and neutralize precursors to OH⁻ radicals such as hydrogen peroxide). Melatonin is a key antioxidant, and in addition to these direct effects, it has indirect antioxidant effects as well. There is evidence to suggest that the night time rise in melatonin may facilitate an increase in antioxidant enzymes helping to remove toxic chemicals from the body.[10]

Topic of Interest #13

The Evolving Picture of Melatonin

Recall from Chapter Seven, that melatonin can help activate your satellite cells and thus help with the repair of muscles following exercise. Well, melatonin plays a major role in fighting damaging free radicals such as OH⁻ as well. Melatonin is produced within the pineal gland. Can you imagine that until just 40 years ago, the pineal gland was thought to play no function of any real significance within the human body? Scientists now know that melatonin may affect physiological processes within every cell in the body. Just like cartilage, as described earlier in the book, melatonin is phylogenetically old. As a molecule, it is possible that it is present in all animals from primitive forms to human beings.

This amazing antioxidant is able to reduce the effects of lipid destruction that has been initiated by a great number of processes, from chemical processes in Alzheimer's disease to those involved in the exposure to ibuprofen, aspirin and alcohol. It is even protective of nuclear DNA (that which is more heavily involved in the hereditary or genetic aspects of a person). It provides protection even in the presence of radiation. Melatonin diminishes the effects of ionizing radiation and thus provides a radioprotective effect. This powerful antioxidant, however, declines with age. After one reaches middle age, its levels in the body are gradually reduced. As Dr. Russel J. Reiter, of the University of Texas Health Science Center observed, ". . . the adage that the older one gets the faster one ages may in part be a consequence of the gradual, albeit persistent, loss of melatonin during aging."[11]

Arthritis and the OH˙ Radical

How is OH˙ involved in arthritis? Reactive oxygen species (ROS) are by-products of cell metabolism. They are normal and indeed necessary for proper biological functioning. Some of these by-products, though, can lead to inflammation with a particularly critical role in joint disease. The problem is that if the amounts or the characteristics of these reactive oxygen species are altered, a variety of diseases can occur. In osteoarthritis there are profound changes to the cartilage matrix. IL-1ß is a primary mover in facilitating the disease process. Its effect is to decrease type 2 collagen and aggrecans (the main proteoglycans in cartilage). It also increases MMP 1 and 3. These metalloproteinases, as we saw earlier, break down cartilage. IL-1ß promotes nitric oxide (NO) production, and this, in turn leads to peroxynitrite (this highly toxic compound that we had just discussed earlier). What happens in rheumatoid arthritis? The cause of rheumatoid arthritis is still unknown. However, reactive oxygen species (ROS) are thought to possibly be involved. In rheumatoid arthritis patients, TNF-α is believed to be the main factor involved in the increased production of ROS.[12]

Many antigens common to both rheumatoid arthritis and osteoarthritis are associated with IgG (immunoglobulin G, a major class of immunoglobulins) in the joints. Immunoglobulins play a key role in the immune system, as they attach to bacteria and other foreign substances and help to destroy them. The IgG within the joints of rheumatoid arthritis and osteoarthritis patients differed significantly from that of normally circulating IgG. There was also a rheumatoid-specific subset of antigens found, and less IgG was found in osteoarthritis than in rheumatoid arthritis joints. Nevertheless, the fact that immune complexes exist in osteoarthritic joints too, and that there are common antigens within *both* diseases have been considered somewhat surprising in light of the earlier notions of osteoarthritis as a "mechanical disorder."[13]

Immune Complexes Can Become Trapped!

It was as far back as research in the 1970's, in which "trapped" immune complexes were actually detected within the joint tissues (e.g., the cartilage, menisci, and ligaments within the joint capsule). Dr. Hugo E. Jasin and colleague explained that there would be the presence of an antigen and then the immune response to it. An antigen is a substance, such as a toxin or bacteria for example, that stimulates the immune system to produce an antibody. However, Dr. Jasin's along with his colleague's research showed that this antigen and antibody pairing could become sequestered in joint tissues. The trapped immune complexes resulted in trapped antigens as well. These complexes of antigens and antibodies were observed to remain in the inflamed joints for long periods of time. If previously exposed to this antigen, then lymphocytes would be sensitized to it, and chronic inflammation would result. Since these immune complexes had been observed in rheumatoid arthritis patients, it was thought that this might help explain why cartilage and tendon deterioration occur in these patients.[14]   As was discussed in Chapter Six, however, in 1985 Dr. Jasin demonstrated that immune complexes were indeed found in *both* rheumatoid arthritis and osteoarthritis patients.

Later, in 1989 Dr. Jasin discussed the immune mechanisms in osteoarthritis. He noted that along with abnormalities in the cartilage structure, there was also synovial, or joint lining, inflammation. This inflammation could range from minimal to severe. He did not think that it would be likely that the initiation of the osteoarthritis inflammation was due to immune processes. Nevertheless, he conjectured that immune responses to cartilage macromolecules could be relevant to the continuance of the inflamed synovial lining in osteoarthritis. Interestingly, he did not discuss the possible sources or origins of this osteoarthritic inflammation because he believed that once the antigen interaction is induced, the inflammatory process follows a "common pathway" (regardless of the specific disease).[15] This pioneering and insightful work on inflammation in osteoarthritis paved the way for a better understanding of the disease process in osteoarthritis.

Trapped Immune Complexes and Toxins

Let's take a look back to the traditional healing practices discussed at the beginning of the chapter. Remaining "open" for a moment, could these trapped immune complexes in any way be likened to trapped "toxins" such as the toxins referred to as "Ama" in ayurvedic medicine? Or perhaps, could the antigen sequestered within the immune complex be considered a "toxin?" Let's come back for a moment to the example of the highly toxic free radical, peroxynitrite. The peroxynitrite that could be formed within the joint capsule is a toxin that contributes to damage. It does so not only in arthritis, but also in many neurodegenerative diseases. Damage by peroxynitrite is done by poisoning cells. It causes them serious harm or cell death. It is obviously of extreme importance to try to prevent peroxynitrite formation and the potential damage it could do to the joint lining and cartilage.

Attempting to understand possible reasons for muscle weakness in rheumatoid arthritis, researchers at the Karolinska Institutet in Sweden conducted an animal study on muscle function in collagen-induced arthritis. The study findings showed that peroxynitrite can impair muscle function. The researchers concluded that impaired contraction of the soleus muscle (a very strong muscle in the back of the calf) was due to changes in the proteins within the muscle fibers caused by peroxynitrite.[16] Muscle weakness is not only common in rheumatoid arthritis, but as we have seen, it is common in osteoarthritis as well. This could prove to be an extraordinary finding in terms of explaining muscle weakness in arthritis.

The fact that there might be toxins that modify and weaken muscle is extremely important. This is why I believe that many people suffering from arthritis may not always be able to benefit optimally from exercise. If inflammation (and toxins) are not being sufficiently controlled, countered, or neutralized through food and supplements, then the exercise will not be as effective. Topical applications and external treatments can partner here to enhance healing. It is very difficult to strengthen muscles that are simultaneously being weakened through destructive chemical processes brought on by the disease of arthritis. So, let's look at some of these topical and manual therapeutics that may work together with healing nutrients and exercises to alleviate menopausal arthritis.

Topical Treatments

Sometimes topical treatments can succeed in addressing inflammation around the joints when the supplements, foods, and herbs do not provide full relief. They may augment the anti-inflammatory effects of the supplements, foods, and herbs by direct application to the specific tissues involved.

---Oils

Oregano oil is a prime example of a topical application that can be quite effective (and it can also be used as a supplement - See Chapter Ten). Oregano oil has anti-inflammatory, antibacterial, and analgesic properties. The oil of oregano can be used topically by rubbing the oil into the skin covering the affected joint. According to Dr. Cass Ingram, a physician and researcher with expertise in the use of oil of oregano in healing, oil of oregano can be used for a wide variety of musculoskeletal conditions. Conditions in which it is considered to be helpful include arthritis, pulled muscles, tendonitis, bursitis, and neuritis.[17] As some of the problems that women may be experiencing as menopausal arthritis may include problems such as pes anserine bursitis (see Chapter 6), this herbal oil is especially helpful.

As Dr. Ingram stressed, the oil *must be from Wild Mediterranean Oregano.* He noted that there are many products on the market labeled as being oregano oil that are not; instead, these products are actually oils derived from thyme or marjoram. It is important to know that many of the oregano oils on the market are derived from "Spanish oregano" which is *not* oregano at all, but rather, thyme. Oil of thyme contains high amounts of thymol which can be toxic. The primary active component of oregano oil is carvacrol. You should make sure that the primary component in the oregano oil that you purchase is carvacrol and that the percentage of carvacrol is listed on the supplement label. It should contain 70% carvacrol.[18] I found this herbal oil to be very healing when applied topically (as directed) to the knee. The Gale Encyclopedia of Alternative Medicine provides a good overview of the safe and effective use of oregano oil both internally and externally.[19]

In Ayurveda, medicated oils are used to release and relax stiff joints, to provide nourishment to the joint tissues, and to clear away toxins that may be trapped within the joint tissues. There are four major oils in Ayurvedic medicine that are used to treat arthritis: Mahanarayan Oil, Narayan Oil, Sahachardi Oil, and Chandanabala-lakshadi Oil. Mahanarayan Oil is used to relieve stiff joints, improve their flexibility, treat muscle fatigue, and stop pain. It also provides skin nutrients. Narayan Oil is used for muscular and joint pain, and it stimulates circulation in the legs. It also helps prevent some of the negative effects of the aging process. Sahachardi Oil is used to treat rheumatoid arthritis. It is particularly effective in cases of muscular and nerve degeneration. Chandanabalalakshadi Oil is used to treat Pitta-type arthritis. This form of arthritis is characterized by inflammation, swelling and burning sensations, and pain that is made worse by heat.[20] On a personal note, I have found Mahanarayan oil to be helpful in reducing the feeling of tendon stiffness.

---*Mud Packs and Balneotherapy*

Mud packs or bathing in mineral waters are not something that many of us, in the United States anyways, think of right away when we are considering treatments for arthritis. However, spa therapies using healing mineral muds and balneotherapy date back thousands of years. Balneotherapy uses bathing as a healing treatment, often in mineral-rich waters or waters with clay or mud. Not only were healing mineral baths an essential aspect of cultures such as the early Greek and Roman, but also of cultures in the East such as ancient Japan. For hundreds of years in Europe, balneotherapy has been touted as effective in curing many diseases. It remains an integral component of mainstream medical practice in many of these countries to include France, Spain, Belgium, and Greece.

Mineral springs and spas have enjoyed some times of popularity in the United States, such as in the late 1800's, and in the 1930's and 1940's. In 1933, The Simon Baruch Research Institute at Saratoga Spa became the first research facility for balneotherapy; at this time it was accepted as a medical practice within the United States. President Franklin Delano Roosevelt had advocated for the new Saratoga Springs Spa in New York prior to being elected as President. Nevertheless, a trend toward scientific, evidence-based practices had already begun toward the end of the nineteenth century. The shift toward rapidly curing disease with modern medications had taken hold within the United States, making balneotherapy seem outdated. The lack of scientific evidence for the use of balneotherapy, and the attractiveness of these new medications, eventually led to the closure of many of the earlier, popular spas.[21]

Fortunately, with renewed interest in these healing methods, scientific research is being conducted. I had discussed earlier in the book, research that showed that mud packs were as effective as hyaluronic acid injections for improving pain in knee osteoarthritis. In this Turkish study, it was found that there was no significant difference between the group receiving the hyaluronic acid injection and the group receiving the mud packs on either functioning and/or pain scores following treatment.[22]

In another Turkish study, the differential effects of balneotherapy (warm mineral baths at 36 degrees centigrade), warm mud packs, and a control group with hot packs (no mud) were compared. The mud packs and hot packs were heated to the same temperature, 42 degrees centigrade. It was found that the distance that the patients could walk without experiencing pain was increased in both the balneotherapy and the mud pack groups, but not in the hot pack group. With regard to pain scores on the WOMAC scale, the hot pack group had an initial decrease in pain, but it was not maintained by the three months post-treatment follow-up as it was in the balneotherapy and mud pack groups. In addition, improvement in pain, physical mobility, and sleep were observed for the balneotherapy and mud pack groups and persisted as long as the follow-up three months later. The hot pack group did not have any change in pain, physical mobility, or sleep.[23]

In a randomized controlled study, osteoarthritis patients received treatment with either mineral-rich mud compresses or mineral-depleted mud compresses. All patients were assessed prior to treatment (consisting of five packs a week for three weeks), at the end of the treatment, and at one-month and three months thereafter. Assessments included self-reported pain, as well as the Lequesne Index of severity of knee osteoarthritis. The Lequesne Index assesses pain as it relates to specific activities and functional tasks. They found that the Dead Sea mud compresses significantly relieved self-reported pain more than the mineral-depleted mud compresses at the end of the three-week treatment period and at the one-month and three-month follow-up periods. In contrast, for the group receiving mineral-depleted mud there was no change or improvement in self-reported knee pain at any time. In fact, the differences in improvement were quite marked, with 72% of patients in the Dead Sea mud group having an improvement in self-reported knee pain, as compared with 33% in the mineral-depleted mud group. The Dead Sea mud-treated group also showed improvement on the Lequesne Index of severity of osteo-arthritis at the end of treatment and one month after.[24]

Is there evidence that mud pack or balneotherapy affect any of the specific chemical processes involved in inflammation and oxidative stress? In an Italian research study, the effects of mud pack therapy on cartilage cell markers were examined in osteoarthritis patients. It was found that 12 daily mud pack treatments (applied for 20 minutes at 40 degrees centigrade, with a 10-12 minute bath at 37-38 degrees centigrade afterwards) resulted in significantly changed cartilage markers. The mud pack treatment group significantly increased in IGF 1 (Insulin-like Growth Factor 1) levels, and significantly decreased in TNF-α levels. The control group showed no change in either of these markers.[25] IGF 1 is a protein that is similar in its structure to insulin. It has a protective effect on cartilage, and it inhibits the metalloproteases that break down cartilage. It also facilitates production of proteoglycans, so vitally important to the cartilage matrix. TNF-α, as described earlier in the book, is involved in activating metalloproteases and increasing inflammation. Decreasing TNF-α is critically important.

Animal studies also point toward the beneficial effects of mud therapy in arthritis. For example, in one such study, Brazilian mud applications were compared with warm water applications and with no treatment for animals that were induced to have chronic arthritis. It was found that after 21 days, the mud treatment reduced leukocyte migration into the synovial membrane and the joint cavity when compared with the water treatment group and the control group. Moreover, there was an increase in collagen, number of cartilage cells, and greater preserved tissue in the animals treated with mud.[26] Similarly, in another animal study of induced arthritis, mud-bath applications decreased inflammation in comparison to the control animals. In addition, the inflammatory cytokines TNF-α and IL-1β were significantly reduced in comparison with the control group animals.[27]

What could account for the effects of the mineral rich mud? It is interesting to consider some of the trace elements found in the Dead Sea mud in the study cited earlier that had compared the mineral-rich versus mineral-depleted compresses. The mineral-rich compresses included manganese, cobalt, boron, copper, zinc, bromine, rubidium and strontium.[28] Are these absorbed to produce a positive effect upon the arthritis process and pain? Studies have demonstrated that there were significant increases in serum concentrations or blood levels of calcium, zinc, bromine, and rubidium in arthritis patients who had bathed within the Dead Sea waters. In addition, an in vitro study showed that substances in mud extracts do have the capability of permeating the full thickness of the human skin, having decisive effects upon how smooth muscle contracts.[29]

In one study of knee osteoarthritis patients, the direct application of the mud pack to the skin was superior in reducing the severity of osteoarthritis compared with the application of mud over an impermeable nylon pack through which the minerals could not penetrate. Both treatments did significantly improve pain and functioning of knee osteoarthritis patients, but the direct application had more marked results. Since both treatments were heated, it could be concluded then, that the better results in the direct mud pack group were due to chemical substances within the mud.[30] Recall from the chapter on muscles and tendons that in one study, elastic tendon energy was proportionate to the mineral content of the tendon. If these minerals are absorbed into the tissues surrounding the joint as research seems to indicate, then perhaps it is not only the muscles, but also the tendons, and muscle-tendon units that are benefiting. This research on balneotherapy and mineral-rich mud pack treatment has provided some provocative and interesting scientific findings.

I tried Dead Sea mud directly applied to my skin with positive results. I bought the Dead Sea mud in bulk, and simply applied it to my knee and muscles around the knee. I did not heat it (it was room temperature), and I still obtained positive results. I left it on my knee for about 15 minutes, and then rinsed it off. My soft tissue pain was much reduced. The chemical substances within the mud seemed to have a direct effect upon some of the more persistent problems with soft tissue pain that I had been experiencing in the area of my shin-bone. It seemed to have a positive effect upon the muscle tissues as well.

Manual and Manipulation Techniques for Arthritis

---Correcting Dysfunctional Energy Patterns

Chinese medical massage, or "tui na" has been used to help alleviate obstructed energy flow. The term "tui na" means to push and grasp, although an extensive array of manipulations that involve actions other than pushing or grasping are employed. The use of massage extends to Chinese self-massage, as well. Techniques for self-massage include rubbing and kneading the body, as well as tapping and pinching. These techniques are used to open up the channels through which the life energy or "qi" flows. It is used for many joints affected by arthritis, to include the knee and shoulder.[31]

---Massage from a Western Standpoint

Massage as viewed from a Western approach serves many diverse functions. First and foremost it is considered to be based within the belief or philosophy of assisting the body in healing itself. Its benefits include positive effects upon mental and emotional well-being, as well as upon the musculoskeletal, lymphatic, circulatory, and other body systems. Massage can be used to relax muscle, decrease sensitivity in myofascial trigger points, and help to move the metabolic wastes or toxins into and through the lymph channels.[32]

---*Alleviating Myofascial Pain*

Many of us unfamiliar with the term "trigger points" may have inadvertently experienced them without knowing what they were. Perhaps when massaging some lotion into your leg (or when receiving a professional massage), you may have at some point noticed an unusually sensitive spot. If it were located within the quadriceps muscle group for example, then satellite trigger points from the quadriceps might have also developed in some of the surrounding muscles (such as semitendinosus or iliopsoas). There is an associated pain pattern from the various trigger points. For example, if a trigger point is within the rectus femoris muscle, then pain would be experienced localized in the front of the knee, and this pain could be experienced as deep within the joint itself.[33] The deep pain in the front part of your knee that you may think is caused by something from within the knee joint, might indeed, have its origin someplace completely different! The pain could be, of course, due to problems internal to the knee such as menisci or ligaments, but it also might *not* be caused by anything within the knee joint at all. Accurate and proper diagnosis is essential.

Trigger points are overly sensitive spots that are prone to heightened irritability or hyperirritability that are located within skeletal muscle. They are not the same thing as the "tender spots" within fibromyalgia syndrome. Unlike the multiple "tender spots" in fibromyalgia, trigger points may be singular or multiple and can be located in any skeletal muscle. This is in contrast to the specific locations characteristic of the fibromyalgia syndrome. Trigger points may also result in *a pattern of referred pain*. This is not the case with fibromyalgia tender spots in which pain is not referred, but is instead caused by a total body increase in sensitivity to pain. Repeated microtraumas (as might occur with joint problems, as we had discussed earlier), or repetitive stress on a particular muscle or muscle group are thought to be two important causes of trigger point development. Joint problems can also result in trigger points. Underuse of some muscles and overuse of others can be sources of trigger points, as well. They may develop, for example, in the quadriceps or calf muscles resulting in restricted movement or lessened range of motion in the knee and in the ankle.[34] Trigger points are located not only in skeletal muscle, but also in its associated fascia to include ligaments and other tissues.[35]

Myofascial pain (pain arising from the fascia that cover and surround muscles) can accompany osteoarthritis. Most medical training with regard to musculoskeletal pain usually focuses on the bones, joints, and surrounding nerves. As a result, many times this source of pain is missed. Myofascial pain results from trigger points in the muscle. In addition to microtraumas as precipitating causes (and also macrotraumas such as pulled muscles), the aging process can cause a loss of flexibility in the myofascial structures and contribute to myofascial pain. Estrogen and thyroid deficiencies (and vitamin and mineral deficiencies) have been implicated, as well. Myofascial pain can lead to joint dysfunction and even joint deterioration.[36] Many invasive treatment strategies have been used (such as injections with local anesthetics and dry needling); nevertheless, there are important non-invasive treatments such as physical therapy and massage.[37]

Dysfunctional muscle does have the ability to contract. The problem is that it does not go back to its normal shape afterwards. This chronic contraction and shortening of the muscle can result in restricted blood flow and a blockage of lymph drainage. Tissue changes occur, to include a decrease in suppleness. The affected muscles may seem to contain bands that feel like ropes or cords. Range of motion is impaired and level of functioning reduced. A non-invasive approach is to determine which muscles are involved in the restricted muscle functioning, identify taut bands and constrictions, and then palpate or massage the regions. In this way, additional constrictions are located. Specific techniques involving targeted palpation and compression are used to "capture" the taut bands. Ischemic compression is then used to soften the trigger points. This can be a complete treatment, although sometimes acupuncture needling may also be used.[38]

Ischemic compression is a massage technique consisting of sustained pressure (which may be maintained between 5 and 15 seconds or possibly longer at times) using the thumb to press down on the muscle. The trigger point area is the focal point of the ischemic compression. Dr. Raymond L. Nimmo is considered to have been a pioneer in this type of soft tissue therapy. He was one of the first practitioners to advocate and develop a theoretical basis for what has evolved into trigger point therapy. Dr. Nimmo had viewed these hypersensitive areas as being "abnormal neurological reflex arcs." He believed that the muscle was in a perpetual state of abnormal contraction (hypertonic muscle). He contended that by extending pressure to the affected muscle, a release of the muscle would occur through the nervous system.[39]

---*Joint Mobilization Techniques*

In Chapter Seven, we discussed passive joint mobilization therapies as one means of helping to restore range of motion and proper joint function. What can joint mobilization do for the ankle joint, for example? The purpose of joint mobilization is to decrease pain and to improve one's mobility. This is accomplished through helping to promote the flexibility of the connective tissues that surround the joint. In a study of older women with a mean age of 70 years, ankle joint mobilization was found to promote body equilibrium (maintaining a stable posture at a steady level) and increase range of motion (the ability to move one's joint freely and optimally within its range of movement). Forty women were randomly assigned to either the control group or the joint mobilization group. Each joint mobilization session lasted for 20 minutes and was performed three times a week over a period of four weeks. The gentle manipulations that are the essence of this type of therapy allowed for significant improvement in the ankle mobilization group in both foot and ankle flexion. Body sway also decreased.[40]

---*Orthopedic Massage - Soft Tissue Therapy*

In terms of my own healing from the pain produced by menopausal arthritis, no other external treatment has been as valuable to me as the form of soft tissue massage used by Thomas Hendrickson, DC and described within his 2003 manual, "Massage for Orthopedic Conditions."[41] Not only did it resolve the pain at the inner, middle of my knee that would just not go away no matter what I did, but it provided an answer as to *why* the pain was there in the first place.

Dr. Hendrickson trained with Lauren Barry, RPT who had formulated a method to correct mechanical dysfunctions in the body by manipulation of the soft tissues and the joints. Of much interest and importance, Lauren Barry had theorized that the soft tissues within the body have a specific relationship and position with regard to other soft tissues and to the accompanying joints. He was able to identify patterns of soft tissue displacement throughout the body. To correct for tissue malposition and dysfunction, he devised a method of manipulating these tissues that involved massage applied in very specific directions. Dr. Hendrickson has built upon the theoretical bases of Lauren Barry and has developed his own technique of manipulation of soft tissues. The basic form of massage is applied perpendicular or transverse to the line of the tissue fibers. The goal is to reposition the soft tissues and bring them back into a normal alignment with each other. In so doing, "twists" or "torsions" of the tissue are corrected, and microscopic adhesions and crosslinks which have formed in distorted patterns are dissolved.[42]

I could actually *feel* these adhesions or crosslinks in the tissues of the inner, medial side of my knee. They were obvious and palpable when I massaged the tissues toward the middle of my knee and away from the outside of my knee. Prior to learning of this technique, I had no idea that these abnormal crosslinks or adhesions were even there. After changing the position of the soft tissues that had migrated out of place, and breaking up or dissolving the microscopic adhesions or crosslinks, the pain in the inner middle side of my knee had disappeared. I was astounded to find such a profound difference in the way my knee felt.

According to Dr. Thomas Hendrickson, one of the causes of knee problems is the positional dysfunctioning of knee muscles. Gracilis, sartorius and semitendinosus tendons, at their attachment site of the pes anserinus, can twist posteriorly or outwardly. So, too, can the medial collateral ligament (MCL). The iliotibial band (ITB) may also move into a posterior position with the lateral collateral ligament (LCL) doing the same. The hamstrings, gastrocnemius and soleus have a tendency to shorten, and then shift inwards toward the midline of the leg.[43]

Could these abnormal changes in position of these muscles, tendons and ligaments be causing what many women experience as pain from menopausal arthritis? I believe that this may, indeed, be the case in many instances. Dr. Hendrickson discussed that many of his older patients with knee pain had been told that they were just getting older. However, most of these patients had knee pain primarily in one knee and as Dr. Hendrickson pointed out, the non-symptomatic knee is just as old as the knee with the problem! He emphasized that prior injuries or accumulated stresses may result in an imbalance in knee alignment and in dysfunction. To have fit and properly functioning knees, one must have proper alignment of the pelvis, feet, and ankles.[44] This form of orthopedic massage is one of the most important external healing techniques that I have encountered.

Topic of Interest #14

Checking the Lower Body for Alignment: Are You Valgus or Varus?

In my research on osteoarthritis, I had come across studies that discussed how the alignment of the lower body as either valgus (knock-kneed), or varus (bow-legged) made a difference in the disease progression of osteoarthritis. I thought that this was indeed interesting but had no relevance to my own situation; I was not either knock-kneed or bow-legged.

However, I was wrong! Although I thought that I looked perfectly normal in alignment, I was very surprised to find out that I had a valgus alignment or knock-kneed alignment (even if not extreme). It turns out, that if in a standing position the knees touch and the ankles do not, then one has a valgus alignment (even if it may be mild enough that one does not actually look "knock-kneed" in appearance). On the other hand, if the ankles touch, and one has more than two finger-widths between the knees, then one is considered to have a varus (or bow-legged) alignment.[45]

Does this matter in terms of osteoarthritis? A review of the literature on knee alignment and the risk for the development and progression of knee osteoarthritis was recently conducted. Although the reviewers of the literature found only limited evidence that knee malalignment may be a factor in the *development* of radiographic osteoarthritis, there was strong evidence found that knee malalignment is a risk factor for the *progression* of osteoarthritis. Specifically, knee valgus alignment is associated with lateral knee compartment osteoarthritis progression, and varus alignment with medial knee osteoarthritis progression.[46]

From a biomechanical perspective, there is a greater load that passes medially rather than laterally even in healthy knees that have a neutral alignment. Varus alignment serves to increase the already present load on the medial compartment of the knee. Valgus alignment is associated with an increased load on the lateral compartment. Nevertheless, unless there is a severe valgus alignment, the medial compartment will often persist in bearing the brunt of the load.[47]

I might be inclined to dismiss my valgus alignment, then, as probably not that contributory to my knee pain if I were only considering osteoarthritis (and menopausal arthritis) from a more traditional medical perspective. However, if one looks at the knee alignment from a more complex and expanded perspective of arthritis, then the valgus alignment does matter.

Dr. Thomas Hendrickson has referred to the valgus malalignment as being "the classic postural dysfunction of the lower extremity."[48] It represents the taxing effects of gravity on the body rendering it into a collapsed position. As such, soft tissues tend to move out of the positions that they should be in with respect to other soft tissues and the surrounding joint, as described earlier.[49] It is quite clear that knee alignment matters, and may have a significant effect upon what might be experienced as menopausal arthritis pain.

Working on Your Arthritis Pain from the "Inside" and the "Outside"

It may not always be possible to eliminate arthritis by internal means; that is, we may not always be able to achieve the results that we want from the foods, herbs, and supplements that we take internally. Sometimes the immune system and your body's overall healing resources are simply overloaded. Fighting arthritis from the outside with external applications and treatment procedures may be needed as a complementary measure to achieve healing.

The combination of using external treatments in healing along with internal treatments has been viewed as important in medical traditions that span hundreds and thousands of years. Moreover, external treatments may not always serve only as supplementary therapeutics. Indeed, as we have seen within this chapter, they can also fulfill a primary purpose of correcting body dysfunction such as soft tissue malalignment, for example. In Chapter Twelve, I will discuss how you can incorporate some of these extremely effective external treatment procedures into your overall plan to heal your menopausal arthritis.

From age-old balneotherapy and mineral-rich mud packs to insightful and innovative orthopedic massage techniques, your options for external healing are rich and plentiful. So, heal "from the inside" with important anti-inflammatory foods, herbs, and supplements, but do not overlook or miss exploring the powerful potential of "healing from the outside!"

Notes for Chapter Nine

[1]Frawley, D. (2000). Ayurvedic healing: A comprehensive guide. (2nd Ed.) Twin Lakes, WI: Lotus Press.

[2]Frank, D., & Flaws, B. (1997). Curing arthritis naturally with Chinese Medicine. Boulder, CO: Blue Poppy Press.

[3]Frawley (2000). Op. Cit.

[4]Amin, A. R., Attur, M., Patel, R. N., Thakker, G. D., Marshall, P. J., Rediske, J., Stuchin, S. A., Patel, I. R., & Abramson, S. B. (1997). Superinduction of Cyclooxygenase-2 activity in human osteoarthritis-affected cartilage: Influence of nitric oxide. *Journal of Clinical Investigation, 99*(6), 1231-1237.

[5]Darlington, L. G., & Stone, T. W. (2001). Antioxidants and fatty acids in the amelioration of rheumatoid arthritis and related disorders. *British Journal of Nutrition, 85*, 251-269.

[6]Reiter, R. J. (2000). Melatonin: Lowering the high price of free radicals. *News in Physiological Sciences, 15*, 246-250.

[7]Ibid.

[8]Afonso, V. , Champy, R., Mitrovic, D., Collin, P., & Lomri, A. (2007). Reactive oxygen species and superoxide dismutases: Role in joint diseases. *Joint Bone Spine, 74*, 324-329.

[9]Henrotin, Y., Kurz, B., & Aigner, T. (2005). Review -- Oxygen and reactive oxygen species in cartilage degradation: friends or foes? *Osteoarthritis and Cartilage, 13*, 643-654.

[10]Reiter (2000). Op. Cit.

[11]Ibid.

[12]Afonso et al. (2007). Op. Cit.

[13]Monach, P. A., Hueber, W., Kessler, B., Tomooka, B. H., BenBarak, M., Simmons, B. P., Wright, J., Thornhill, T. S., Monestier, M., Ploegh, H., Robinson, W. H., Mathis, D., & Benoist, C. (2009). A broad screen for targets of immune complexes decorating arthritic joints highlights deposition of nucleosomes in rheumatoid arthritis. *Proceedings of the National Academy of Sciences, 106*(37), 15867-15872. doi: 10.1073/pnas.0908032106

[14]Jasin, H. E., & Cooke, T. D. (1978). The inflammatory role of immune complexes trapped in joint collagenous tissues. *Clinical and Experimental Immunology, 33*, 416-424.

[15]Jasin, H. E. (1989). Immune mechanisms in osteoarthritis. *Seminars in Arthritis and Rheumatism, 18(4)*, 86-90.

[16]Yamada, T., Place, N., Kosterina, N., Ostberg, T., Zhang, S. J., Grundtman, C., Erlandsson-Harris, H., Lundberg, I. E., Glenmark, B., Bruton, J. D., & Westerblad, H. (2009). Impaired myofibrillar function in the soleus muscle of mice with collagen-induced arthritis. *Arthritis and Rheumatism, 60* (11), 3280-3289.

[17]Ingram, C. (2001). *The cure is in the cupboard: How to use oregano for better health.* Buffalo Grove, IL: Knowledge House.

[18]Ibid.

[19]Oregano essential oil. In L. J. Fundukian (Ed.) (2009). *The Gale encyclopedia of alternative medicine* (3rd ed.) (pp. 1638-1641). Detroit: Gale.

[20]Frawley (2000). Op. Cit.

[21]Altman, N. (2000). *Healing springs: The ultimate guide to taking the waters.* Rochester, VT: Healing Arts Press.

[22]Bostan, B., Sen, U., Günes, T., Sahin, S.A., Sen, C., Erdem, M., & Erkorkmaz, U. (2010). Comparison of intra-articular hyaluronic acid injections and mud-pack therapy in the treatment of knee osteoarthritis. *Acta Orthopaedica et Traumatologica Turcica, 44*(1), 42-47. doi: 10.1016/j.jbspin.2006.03.009

[23]Evcik, D., Kavuncu, V., Yeter, A., & Yigit, I. (2007). The efficacy of balneotherapy and mud-pack therapy in patients with knee osteoarthritis. *Joint Bone Spine, 74*, 60-65.

[24]Flusser, D., Abu-Shakra, M., Friger, M., Codish, S., & Sukenik, S. (2002). Therapy with mud compresses for knee osteoarthritis: Comparison of natural mud preparations with mineral-depleted mud. *Journal of Clinical Rheumatology, 8*(4), 197-203.

[25]Bellometti, S., Cecchettin, M., & Galzigna, L. (1997). Mud pack therapy in osteoarthrosis. Changes in serum levels of chondrocyte markers. *Clinica Chimica Acta, 268*, 101-106.

[26]Britschka, Z. M., Teodoro, W. R., Velosa, A. P., & de Mello, S. B. (2007). The efficacy of Brazilian black mud treatment in chronic experimental arthritis. *Rheumatology International, 28*(1), 39-45.

[27]Cozzi, F., Carrara, M., Sfriso, P., Todesco, S., & Cima, L. (2004). Anti-inflammatory effect of mud-bath applications on adjuvant arthritis in rats. *Clinical and Experimental Rheumatology, 22*(6), 763-766.

[28]Flusser et al. (2002). Op. Cit.

[29]Fioravanti, A., Cantarini, L., Guidelli, G. M., & Galeazzi, M. (2011). Mechanisms of action of spa therapies in rheumatic diseases: What scientific evidence is there? *Rheumatology International, 31*, 1-8.

[30]Odabasi, E., Turan, M., Erdem, H., & Tekbas, F. (2008). Does mud pack treatment have any chemical effect? A randomized controlled clinical study. *Journal of Alternative and Complementary Medicine, 14*(5), 559-565.

[31]Frank et al. (1997). Op. Cit.

[32]Freeman, L. (2009). *Mosby's complementary & alternative medicine: A research-based approach* (3rd Ed.). St. Louis, MO: Mosby Elsevier.

[33]Finando, D., & Finando, S. (2005). *Trigger point therapy for myofascial pain: The practice of informed touch.* Rochester, VT: Healing Arts Press.

[34]Alvarez, D. J., & Rockwell, P. G. (2002). Trigger points: Diagnosis and management. *American Family Physician, 65*(4), 653-661.

[35]Finando et al. (2005). Op. Cit.

[36]Yap, E.-C. (2007). Myofascial pain - An overview. *Annals of the Academy of Medicine Singapore, 36*, 43-48.

[37]Lavelle, E. D., Lavelle, W., & Smith, H. S. (2007). Myofascial trigger points. *Anesthesiology Clinics, 25*(4), 841-851.

[38]Finando et al. (2005). Op. Cit.

[39]Hains, G. (2002). Locating and treating low back pain of myofascial origin by ischemic compression. *Journal of the Canadian Chiropractic Association, 46*(4), 257-264.

[40]Gong, W., Park, G. D., & Ma, S. (2011). The influence of ankle joint mobilization on ROM of the ankle joint and maintenance of equilibrium in elderly women. *Journal of Physical Therapy Science, 23*, 217-219.

[41]Hendrickson, T. (2003). *Massage for orthopedic conditions.* Philadelphia, PA: Lippincott Williams & Wilkins.

[42]Ibid.

[43]Ibid.

[44]Ibid

[45]Ibid.

[46]Tanamas, S., Hanna, F. S., Cicuttini, F. M., Wluka, A. E., Berry, P, & Urquhart, D. M. (2009). Does knee malalignment increase the risk of development and progression of knee osteoarthritis? *Arthritis & Rheumatism, 61*(4), 459-467. doi: 10.1002/art.24336

[47]Sharma, L., Song, J., Dunlop, D., Felson, D., Lewis, C. E., Segal, N., Torner, J., Cooke, D. V., Heitpas, J., Lynch, J., & Nevitt, M. (2010). Varus and valgus alignment and incident and progressive knee osteoarthritis. *Annals of the Rheumatic Diseases, 69*(11), 1940-1945. doi: 10.1136/ard.2010.129742

[48]Hendrickson (2003). Op. Cit.

[49]Ibid.

Chapter Ten

Food, Supplements, and Herbs for Menopausal Arthritis

Powerful Partners in Fighting Menopausal Arthritis

Food is good medicine, of course. However, sometimes we just do not have the needed information to know what foods (and nutritional supplements) can help us get rid of our arthritis. Herbs, too, can have dramatic effects on arthritis symptoms. Much of what we learn about herbs may be through the writings of traditional herbalists whose knowledge base stems from the time-honored practice of empirical observation; that is, the reported experiences of which herbs work for particular ailments. This is fine for many of us who are inclined toward alternative medicine and the non-Western healing methods in which vital information has often been gained in this manner. Medicine of earlier times, and traditional medicine practices, were based upon the experiences of healing and the collected observations of what worked. They were not based upon experimental, scientific studies.

However, for many of us, we want to see the "proof," the scientific evidence. So, as such, this chapter will look at herbs, foods, and supplements that research shows may be effective for arthritis. Since information on supplements to help alleviate arthritis is often not accompanied by scientific reviews of how effective individual supplements are, I will try to fill that gap within this chapter. We will look at the scientific studies and what they have found. With this information, you can begin to eat foods and take herbal and vitamin supplements that, based upon research, may be able to decrease your symptoms of arthritis. These foods, herbs, and supplements have been found to help check inflammation, change your metabolism, and reduce arthritis symptoms.

Good nutrition using key foods, herbs, and supplements will go a long way in helping to alleviate menopausal arthritis, even prior to any weight loss (if weight loss is indicated). Of course, the advice holds throughout this book that you should consult first with your physician or medical doctor to determine what interventions are appropriate for you. It is important to know whether the supplements, vitamins, foods, and exercises within this program are suitable for you and any disorders that you may be experiencing.

Vitamins, Minerals, and Phytonutrients

Vitamin K: Its Newly Discovered Role in Fighting Arthritis

In addition to the scientific research on hormones and arthritis in menopause, important new studies point toward a dynamic connection between some foods and supplements and cartilage health. For example, did you know that vitamin K intake may play an important role in protecting one from hand and knee arthritis? This is what a research team found in the Framingham Offspring Study. Osteoarthritis, joint space narrowing, and osteophytes (bony outgrowths) of the hand were significantly reduced with increased vitamin K intake levels. Additionally, knee bone spurs or bony outgrowths (and the number of knee joints afflicted with them) were decreased as vitamin K intake levels increased.[1] Moreover, in a study conducted out of the University of Tokyo, researchers found that the greater the vitamin K intake within the elderly population examined, the less presence of osteoarthritis of the knee. In fact, these researchers even found less knee joint space narrowing with greater vitamin K intake.[2] Vitamin K is found in many dark green plant sources to include vegetables such as kale, Swiss chard, broccoli, and fresh parsley. A simple dietary change could go a long way in promoting healing from osteoarthritis!

Niacinamide -- Shown To Be Effective Long Ago, but Often Overlooked

Over fifty years ago, Dr. William Kaufman discovered that high doses of niacinamide, a form of vitamin B-3, helped his patients to be free from osteoarthritis and rheumatoid arthritis pain. The observation that niacinamide helped alleviate arthritis was a chance discovery. In a study of 150 patients being treated for a deficiency in niacin (which Dr. Kaufman termed "aniacinamidosis"), he noticed that arthritis symptoms also improved.

The niacinamide deficiency that Dr. Kaufman observed in his patients prior to 1943 included changes in skin texture, subcutaneous swellings, liver tenderness and enlargement, and tenderness of cartilage and muscle to pressure, to name just a few of the manifestations of deficiency. Between 1945 and 1947, Dr. Kaufman performed a further study using niacinamide therapy for 455 patients (both male and female) in his private practice. In treating these patients he found that it did not matter what other diseases the patients had (e.g., gallbladder disease, irritable colon, duodenal ulcer, postmenopausal osteoarthritis, among many ailments) *the joint dysfunction responded to the niacinamide in a predictable manner of improvement.* In contrast, for those who did not undergo treatment with niacinamide, joint deterioration seemed to exceed the process of joint repair. However, if the joint damage or deformation was too advanced, he believed that it might be beyond repair through niacinamide therapy. To determine this, he advised that an adequate trial period would be needed. Dr. Kaufman found that the best way to administer niacinamide was in smaller doses across the entire day. So, for example, he emphasized that 300 mg. of niacinamide taken three times a day, was not as therapeutic as 150 mg. taken 6 times a day (every three hours).[3] I have included within the Appendix a source for niacinamide in 100 mg. tablets, as most that are commonly available in retail stores contain a much higher dose of 500 mg. (or 250 mg.) per tablet.

The connection between alleviation of joint pain and niacinamide was clear from his careful and meticulously recorded clinical observations of his private patients. Nevertheless, it was not until 1996 that a randomized, controlled trial of niacinamide confirmed Dr. Kaufman's earlier findings.[4] In an experimentally controlled study out of the Office of Alternative Medicine of the National Institutes of Health (NIH), the findings indicated that niacinamide *did* improve osteoarthritis. The researchers found that it improved the flexibility of the joints and that it reduced inflammation in comparison with the control group without supplementation. Moreover, those who had taken niacinamide as a supplement were able to reduce their use of anti-inflammatory medications compared to those who had not received the niacinmide.[5] It has also been shown that niacinamide was able to suppress some of the chemical processes of cytokines that contribute to osteoarthritis.[6]

Information on niacinamide from the Natural Medicines Comprehensive Database provided by the U.S. National Library of Medicine (National Institutes of Health) outlines the benefits and uses of niacinamide and provides guidelines for proper dosage. It is important to note here that the two forms of B-3, niacin and niacinamide, work differently in high doses within the body and are used for different health problems. Since large doses can cause serious side effects (especially so for people with certain medical conditions), following the guidelines of NIH for usage is important.[7] Likewise, it would also be important to consult with your medical doctor with regard to whether taking niacinamide is appropriate for you.

Vitamin D -- Muscle Activator and Inflammation Reducer

Vitamin D is an extremely important vitamin, and deficiencies of it are higher in menopausal women due to loss of estrogen. This is because there are changes in vitamin D synthesis following estrogen loss in menopause. As a result, postmenopausal women are at increased risk for bone loss, hypertension, malignancy, and diabetes. Deficiencies of vitamin D in postmenopausal women may lead to muscle weakness, postural instability and increased falls, and osteoporotic bone fractures. There is even some evidence to suggest that a deficiency in vitamin D may increase the risk for cognitive impairment.[8]

Vitamin D is important in the body's immune responses. It has been shown to modulate the activities of immune cells within the body. Blood levels of vitamin D have been found to be lower in several autoimmune diseases such as systemic lupus erythematosus and type 1 diabetes. Moreover, lower levels of vitamin D were associated with higher levels of disease activity in rheumatoid arthritis.[9]

Is vitamin D actually involved in the physiology of the disease process in osteoarthritis? One animal research study looking specifically at chronic arthritis found that the vitamin D receptors were important in curtailing inflammation. If there were no signals from vitamin D receptors, inflammation increased and so did cartilage destruction and bone erosion. A lack of vitamin D receptors in cells led to an over-receptiveness to TNF (tumor necrosis factor) stimulation and to cytokine production. An overproduction of TNF, as discussed earlier, can lead to degradation of the cartilage matrix.[10]

As discussed in Chapter Four, ensuring muscle health is critical in helping to prevent and alleviate symptoms of menopausal arthritis. It is very important to note that skeletal muscle has been found to contain vitamin D receptors; for muscles to optimally function they may, thus, require vitamin D. Muscle weakness is one of the primary signs of a deficiency of this vitamin.[11] Supplementation with vitamin D has been found to improve muscle performance on tests, reduce falls, and it is hypothesized that it may have an impact upon the actual composition of the muscle fibers.[12]

In one study of elderly adults, there was a relationship between fatty degeneration of the thigh muscles and vitamin D deficiency. Low levels of vitamin D were directly associated with higher infiltration of fat into the muscles. In fact, one of the thigh muscles observed had complete fatty degeneration! The fatty degeneration of the muscles was also associated with problems in balance and gait.[13] This fat infiltration into muscle has possibly been an unseen or overlooked problem in the elderly. The negative effects upon balance and gait are especially important. Many times, we may think more toward the neurological aspects of balance; we may not fully apprehend how devastating something like fat infiltration into muscle can be to older people's ability to navigate the environment.

Linkages between patients' symptoms of general muscle weakness, muscle aches and pains, and vitamin D deficiency have also been reported. Vitamin D is critical to neuromuscular functioning. Within the skeletal muscle cells, it helps facilitate actions involving calcium transport, protein synthesis, and muscle contraction. Body sway (or the oscillation of the body when standing erect) is a neuromuscular function. Vitamin D supplementation has been shown to help lessen body sway and to help in reducing falls.[14]

In a German study of 242 community-dwelling older people, the effects of vitamin D and calcium supplementation were explored with regard to the incidence of falling. Specifically, the researchers were looking at first incidences of falling among the elderly. In comparison with calcium only supplementation, calcium plus vitamin D was far more effective in reducing the number of falls. There was a decrease in first falls of 39% at 20 months of supplementation. Quadriceps strength also increased, and there was a 28% decrease in body sway.[15] In a review of the literature, it has been suggested that a dose of at least 800 IU per day would be important to provide postmenopausal women the most beneficial effect upon bone and muscle health.[16]

Finally, vitamin D levels may be related to joint pain in postmenopausal women. Vitamin D is converted by the liver into 25-hydroxyvitamin D - [25(OH)D]. In a study conducted out of the Los Angeles Biomedical Research Institute at Harbor/UCLA Medical Center, lower blood levels of 25(OH)D were related to greater joint pain in these postmenopausal women.[17] The main circulating form of vitamin D within the body is 25(OH)D, and its level is used to determine vitamin D status. As previously discussed, joint pain is experienced widely by women in menopause. Vitamin D may be a very helpful supplement to reduce joint pain in conjunction with anti-inflammatory supplements.

Other Vitamins

I have focused upon vitamins D, K, and niacinamide as there are some solid research findings behind these vitamins in their effects upon inflammation and arthritis. Vitamins C, E, A and minerals such as selenium are antioxidants. In theory, they might seem to have potential in providing beneficial effects upon arthritis. However, a recent review of randomized clinical trials found contradictory findings for vitamin E, and no compelling evidence for any positive effects of selenium, vitamin A, or vitamin C.[18] Personally, I have found selenium to be helpful in menopausal arthritis. Perhaps part of the effectiveness that I perceive with selenium is due to its association with muscle strength. For example, in the large InCHIANTI study of older community dwelling adults (age 65 years or older), researchers explored the relationship between skeletal muscle strength and older adult's selenium levels. They assessed hip flexion, grip, and knee extension strength and measured the participants' plasma selenium levels. Those adults in the bottom most quartile of plasma selenium were at a significantly greater risk for lower hip and knee flexion strength, and there was a trend toward lower grip strength. This was found after adjusting for other factors such as age, gender, body mass index, and chronic disease.[19] As discussed earlier in the book, the importance of muscle strength in preventing or correcting menopausal arthritis symptoms cannot be overstated! In light of this marked effect of selenium on muscle, it is a very important mineral to consider including in your healing plan.

I also take supplements of vitamin C, E (d-alpha tocopherol *plus mixed tocopherols*) and vitamin A (from fish oil) as they help to provide a strong nutritional ground base for healing. In addition, I take a vitamin B complex supplement (50 mg.), plus small doses of niacinamide (100 mg.) several times a day. As per Dr. William Kaufman's findings noted earlier in this chapter, I do notice a difference in my menopausal arthritis symptoms with improvement using niacinamide.

Resveratrol (and Other Polyphenols) -- Formidable Inflammation Fighters

I'm sure most people have heard of resveratrol, the polyphenol found in grapes and red wine that is a powerful antioxidant. It is often associated with its heart protective effects.[20,21] However, recent research has demonstrated that it may protect your cartilage cells by suppressing the damaging inflammatory chemicals and cell destruction mediators within arthritis.[22] Resveratrol protects against the inflammatory cytokine IL-1-beta's destructive effects by preventing cartilage cell destruction. This is accomplished partly through resveratrol's inhibition of the process in which COX-2 facilitates the synthesis of prostaglandin E2.[23] In addition, remember the connection between obesity and arthritis regarding the association with proinflammatory cytokines? Well, in one animal study, resveratrol helped suppress some of the production of visceral fat and the production of inflammatory cytokines such as TNFα and IL-6 in adipose tissue.[24]

Resveratrol is a polyphenolic compound; these compounds are antioxidants found in many foods such as wine, tea, chocolate, artichokes, dark plums, and cherries, for example. In a study in which 21 polyphenolic compounds were tested, resveratrol (as well as p-coumaric acid and quercetin) were the most effective in reducing production of interleukin-6 (IL-6).[25] IL-6 as you may recall is often a major player in the proinflammatory process. IL-6 in the synovial, or joint fluid, has been associated with synovial inflammation in osteoarthritis patients.[26]

Moreover, resveratrol, p-coumaric acid, and quercetin have been shown to increase adiponectin levels.[27] As low adiponectin levels (as noted earlier) have been found to be associated with metabolic syndrome, these are important supplements to consider. Recall that it was the ratio between adiponectin and leptin that was important in knee osteoarthritis, as we had previously seen in the research literature. Higher levels of adiponectin in comparison to leptin were associated with less pain. Quercetin (as a bioactive ingredient in an extract from grape powder) has also been found to lessen the inflammation associated with obesity. It helped to reduce inflammation in macrophages (the large, white blood cells that help fight off bacteria and other foreign invaders) and to help prevent insulin resistance in adipose tissues that is mediated by these macrophages.[28]

Where do you find some of these polyphenolic compounds in food? One can find p-coumaric acid in peanuts, garlic, tomatoes, and carrots, for example, and quercetin can be found in a wide variety of foods such as onions (especially red onions) and red grapes.

Tomatoes, broccoli, and raspberries, also are all high in quercetin. Interestingly as a side note, there is a very good reason (among others of course) to buy organic tomatoes. Organically grown tomatoes have been found to contain a whopping 79% more quercetin than tomatoes that were grown conventionally! Moreover, kaempferol (and we will discuss this amazing flavonoid next), was 97% higher in organic tomatoes than in conventional tomatoes![29]

Some herbs and supplements work better when they are used in combination. For example, if resveratrol is combined with curcumin (this is the major component in the spice turmeric so commonly used in Indian curries, etc.) you reap even greater healing effects upon arthritis according to one research study. There was a synergistic effect (action when together is more powerful than either singularly) between these two antioxidants. When acting together they inhibited interleukin-1 induced destruction of articular cartilage cells.[30] Thus, taking these together could go a long way in promoting survival of your joints' cartilage cells.

Kaempferol – A Virtual Pharmacy in a Flavonoid

Flavonoids are chemicals found in food that help prevent oxidative damage to cells within your body. Oxidative damage occurs when the body is not able to recover well from the effects of oxidation (the reaction of the cells to oxygen). This process has been likened to "rust" within the body, as we had noted earlier. Flavonoids are phytonutrients (plant nutrients) that have anti-inflammatory effects. One of these flavonoids, kaempferol, found in many foods (e.g., broccoli, cabbage, kale, leeks, beans, and strawberries) could be thought of as a pharmacy at your fingertips! For example, many studies have shown that kaempferol exhibits a vast array of pharmacological actions to include not only being anti-inflammatory and antioxidant, but also anticancer, cardioprotective, neuroprotective, analgesic, antimicrobial, anti-allergic, and anti-osteoporotic! Kaempferol provides anti-inflammatory actions that can help rein in some of the destructive processes in osteoarthritis. Moreover, it has neuroprotective actions that, as you may recall from our discussion earlier, may be critical in preventing and reversing menopausal arthritis. It is also naturally analgesic and wards off osteoporosis.[31] You can see why I think of kaempferol as a virtual pharmacy in and of itself!

Procyanidins -- A Flavonoid Group That May Help Balance Your Cytokines

Another group of flavonoids, the procyanidins, also increases adiponectin levels. So where do you find this beneficial flavonoid? Happy to say, in foods that many people enjoy eating such as chocolate and apples! However, be aware that the content of procyanidins varies by apple with Red Delicious and Granny Smith containing high amounts and Golden Delicious and McIntosh with much lower amounts.[32] Animal research has shown that grape-seed procyanidin extract significantly increased adiponectin and decreased the proinflammatory cytokines interleukin-6 and TNF-alpha in white adipose tissue and muscle.[33]

This effect on interleukin-6 and the increased production of adiponectin were also confirmed in a laboratory. In an "in vitro" study, grape-seed procyanidins were cultured together with human fat cells and macrophage-like cell lines. The grape-seed procyanidins improved adiponectin levels. Increases in adiponectin may be of help in fighting low-grade inflammatory diseases such as obesity and type 2 diabetes.[34] Laboratory and animal research studies show that cocoa, another procyanidin, is an antioxidant and immune system modulator.[35] In addition, the proinflammatory cytokine IL-2 was found to be inhibited by 75% through the administration of cocoa extract in an "in vitro" laboratory study on cocoa and immune system responses.[36] Keep in mind that dark chocolate is the highest in procyanidins when shopping for chocolate to provide these beneficial effects.

Foods and Spices -- From Pomegranates and Cherries to Ginger and Turmeric

The Protective Effects of Pomegranate

Another potentially important nutritional contribution to fighting arthritis is pomegranate. This ancient fruit has long been praised for its beneficial effects and was thought to promote fertility, abundance, and good luck. It has been used in Ayurvedic medicine in many ways, for example as a remedy for ailments such as ulcers and as a blood tonic. In addition, in the Unani medicine practiced in the

Middle East and India it has been used to treat diabetes.[37] With regard to healing arthritis, it has been found to inhibit the activity of Interleukin-1ß, a proinflammatory cytokine. IL-1ß is actively involved in the promotion of mediating chemicals of cartilage breakdown. Pomegranate extract inhibited the ability for IL-1ß to activate chemicals which cause degenerative changes in cartilage cells.[38] In one animal study in which joint cartilage loss was produced as an experimental condition, researchers found evidence that pomegranate extract provided significant protection from cartilage cell damage. Proteoglycans were less disturbed in the groups receiving pomegranate juice. Proteoglycans, as emphasized earlier, are important for smooth joint movement. Also in this study, there was no presence of inflammatory cells or abnormal cell proliferation in the synovial fluid of the groups receiving high levels of pomegranate juice.[39]

Of importance as well, an animal study conducted by researchers at Case Western Reserve University, explored the effect of pomegranate extract upon collagen-induced arthritis. Pomegranate consumption impressively lessened the incidence of this arthritis, and it delayed onset as well.[40] Pomegranate is a seasonal fruit, and its season of growth in the Northern Hemisphere is from September to February. However, you can buy pomegranate extracts and juices in the off-season (see Appendix).

Cherries - Natural Cox 1 and 2 Inhibitors

Cherries are a nutritionally dense food to include important nutrients such as anthocyanins, quercetin, and carotenoids. They also contain melatonin. As discussed in Chapter Seven, melatonin can assist in the activation of satellite cells to repair muscle after exercise. In addition, as noted in Chapter Nine, melatonin plays a major role in fighting off damaging free radicals such as OH˙.

Cherries have been found to inhibit both COX-1 and COX-2 enzymes (these are the enzymes that are responsible for stimulating prostaglandin release and facilitating the inflammation process). They also come with a whole host of antioxidant and anti-carcinogenic effects.[41] Both sweet and tart cherries are abundant in phenolic compounds such as anthocyanins (which impart to them their red color).

The anthocyanins in cherries have marked anti-inflammatory effects through their inhibition of cyclooxygenase (COX) within the body. In both animal and human studies, cherries have shown anti-inflammatory effects. In a study conducted by the U.S. Department of Agriculture and the University of California at Davis, the participants found that after 28 days of daily consumption of cherries that their CRP or C-reactive protein dropped by 25%! CRP, as noted earlier, is an indicator of inflammation. Cherry consumption also decreased nitric oxide (NO) production. Interestingly, this effect upon circulating CRP and NO occurred in 12 of the 18 participants (with six of the participants unaffected). So, there is variability in how people respond to cherries with regard to fighting inflammation.[42] This is an important point, because any supplement taken may have greater or lesser effects depending upon your own biology, physiology, and environmental circumstances (to include diet, stress, etc.). That is why it is important to try many different supplements and combinations until you find those that will work most optimally for you. As such, cherries have great potential to help with menopausal arthritis, however. Also of importance to women concerned with insulin levels, cherries have a low glycemic response.[43] As so many menopausal women are burdened with metabolic syndrome, it is good to know that glucose and insulin levels were not affected by cherry consumption.

The Benefits of Oily Fish and Fish Oils

Fish with a high fat content or oil content can help reduce cytokines in your body as can supplements of fish oil. For example, it was found that supplementation with omega-3 fatty acids, but not omega-6 fatty acids, decreased activity in joint cartilage that could lead to cartilage deterioration.[44] Omega-3 fatty acids are found in abundance in fish oils and some vegetable oils such as flax seed oil. In fact, flax seed oil supplements have been found to decrease inflammatory cytokines in healthy adults. Unfortunately, in people with rheumatoid arthritis and insulin resistance, the chain of reactions needed to process this oil (and alpha-linoleic acid Omega-3) does not function optimally. Thus, if you are suffering from either of these conditions, using flax seed oil as your Omega-3 source to decrease inflammation may not work. As such, I will focus on the benefits of fish and krill oil as Omega-3 fatty acid sources.

The other major essential fatty acid group, in addition to Omega-3 fatty acids, consists of the Omega-6 fatty acids. Linoleic acid (an Omega-6 fatty acid) is primarily obtained from vegetable oils in the American diet (oils such as sunflower, safflower, and corn oil, for example). A key point with regard to the balance between these two types of essential fatty acids is important to stress here: Omega-3 supplementation is even more effective if the levels of Omega-6 fatty acids are low.[45]

Looking at the benefits of fish oil on arthritis, some animal studies have found that fish oil decreased production of interleukin-6, interleukin 1ß, and tumor necrosis factor-α by macrophages. On the other hand, studies in humans are mixed. Some studies in humans have shown a decrease in the inflammatory cytokines TNF, IL-1 and IL-6, but other studies have not demonstrated much of an effect on inflammatory cytokine production. Importantly, the doses of Omega-3 oil used and differences among the participants within the studies (along with other factors) may have contributed to some of the variations in effects that have been found.[46]

Some studies have shown that krill oil is beneficial for reducing symptoms of arthritis. Krill are very small, shrimp-like sea crustaceans that have been used as a food (e.g., in soups and noodle dishes) in many Asian countries for hundreds of years. In a randomized, double-blind, placebo controlled study, it was found that the group of people supplemented with krill oil (in comparison to the control group) had significantly reduced C-reactive protein or CRP (a marker of inflammation). In fact, by 30 days into the treatment CRP had been reduced by 30.9%. As the length of time of taking krill oil increased, the difference between the two groups became even more pronounced and significant. Those taking krill oil also had lower osteoarthritis symptom scores (with a 28.9% reduction in pain, a 20.2% reduction in stiffness, and a 22.8% reduction in functional impairment). It was concluded that a daily dose of krill oil of 300 mg. significantly reduced inflammation and arthritis symptoms within a period of just 7 to 14 days.[47]

Is krill oil better than fish oil for alleviating arthritis symptoms? A very interesting animal study of collagen-induced arthritis examined the effects of krill oil versus fish oil on arthritis scores. The EPA (eicosapentaenoic acid) and DHA (docosahexaenoic acid) within the fish oil was comparable in amount to that within the krill oil. EPA and DHA are precursors to some important eicosanoids which act as inflammation reducers within the body. Both the fish oil and the krill oil diets significantly reduced arthritis scores and abnormal tissue measures. Only krill oil, though, was found to significantly lower the arthritis score in the later phases of this study. The krill oil diet was significantly more effective than the control diet in reducing infiltration of cytokines into the joint and synovial layer. Interestingly, krill oil did not have a direct regulating effect upon cytokines; fish oil, in contrast, increased the levels of IL-1 alpha and IL-13 which can act as anti-inflammatory cytokines.[48]

There are some studies with cartilage explants (tissue removed from human and from bovine osteoarthritic cartilage that have been placed into a laboratory culture medium) that have demonstrated that Omega-3 fatty acids have considerable potential for preventing cartilage breakdown and reducing inflammation.[49,50] It is important to note, however, that the findings of "in vitro" studies may not necessarily apply to "in vivo" conditions. Within the human body, there are obviously many other chemical and biological processes occurring as well that may influence how Omega-3 fatty acids work. In sum, krill oil and fish oil seem to have beneficial, but different effects upon inflammation and arthritis symptoms. It would seem, then, that including both in one's diet might be of benefit in addressing menopausal arthritis.

Ginger

Ginger has long been used for thousands of years in traditional medicine to help stem inflammation. Ginger works in countering inflammation through the inhibition of COX-1 and COX-2. It has also been shown to suppress leukotriene synthesis. In fact, it has even been found that ginger can intervene in the biochemical processes of inflammation through inhibiting genes that encode for cytokines and

COX-2.[51] The scientific evidence for ginger's effectiveness, however, has been mixed with not all studies reporting clear, positive effects.[52,53] Importantly, though, one study did show reduced pain in knee osteoarthritis patients who consumed a ginger extract compared with a control group that did not receive the supplement. Those who took ginger had significantly reduced knee pain on standing and after walking.[54] It also helps to increase insulin sensitivity, as noted below in the discussion of curcumin.

In another study using animal research, the effects of red ginger on arthritis were examined. Red ginger has been used as a pain reliever in Indonesian traditional medicine for arthritis. In this animal study, it was found that red ginger had a strong suppressive effect upon both acute and chronic inflammation. The red ginger extract seemed to reduce inflammation, at least in part, by reducing macrophage activity.[55] Ginger can cause mild stomach upset in some people, so combining it with adequate food intake might lessen this problem. I use it in Chinese cooking, and also as a supplement (See Appendix).

Turmeric and Its Active Ingredient Curcumin

This is by far one of the most important supplements to use in healing from menopausal arthritis. Curcumin is a major element in the spice, turmeric. It imparts the orange-yellow color to the spice. It has been used in India from ancient times to treat inflammation, as well as a range of ailments such as rheumatism, body aches, and liver disorders.[56] Curcumin possesses both antioxidant and anti-inflammatory capabilities. In recent animal research, curcumin was found to show strong anti-inflammatory activity through lowering TNF-alpha and IL-1beta. Tumor necrosis factor-alpha (TNF-alpha) and IL-1 are proinflammatory cytokines involved in the inflammation process of arthritis as noted in Chapter Two. The reduction of these two cytokines through the actions of curcumin is similar to the effect discussed earlier with regard to resveratrol.

Curcumin also inhibited PGE2 production and COX-2.[57] As previously noted, COX-2 speeds up or increases the rate of production of PGE2, and PGE2 facilitates cartilage destruction in osteoarthritis. In addition, as discussed earlier, leptin facilitates the production of proinflammatory cytokines. In one study in which leptin produced the proinflammatory cytokine, IL-8, curcumin was shown to effectively block IL-8 expression.[58] Research shows that curcumin is often not absorbed well and is metabolized and eliminated rapidly by the body. Nevertheless, its ability to be therapeutic against arthritis and many diseases such as cancer, cardiovascular, and neurological diseases has been verified.[59]

Research shows that curcumin can affect the activation of T cells, B cells, macrophages, neutrophils, and other critical cells within the immune response. It also inhibits expression of a whole host of proinflammatory cytokines, such as TNF, IL-1, IL-2, IL-6, IL-8, and IL-12.[60] Moreover, researchers at The University of Texas, Department of Experimental Therapeutics have written that *curcumin actually shows actions that are similar to new pharmaceutical drugs that block tumor necrosis factor.* They also stress that there is recent, growing evidence to suggest that "multi-targeted therapy" is superior to "mono-targeted therapy."[61] As you can see, curcumin wields its anti-inflammatory effects upon a wide range of proinflammatory cytokines!

Not only does it act upon proinflammatory cytokines, but very importantly it has an effect upon leptin, too. As discussed earlier in the book, higher leptin levels have been found in the joint tissues of people with osteoarthritis. Research shows that curcumin suppresses proinflammatory nuclear factor-kappa B, and intervenes in several other processes that lead to the *downregulation of leptin*, as well as other adipokines. Nuclear factor-kappa B is a "rapid response" transcription factor (this is a protein that determines whether a gene is "switched on" or "switched off") which is in cells that express inflammatory actions. Nuclear factor-kappa B, thus, controls whether certain cytokines and other molecules and proteins within the immune system will be expressed. Through suppressing nuclear factor kappa-B, there is a downregulation and decrease in leptin (and other adipokines).[62] Recall the yin and yang relationship of leptin and insulin discussed in Chapter Two. Ginger has been found to increase insulin sensitivity.[63] Thus the use of curcumin and ginger may be very beneficial in reducing metabolic syndrome and menopausal arthritis.

Oregano (Wild Mediterranean with 70% Carvacrol)

This spice and herb has been studied primarily with regard to its antibacterial properties. Much anecdotal evidence has been documented for its prevention and cure of a variety of diseases and disorders.[64] However, some very important scientific research on oregano oil, and its primary constituent carvacrol, has emerged which is of relevance to arthritis. A research team out of the Institute of Infectious Diseases and Immunology of Utrecht University has documented some important roles in the immune system for oregano oil. Their research findings showed that carvacrol (obtained from oregano) is a strong coinducer of stress proteins.[65] What does this mean, and why is it important?

Stress proteins are up-regulated by tissues where there is inflammation present. As such, they may provide a "sensor system," so to speak, to identify a condition of inflammation. Heat shock proteins (Hsp) belong to this category of stress proteins. They are produced in response to a variety of stressors in the environment to include infection and inflammation. They play an important role in the immune system by binding antigens, or forming a chemical bond with antigens (substances that produce an immune response) and handing them over to the immune system. Hsp70 is particularly important in this regard.

Carvacrol was found to be a coinducer of stress proteins. This is important, because it means that the increase in heat shock proteins associated with carvacrol will only occur along with a genuine stress signal. Carvacrol, thus, appeared as a strong and impressive enhancer of Hsp70 that was induced by stress; carvacrol did not enhance Hsp70 in the absence of stress. The authors concluded that their findings suggested a role for carvacrol in the development of nutraceuticals that have the potential to support immune regulation.

As discussed in Chapter Nine, oregano oil is also beneficial in external applications. As was stressed in Chapter Nine, the oil *must be from Wild Mediterranean Oregano*. There are many products on the market labeled as being oregano oil that are not; instead, these products are actually oils derived from thyme or marjoram. Oil of thyme contains high amounts of thymol which can be toxic. The primary active component of oregano oil is carvacrol. You should make sure that the primary component in the oregano oil that you purchase is carvacrol, and that the percentage of carvacrol (it should be 70%) is listed on the supplement label.[66] As noted in the last chapter, the Gale Encyclopedia of Alternative Medicine provides a comprehensive overview of essential guidelines for the safe use of oregano oil.[67]

Two Herbs with Research Behind Them: Cat's Claw and Boswellia

Cat's Claw

Cat's Claw (Uncaria tomentosa) is an Amazonian herb named after the resemblance of its thorns to the claws of a cat. In a recent review of antioxidant and anti-inflammatory dietary supplements, supportive evidence was found for Cat's Claw in three studies of the herb either singularly or in combination (e.g., with another herb such as maca) in alleviating osteoarthritis symptoms.[68] In one study with knee osteoarthritis patients, pain with use of the joints and both medical and patient assessments of pain were significantly reduced. Moreover, the herb acted quickly, and results were obtained within one week of using cat's claw.[69] The way in which cat's claw appears to work is through inhibiting TNF-alpha and acting as an antioxidant.[70]

In a study examining human cartilage samples, it was found that an extract derived from cat's claw and the medicinal herb Lepidium meyenii, commonly known as maca, worked together in their effect. This combination of herbs even protected chondrocytes from the destructive effects of IL-1ß, restoring chondrocyte cells to normal production levels.[71] In another animal study, Cat's Claw shielded cells from oxidative stress, or the so-called "rust" in the body's cells. There is clear scientific evidence for both an antioxidant and an anti-inflammatory effect of Cat's Claw.[72]

Boswellia

Boswellia (also known as frankincense) is a traditional herb derived from the gum resin of Boswellia serrata. The Boswellia serrata tree is moderate to large in size and grows in India, Northern

Africa, and the Middle East. To obtain the herb, bark is stripped away to uncover a gummy substance, the resin. It is a major healing agent in Ayurvedic medicine and has been used not only as an anti-arthritic agent, but also as an astringent and diuretic. Research shows that Boswellia is a powerful anti-inflammatory herb with much potential to help in fighting arthritis. One particular Boswellia extract used in research, Aflapin (a formula which increases its bioavailability), had much benefit in protecting the joint from cartilage damage and in providing anti-arthritic actions.[73] Also, in a study of the effects of Boswellia serrata on knee osteoarthritis, it was found that those consuming the gum resin had significantly less knee pain, knee swelling, and significantly increased ability to flex the knee and to walk greater distances.[74]

The exact anti-inflammatory actions of Boswellia are currently debated. Some research has pointed toward suppression of leukotriene. However, one current assessment connected the inhibition of prostaglandin E to its anti-inflammatory effects. This particular review emphasized its importance as a potential alternative to NSAIDs which are associated with significant gastrointestinal and cardiovascular adverse effects.[75] Some studies show that Boswellia decreases TNF-alpha and the inflammatory cytokines IL-1, IL-2, IL-4, and IL-6. Boswellia extract has been found to be helpful, not only in osteoarthritis, but also diseases such as rheumatoid arthritis, ulcerative colitis, and Crohn's disease.[76]

Supplements -- Boosting Levels of Key Vitamins, Minerals, Polyphenols, and Herbs

Many of the foods, herbs, vitamins, and minerals described above can be obtained in supplement form. Most of the supplements that I use consist of these vitamins and herbs which provide key antioxidants and phytonutrients. I also take Zyflamend; this is an herbal supplement that contains some of the above nutrients such as ginger and turmeric, and some herbs not included within this chapter's review. Although one review of the literature did not find enough evidence to support recommendation of Zyflamend's use for osteoarthritis,[77] I have found it to be very helpful in reducing my menopausal arthritis symptoms. Interestingly, much of the research on Zyflamend points toward its beneficial effects in the treatment of prostate cancer. Research out of the University of Texas MD Anderson Cancer Center found that Zyflamend is able to inhibit prostate cancer cell growth.[78] In addition, research out of Columbia University Medical Center also demonstrated an anti-cancer effect of Zyflamend on prostate cancer cells. These researchers had noted that many studies have pointed toward Eastern diets as possibly protective against prostate cancer. Since Zyflamend contains 10 botanical ingredients common to the Eastern diet, they were particularly interested in what effect it might have on cancer cells. They thought that a supplement with a "diverse chemical profile" might yield information concerning the benefits of an Eastern diet better than would supplements of individual components alone. What they found was that each component in Zyflamend was able to influence arachidonic acid metabolism. Zyflamend further inhibited COX-1 and COX-2, and induced cell death in prostate cancer cells.[79]

As discussed in Chapter Two, arachidonic acid is a facilitator of prostaglandins and inflammation. In addition, COX-2 expedites production of prostaglandin E2 which is destructive to cartilage in osteoarthritis. Although studies may not have demonstrated Zyflamend's positive effect upon arthritis as of yet, I suspect that the positive benefits that I obtain may be related to some of these effects upon inflammation. I consider Zyflamend to be one of the key supplements in my own healing plan.

I try to consume all of the supplements that I take in moderate quantities, but I include a wide range of supplements. I also try to combine any supplements with food forms that contain the actual nutrient(s) being taken in supplement form. For example, if I take vitamin E and selenium, I try to take them with food that contains both the vitamin and the mineral (such as mixed nuts, for example). If I take vitamin C, I combine it with a fruit such as strawberries, or a meal containing red bell peppers, for example, both of which are rich in vitamin C. The reason for this is that these nutrients may have a synergistic effect with phytochemicals and nutrients that exist naturally within their food sources. Scientists have attempted to isolate compounds within fruits or vegetables (e.g., quercetin, carotenoids, etc.) believing that they may be the most important or active elements in promoting health. However, research is beginning to point toward the critical importance of the effects of complex mixtures of nutrients that provide synergistic benefits not obtainable through isolated nutrients.[80]

Glucosamine and Chondroitin: Popular Supplements, but Are They Actually Effective in Alleviating Osteoarthritis Symptoms?

I would guess that there are probably very few people who are suffering from menopausal arthritis who haven't tried using glucosamine and/or chondroitin to alleviate symptoms. These have become increasingly used over the past decade, and they are widely available as over the counter treatments. Many general practitioners and rheumatologists prescribe their use based upon recommended guidelines. They are thought to supply elements needed by the cartilage to compensate for loss due to osteoarthritis. For example, chondroitin possesses hydrocolloid properties (gel-like when combined with water) which act in ways very similar to the properties that allow cartilage to resist compression.

Glucosamine, an amino sugar, stands as a building block for the glycosaminoglycans, critical components of cartilage. The thinking is that these ingested supplements, which are partially absorbed in the intestine, will make their way into the joints themselves. But, do they, and are they really effective in alleviating arthritis? Research has yielded mixed results. The studies on glucosamine and chondroitin have been dissimilar in some areas such as using different glucosamine preparations (glucosamine sulfate versus glucosamine hydrochloride). The designs of the studies have also been criticized for flaws in methodological procedures (such as not providing enough concealment of the treatment that the participants are receiving).[81]

A recent, very large meta-analysis conducted by Simon Wandel and colleagues at the Institute of Social and Preventative Medicine at the University of Bern, Switzerland, does raise serious questions about the efficacy of glucosamine/chondroitin supplementation for arthritis. The principal findings of their meta-analysis did not show glucosamine and chondroitin to be effective in osteoarthritis of the hip and knee. In a comprehensive analysis, they examined twelve research reports consisting of 10 experimental trials to include 3,803 patients. These participants were either randomized to the treatment group or to the control/placebo group. They concluded that there was no significant reduction in pain or joint space narrowing in participants who used glucosamine, chondroitin, or their combination when compared with the placebo groups.[82]

A Word About Water: Why You May Want to Shun Tap Water

One thing of which many may be unaware is that an over-exposure to fluoride in our drinking water could lead to problems that mimic arthritis. For example, fluoride had originally been thought to help reduce osteoporosis by strengthening the bone. However, research showed that bone after fluoride use was denser, but *not* necessarily stronger. Some of the side effects of using fluoride therapy for osteoporosis included stress fractures, and importantly, *severe joint pain in the lower limbs.*[83] If fluoride therapy for osteoporosis can do this, actually mimic arthritis pain, what about our consumption of fluoridated tap water?

Here is a very interesting example of a woman who became a victim of skeletal fluorosis (excessive intake of fluorine) from drinking brewed tea. The fluorine, in this case, was thought to come from the plant source, the tea. The researchers noted that many teas from the plant Camellia sinensis, such as the orange pekoe tea that this woman was drinking, contain high levels of fluorine. She consumed 1-2 gallons of instant tea per day over several decades. Her fluoride ion levels were high, and she was unresponsive to vitamin D supplementation. Only after she discontinued drinking her tea, and continued with vitamin D2 supplementation did her pain resolve.[84]

It is important to note, however, that these researchers apparently did not directly measure the fluoride within her drinking water. Instead, they reported an estimate of what the additional fluoridated water would add to the total fluorine levels had the water been fluoridated at "optimal" levels. Thus, one would have to keep open the possibility that her water could possibly have deviated from normal fluoridation levels and may have been high in fluoride itself.

The important takeaway point here, though, is that fluorine in water (and other sources) if it builds up excessively in the body, could cause joint pain. I eliminated the use of all tap water except in washing dishes. We even cook our food in non-tap water. To be sure that you eliminate all possible sources of joint pain, use a high-quality water filter to remove fluoride (and chlorine and other toxic elements), or buy bottled water that is from known sources with the contents well-documented.

Foods, Herbs, and Supplements in Sum

There is a wealth of natural foods, supplements, herbs, and vitamins to help heal your arthritis. This summary of some of the more prominent ones backed by scientific research is intended to provide you with a base. I have found that these foods, herbs, vitamins, and supplements can go a long way in alleviating arthritis, even before any weight loss is achieved (if weight loss is indeed indicated). They also provide an excellent base for the vital muscle-tendon-bone strengthening effects of our exercise program. This nutritional base is a launching point from which you can begin to heal from menopausal arthritis. It is also a fulcrum from which you may balance your health and sustain your freedom from menopausal arthritis. Your nutritional base is your pillar of power that will make all of the other interventions succeed at their peak potential.

Notes for Chapter Ten

[1]Neogi, T. , Booth, S. L., Zhang, Y. Q., Jacques, P. F., Terkeltaub, R., Aliabadi, P., & Felson, D. T. (2006). Low vitamin K status is associated with osteoarthritis in the hand and knee. *Arthritis & Rheumatism, 54*(4), 1255-1261.

[2]Oka, H., Akune, T., Muraki, S., En-yo, Y., Yoshida, M., Saika, A., Sasaki, S., Nakamura, K., Kawaguchi, H., &Yoshimura, N. (2009). Association of low dietary vitamin K intake with radiographic knee osteoarthritis in the Japanese elderly population: Dietary survey in a population-based cohort of the ROAD study. *Journal of Orthopaedic Science, 14*(6), 687-692.

[3]Kaufman, W. (1949). *The common form of joint dysfunction.* Brattleboro, VT: E. L. Hildreth.

[4]Saul, A. W. (2003). The pioneering work of William Kaufman: Arthritis and ADHD. *Journal of Orthomolecular Medicine, 18*(1), 29-32.

[5]Jonas, W. B., Rapoza, C. P., & Blair, W. F. (1996). The effect of niacinamide on osteoarthritis: A pilot study. *Inflammation Research, 45*(7), 330-334.

[6]McCarty, M. F., & Russell, A. L. (1999). Niacinamide therapy for osteoarthritis - does it inhibit nitric oxide synthase induction by interleukin 1 in chondrocytes? *Medical Hypotheses, 53*(4), 350-360.

[7]Natural Medicines Comprehensive Database. Consumer Version (2011, August 1). Niacin and Niacinamide (Vitamin B3). Retrieved from http://www.nlm.nih.gov/medlineplus/druginfo/natural/924.html (MedlinePlus -- U.S. National Library of Medicine, National Institutes of Health)

[8]Munir, J., & Birge, S. J. (2008). Vitamin D deficiency in pre- and postmenopausal women. *Menopause Management, 17*(5), 10-21.

[9]Cutolo, M., Plebani, M., Shoenfeld, Y., Adorini, L., & Tincani, A. (2011). Vitamin D endocrine system and the immune response in rheumatic diseases. *Vitamins and Hormones, 86*, 327-351.

[10]Zwerina, K., Baum, W., Axmann, R., Heiland, G. R. Distler, J. H., Smolen, J., Hayer, S., Zwerina, J., & Schett, G. (2011). Vitamin D receptor regulates TNF-mediated arthritis. *Annals of the Rheumatic Diseases, 70*(6), 1122-1129.

[11]Munir et al. (2008). Op. Cit.

[12]Ceglia, L. (2009). Vitamin D and its role in skeletal muscle. *Current Opinion in Clinical Nutrition and Metabolic Care, 12*(6), 628-633.

[13]Tagliafico, A. S. , Ameri, P., Bovio, M., Puntoni, M., Capaccio, E., Murialdo, G., & Martinoli, C. (2010). Relationship between fatty degeneration of thigh muscles and vitamin D status in the elderly: A preliminary MRI study. *American Journal of Roentgenology, 194*(3), 728-734.

[14]Pedrosa, M. A., & Castro, M. L. (2005). Role of vitamin D in neuro-muscular function. *Arquivos Brasileiros de Endocrinologia & Metabologia, 49*(4), 495-502.

[15]Pfeifer, M., Begerow, B., Minne, H. W., Suppan, K., Fahrleitner-Pammer, A., & Dobnig, H. (2009). Effects of a long-term vitamin D and calcium supplementation on falls and parameters of muscle function in community-dwelling older individuals. *Osteoporosis International, 20*(2), 315-322.

[16]Bischoff-Ferrari, H. A., & Staehelin, H. B. (2008). Importance of vitamin D and calcium at older age. *International Journal for Vitamin and Nutrition Research, 78*(6), 286-292.

[17]Chlebowski, R. T., Johnson, K. C., Lane, D., Pettinger, M., Kooperberg, C. L., Wactawski-Wende, J., Rohan, T., O'Sullivan, M. J., Yasmeen, S., Hiatt, R. A., Shikany, J. M., Vitolins, M., Khandekar, J., & Hubbell, F. A. (2011). 25-hydroxyvitamin D concentration, vitamin D intake and joint symptoms in postmenopausal women. *Maturitas, 68*(1), 73-78.

[18]Canter, P. H., Wider, B., & Ernst, E. (2007). The antioxidant vitamins A, C, E and selenium in the treatment of arthritis: A systematic review of randomized clinical trials. *Rheumatology, 46*(8), 1223-1233.

[19]Lauretani, F., Semba, R. D., Bandinelli, S., Ray, A. L., Guralnik, J. M., & Ferrucci, L. (2007). Association of low plasma selenium concentrations with poor muscle strength in older community-dwelling adults: The InCHIANTI Study. *American Journal of Clinical Nutrition, 86*(2), 347-352.

[20]Bertelli, A. A., & Das, D. K. (2009). Grapes, wines, resveratrol, and heart health. *Journal of Cardiovascular Pharmacology, 54*(6), 468-476.

[21]Huang, P. H., Chen, Y. H., Tsai, H. Y., Chen, J. S., Wu, T. C., Lin, F. Y., Sata, M., Chen, J. W., & Lin, S. J. (2010). Intake of red wine increases the number and functional capacity of circulating endothelial progenitor cells by enhancing nitric oxide bioavailability. *Arteriosclerosis, Thrombosis, and Vascular Biology, 30*(4), 869-877.

[22]Khalifé, S., & Zafarullah, M. (2011). Molecular targets of natural health products in arthritis. *Arthritis Research & Therapy, 13*(1), 102. Advance online publication. PMID: 21345249

[23]Dave, M., Attur, M., Palmer, G., Al-Mussawir, H. E., Kennish, L., Patel, J., & Abramson, S. B. (2008). The antioxidant resveratrol protects against chondrocyte apoptosis via effects on mitochondrial polarization and ATP production. *Arthritis & Rheumatism, 58*(9), 2786-2797.

[24]Kim, S., Jin, Y., Choi, Y., & Park, T. (2011). Resveratrol exerts anti-obesity effects via mechanisms involving down-regulation of adipogenic and inflammatory processes in mice. *Biochemical Pharmacology, 81*(11), 1343-1351. doi: 10.1016/j.bcp.2011.03.012

[25]Yen, G. C., Chen, Y. C., Chang, W. T., & Hsu, C. L. (2011). Effects of polyphenolic compounds on tumor necrosis factor-_ (TNF-_)-induced changes of adipokines and oxidative stress in 3T3-L1 adipocytes. *Journal of Agricultural and Food Chemistry, 59*(2), 546-551.

[22]Pearle, A. D., Scanzello, C. R., George, S., Mandl, L. A., DiCarlo, E. F., Peterson, M., Sculco,T. P., & Crow, M. K. (2007). Elevated high-sensitivity C-reactive protein levels are associated with local inflammatory findings in patients with osteoarthritis. *Osteoarthritis and Cartilage, 15*(5), 516-523.

[27]Yen et al. (2011). Op. Cit.

[28]Overman, A., Chuang, C. C., & McIntosh, M. (2011). Quercetin attenuates inflammation in human macrophages and adipocytes exposed to macrophage-conditioned media. *International Journal of Obesity, 35*(9), 1165-1172. doi: 10.1038/ijo.2010.272.

[29]Mitchell, A. E., Hong, Y. J., Koh, E., Barrett, D. M., Bryant, D. E., Denison, R. F., & Kaffka, S. (2007). Ten-year comparison of the influence of organic and conventional crop management practices on the content of flavonoids in tomatoes. *Journal of Agricultural and Food Chemistry, 55*(15), 6154-6159.

[30]Csaki, C., Mobasheri, A., & Shakibaei, M. (2009). Synergistic chondoroprotective effects of curcumin and resveratrol in human articular chondrocytes: inhibition of IL-1beta-induced NF-kappaB-mediated inflammation and apoptosis. *Arthritis Research and Therapy, 11*(6), R165.

[31]Calderón-Montaño, J. M., Burgos-Morón, E., Pérez-Guerrero, C., & López-Lázaro, M. (2011). A review on the dietary flavonoid kaempferol. *Mini Reviews in Medicinal Chemistry, 11*(4), 298-344.

[32]Hammerstone, J. F., Lazarus, S. A., & Schmitz, H. H. (2000). Procyanidin content and variation in some commonly consumed foods. *Journal of Nutrition, 130*(8), 2086S-2092S.

[33]Terra, X., Pallarés, V., Ardèvol, A., Bladé, C., Fernández-Larrea, J., Pujadas, G., Salvadó, J., Arola, L., & Blay, M. (2011). Modulatory effect of grape-seed procyanidins on local and systemic inflammation in diet-induced obesity rats. *Journal of Nutritional Biochemistry, 22*(4), 380-387.

[34] Chacón, M. R., Ceperuelo-Mallafré, V., Maymó-Masip, E., Mateo-Sanz, J. M., Arola, L., Guitiérrez, C., Fernandez-Real, J. M, Ardèvol, A., Simón, I., & Vendrell, J. (2009). Grape-seed procyanidins modulate inflammation on human differentiated adipocytes in vitro. *Cytokine, 47*(2), 137-142.

[35]Ramiro-Puig, E., & Castell, M. (2009). Cocoa: Antioxidant and immunomodulator. *British Journal of Nutrition, 101*(7), 931-940.

[36]Ramiro, E., Franch, A., Castellote, C., Andrés-Lacueva, C., Izquierdo-Pulido, M., & Castell, M. (2005). Effect of Theobroma cacao flavonoids on immune activation of lymphoid cell line. *British Journal of Nutrition, 93*(6), 859-866.

[37]Jurenka, J. (2008). Therapeutic applications of pomegranate (Punica granatum L.): A review. *Alternative Medicine Review, 13*(2), 128-144.

[38]Rasheed, Z., Akhtar, N., & Haqqi, T. M. (2010). Pomegranate extract inhibits the interleukin-1β-induced activation of MKK-3, p38_-MAPK and transcription factor RUNX-2 in human chrondrocytes. *Arthritis Research & Therapy, 12*(5), R195.

[39]Hadipour-Jahromy, M., & Mozaffari-Kermani, R. (2010). Chondroprotective effects of pomegranate juice on monoiodoacetate-induced osteoarthritis of the knee joint of mice. *Phytotherapy Research, 24*(2), 182-185.

[40]Shukla, M., Gupta, K., Rasheed, Z., Khan, K. A., & Haqqi, T. M. (2008). Consumption of hydrolyzable tannins-rich pomegranate extract suppresses inflammation and joint damage in rheumatoid arthritis. *Nutrition, 24*(7-8), 733-743.

[41]McCune, L. M., Kubota, C., Stendell-Hollis, N. R., & Thomson, C. A. (2011). Cherries and health: A review. *Critical Reviews in Food Science and Nutrition, 51*(1), 1-12.

[42]Kelley, D. S., Rasooly, R., Jacob, R. A., Kader, A. A., & Mackey, B. E. (2006). Consumption of Bing sweet cherries lowers circulating concentrations of inflammation markers in health men and women. *Journal of Nutrition, 136*(4), 981-986.

[43]McCune et al. (2011). Op. Cit.

[44]Tattersall, A. L., & Wilkins, R. J. (2008). Effects of hexosamines and omega-3/omega-6 fatty acids on pH regulation by interleukin 1-treated isolated bovine articular chondrocytes. *Pflügers Archiv, 456*(3), 501-506.

[45]Johnson, K. (2011). Nutritional interventions in rheumatology. In R. Horwitz & D. Muller (Eds.), *Integrative rheumatology* (pp. 6-22). New York: Oxford University Press.

[46]Calder, P. C. (2011). Polyunsaturated fatty acids, inflammatory processes and rheumatoid arthritis. In R. Horwitz & D. Muller (Eds.), *Integrative rheumatology* (pp. 23-46). New York: Oxford University Press.

[47]Deutsch, L. (2007). Evaluation of the effect of Neptune Krill Oil on chronic inflammation and arthritic symptoms. *Journal of the American College of Nutrition, 26*(1), 39-48.

[48]Ierna, M., Kerr, A., Scales, H., Berge, K., & Griinari, M. (2010). Supplementation of diet with krill oil protects against experimental rheumatoid arthritis. *BMC Musculoskeletal Disorders, 29*(11), 136.

[49]Curtis, C. L., Rees, S. G., Little, C. B., Flannery, C. R., Hughes, C. E., Wilson, C., Dent, C. M., Otterness, I. G., Harwood, J. L., & Caterson, B. (2002). Pathologic indicators of degradation and inflammation in human osteoarthritic cartilage are abrogated by exposure to n-3 fatty acids. *Arthritis & Rheumatism, 46*(6), 1544-1553.

[50]Wann, A. K., Mistry, J., Blain, E. J., Michael-Titus, A. T., & Knight, M. M. (2010). Eicosapentaenoic acid and docosahexaenoic acid reduce interleukin-1ß-mediated cartilage degradation. *Arthritis Research & Therapy, 12*(6), R207.

[51]Grzanna, R., Lindmark, L., & Frondoza, C. G., (2005). Ginger -- an herbal medicinal product with broad anti-inflammatory actions. *Journal of Medicinal Food, 8*(2), 125-132.

[52]Hoffman, T. (2007). Ginger: An ancient remedy and modern miracle drug. *Hawaii Medical Journal, 66*(12), 326-327.

[53]Bliddal, H., Rosetzsky, A., Schlichting, P., Weidner, M. S., Andersen, L. A., Ibfelt, H. H., Christensen, K., Jensen, O. N., & Barslev, J. (2000). A randomized, placebo-controlled, cross-over study of ginger extracts and ibuprofen in osteoarthritis. *Osteoarthritis and Cartilage, 8*(1), 9-12.

[54]Altman, R. D., & Marcussen, K. C. (2001). Effects of a ginger extract on knee pain in patients with osteoarthritis. *Arthritis & Rheumatism, 44*(11), 2531-2538.

[55]Shimoda, H., Shan, S. J., Tanaka, J., Seki, A., Seo, J. W., Kasajima, N., Tamura, S., Ke, Y., & Murakami, N. (2010). Anti-inflammatory properties of red ginger (Zingiber officinale var. Rubra) extract and suppression of nitric oxide production by its constituents. *Journal of Medicinal Food, 13*(1), 156-162.

[56]Pari, L., Tewas, D., & Eckel, J. (2008). Role of curcumin in health and disease. *Archives of Physiology and Biochemistry, 114*(2), 127-149.

[57]Moon, D. O., Kim, M. O., Choi, Y. H., Park, Y. M., & Kim, G. Y. (2010). Curcumin attenuates inflammatory response in IL-1beta-induced human synovial fibroblasts and collagen-induced arthritis in mouse model. *International Immunopharmacology, 10*(5), 605-610.

[58]Tong, K. M., Shieh, D. C., Chen, C. P., Tzeng, C. Y., Wang, S. P., Huang, K. C., Chiu, Y. C., Fong, Y. C., & Tang, C. H. (2008). Leptin induces IL-8 expression via leptin receptor, IRS-1, P13K, Akt cascade and promotion of NF-kappaB/p300 binding in human synovial fibroblasts. *Cellular Signalling, 20*(8), 1478-1488.

[59]Anand, P., Kunnumakkara, A. B., Newman, R. A., & Aggarwal, B. B. (2007). Bioavailability of curcumin: Problems and promises. *Molecular Pharmaceutics, 4*(6), 807-818.

[60]Jagetia, G. C., & Aggarwal, B. B. (2007). "Spicing up" of the immune system by curcumin. *Journal of Clinical Immunology, 27*(1), 19-35.

[61]Aggarwal, B. B., Sundaram, C., Malani, N., & Ichikawa, H. (2007). Curcumin: the Indian solid gold. *Advances in Experimental Medicine and Biology, 595*, 1-75.

[62]Aggarwal, B. B. (2010). Targeting inflammation-induced obesity and metabolic diseases by curcumin and other nutraceuticals. *Annual Review of Nutrition, 30*, 173-199. doi: 10.1146/annurev.nutr.012809.104755

[63] Al-Suhaimi, E. A., Al-Riziza, N. A., & Al-Essa, R. A. (2011). Physiological and therapeutical roles of ginger and turmeric on endocrine functions. *American Journal of Chinese Medicine, 39*(2), 215-231.

[64] Ingram, C. (2001). *The cure is in the cupboard: How to use oregano for better health.* Buffalo Grove, IL: Knowledge House.

[65] Wieten, L., van der Zee, R., Spiering, R., Wagenaar-Hilbers, J., van Kooten, P., Broere, F., & van Eden, W. (2010). A novel heat-shock protein coinducer boosts stress protein Hsp70 to activate T cell regulation of inflammation in autoimmune arthritis. *Arthritis & Rheumatism, 62*(4), 1026-1035. doi: 10.1002/art.27344

[66] Ingram (2001). Op. Cit.

[67] Oregano essential oil. In L. J. Fundukian (Ed.) (2009). *The Gale encyclopedia of alternative medicine (3rd ed.)* (pp. 1638-1641). Detroit: Gale.

[68] Rosenbaum, C. C., O'Mathúna, D. P., Chavez, M., & Shields, K. (2010). Antioxidants and antiinflammatory dietary supplements for osteoarthritis and rheumatoid arthritis. *Alternative Therapies in Health and Medicine, 16*(2), 32-40.

[69] Piscoya, J., Rodriguez, Z., Bustamante, S. A., Okuhama, N. N., Miller, M. J., & Sandoval, M. (2001). Efficacy and safety of freeze-dried cat's claw in osteoarthritis of the knee: Mechanisms of action of the species Uncaria guianensis. *Inflammation Research, 50*(9), 442-448.

[70] Hardin, S. R. (2007). Cat's claw: An Amazonian vine decreases inflammation in osteoarthritis. *Complementary Therapies in Clinical Practice, 13*(1), 25-28.

[71] Miller, M. J., Ahmed, S., Bobrowski, P., & Haqqi, T. M. (2006). The chrondroprotective actions of a natural product are associated with the activation of IGF-1 production by human chondrocytes despite the presence of IL-1beta. *BMC Complementary and Alternative Medicine, 7*(6), 13.

[72] Sandoval-Chacón, M., Thompson, J. H., Zhang, X. J., Liu, X., Mannick, E. E., Sadowska-Krowicka, H., Charbonnet, R. M., Clark, D. A., & Miller, M. J. (1998). Antiinflammatory actions of cat's claw: the role of NF-kappaB. *Alimentary Pharmacology &Therapeutics, 12*(12), 1279-1289.

[73] Sengupta, K., Kolla, J. N., Krishnaraju, A. V., Yalamanchili, N., Rao, C. V., Golakoti, T., Raychaudhuri, S., & Raychaudhuri, S. P. (2011). Cellular and molecular mechanisms of anti-inflammatory effect of Aflapin: A novel Boswellia serrata extract. *Molecular and Cellular Biochemistry, 354*(1-2), 189-197.

[74] Kimmatkar, N., Thawani, V., Hingorani, L., & Khiyani, R. (2003). Efficacy and tolerability of Boswellia serrata extract in treatment of osteoarthritis of knee -- a randomized double blind placebo controlled trial. *Phytomedicine, 10*(1), 3-7.

[75] Abdel-Tawab, M. Werz, O., & Schubert-Zsilavecz, M. (2011). Boswellia serrata: an overall assessment of in vitro, preclinical, pharmacokinetic and clinical data. *Clinical Pharmacokinetics, 50*(6), 349-369.

[76]Ammon, H. P. (2010). Modulation of the immune system by Boswellia serrata extracts and boswellic acids. *Phytomedicine, 17*(11), 862-867.

[77]Rosenbaum et al. (2010). Op. Cit.

[78]Yang, P., Cartwright, C., Chan, D., Vijjeswarapu, M., Ding, J., & Newman, R. A. (2007). Zyflamend-mediated inhibition of human prostate cancer PC3 proliferation: Effects on 12-LOX and Rb protein phosphorylation. *Cancer Biology and Therapy, 6*(2), 228-236.

[79]Bemis, D. L., Capodice, J. L., Anastasiadis, A. G., Katz, A. E., & Buttyan, R. (2005). Zyflamend, a unique herbal preparation with nonselective COX inhibitory activity, induces apoptosis of prostate cancer cells that lack COX-2 expression. *Nutrition and Cancer, 52*(2), 202-212.

[80]Bouayed, J., & Bohn, T. (2010). Exogenous antioxidants - Double-edged swords in cellular redox state: Health beneficial effects at physiologic doses versus deleterious effects at high doses. *Oxidative Medicine and Cellular Longevity, 3*(4), 228-237

[81]Kolasinski, S. L. (2011). Dietary supplements in rheumatologic disorders. In R. Horwitz & D. Muller (Eds.), *Integrative rheumatology* (pp. 75-92). New York: Oxford University Press.

[82]Wandel, S., Jüni, P., Tendal, B., Nüesch, E., Villiger, P. M., Welton, N. J., Reichenbach, S., & Trelle, S. (2010). Effects of glucosamine, chondroitin, or placebo in patients with osteoarthritis of hip or knee: Network meta-analysis. *BMJ, 341*, c4675. doi:10.1136/bmj.c4675

[83]Laroche, M., & Mazières, B. (1991). Side-effects of fluoride therapy. *Baillieres Clinical Rheumatology, 5*(1), 61-76.

[84]Izuora, K., Twombly, J. G., Whitford, G. M., Demertzis, J., Pacifici, R. & Whyte, M. P. (2011). Skeletal fluorosis from brewed tea. *Journal of Clinical Endocrinology and Metabolism, 96*(8), 2318-2324.

Chapter Eleven

Menopausal Arthritis, Pain, and Emotions

--- ◻ ---

Precursors of Pain and Physical Disorders

In most conventional approaches toward treating arthritis, pain is thought of as being a result of the disease process. For example, pain may be a result of inflammation or muscular dysfunction, etc. Pain is seldom considered to be a precipitating factor, something actually involved in the formation or onset of arthritis. However, as noted in Chapter Six, it is well established now that people's emotional states can affect immune functions.

With an eye toward possible psychological precursors to arthritis pain, we can approach healing from multiple perspectives. However, I must stress that the most vital aspects to healing menopausal arthritis, the heart of this healing program, remain the following: (1) what we take into our bodies in terms of anti-inflammatory herbs, supplements, vitamins, and foods, (2) what we do with our bodies in terms of effective exercise (and healthful weight loss, if needed), (3) what we apply to our bodies in terms of external therapies such as orthopedic massage, healing oils, and other preparations, and (4) what we do as positive adaptations to everyday living and functions (such as wearing shoes with flexible soles and walking erectly with correct posture).

An additional aspect that may be very important is how psychological factors are involved in arthritis. This chapter will discuss why psychological factors may be involved in some of the processes of arthritis. It will also focus upon a fifth aspect of healing (in addition to the four noted above), and that is what we do in terms of addressing emotions, fostering positive feeling states, and reducing stress. In the final chapter, "Putting It All Together for Your Own Healing," I will discuss all of these as part of a total plan. For now, though, let's look at some of the ways that psychological pain might lead to arthritis pain.

Psychological pain (e.g., caused by trauma, stress) can lead to anxiety and/or depression and related disorders. Psychological pain, trauma, and stress may be rooted in past experiences or in present ones, or both. Indeed, the pain, stress (and other psychological outcomes such as depression and anxiety) could also be a result of the experience of the disease of arthritis itself. Whether one can successfully reduce stress through yoga training, Tai Chi exercise, and other stress-alleviating practices not based in psychological theory, really depends much upon these three factors: (1) how deeply rooted the causative stressors are (i.e., at what point in one's development as a person it occurred), (2) how severe the stressors were then and are presently, and (3) one's own inherent resilience in coping with psychological (and physical) stressors. This resilience may be facilitated through one's belief systems (e.g., spiritual or religious beliefs, positive psychology, etc.) or other approaches (e.g., social support, or positive coping strategies that allow one to adapt effectively).

Generally stated, if the stressors are severe and deeply rooted in childhood trauma (or trauma experienced in adulthood or both), then a treatment or intervention such as psychotherapy may be beneficial. If, on the other hand, the stressors are less severe and less based in character or personality disorders, then other types of stress reduction (e.g., exercise, relaxation techniques, etc.) may sometimes suffice. Within this chapter, I will discuss research that highlights some of the ways that psychological pain and stressors could potentially create disease (in this case, arthritis), and some of the ways that one might try to alleviate stressors and psychological manifestations such as anxiety and depression.

Will reducing stress, anxiety, and/or depression help alleviate arthritis symptoms? There is simply not enough research on this to be able to answer this question. Nevertheless, while we wait for science to bring some answers, a reduction in chronic stress and anxiety would certainly seem to provide a better base for overall healing to occur. This is just common sense. So, even if interventions to decrease stress and anxiety do not end up having a direct impact upon arthritis pain, there are most certainly other dimensions of importance to healing that are affected (e.g., improved sleep, better digestion with improved assimilation of nutrients, improved social functioning, etc.). The positive effects in these areas will all decidedly contribute to improved healing of menopausal arthritis and other physical dysfunctions, as well.

Can Childhood Trauma Contribute to Chronic Disease In Adulthood? -- Some Compelling Findings

As you may recall from research cited within Chapter Six, childhood stressors were found to be significantly associated with the onset of arthritis in adulthood. This is important to keep in mind, as stressors from the past can affect one's current physical functioning. Indeed, it has been suggested that childhood abuse may result in long-term changes in hypothalamic-pituitary-adrenocortical activities in the body. The hypothalamic-pituitary-adrenal (HPA) axis could not be more important to your functioning. The activities of the HPA axis influence and control how you react to stress, the workings of your immune system, experience of moods and emotions, and bodily processes such as digestion, just to name a few of the critical processes it affects. For example, in women with chronic pain, the experience of childhood maltreatment has been associated with higher cortisol levels.[1] Cortisol is a stress hormone produced by the adrenal gland and released through the functions of the hypothalamus. These findings contribute to the evidence that abuse as a child can have long-lasting effects upon the activities of the hypothalamic-pituitary-adrenal axis.

Moreover, the neuropeptide oxytocin (one of many molecules used by nerve cells to communicate with each other) is released by the posterior pituitary gland. It has been found to occur in lower concentrations in women with a history of childhood abuse. Researchers at Emory University found that women who had experienced any kind of child maltreatment showed significantly lower oxytocin levels in their cerebrospinal fluid than did women with no exposure to maltreatment. As the number of types of maltreatment (e.g., emotional abuse, physical abuse, and emotional neglect) increased, the concentration of oxytocin significantly decreased. Childhood emotional abuse showed a very strong effect in terms of lowered oxytocin levels in adulthood.[2] Why is oxytocin important? This signaling molecule is intricately involved in social affiliation, attachment, and social support. It is also involved in the development of maternal behavior and trust. Moreover, it is involved in helping to protect humans from stress.[3,4]

Findings from animal research show that oxytocin gates or puts a stop to fear responses through outputs from the central amygdala.[5] In fact, animal research has demonstrated that oxytocin reduces anxiety.[6] If fear responses are less able to be mitigated or lessened in a person, then anxiety must decidedly increase as a result. Childhood stressors (which, of course childhood abuse is one) were linked to the onset of arthritis in adulthood.[7] Childhood abuse was linked to lowered oxytocin levels in adults.[8] When one has a lowered oxytocin level, the ability to counter fear is decreased and anxiety may increase.

Childhood Stressors and the Onset of Arthritis in Adulthood

The strong association of the onset of arthritis in adulthood and childhood stressors is something that is important to consider in healing.[9] However, it is beyond the scope of this book to address specific interventions to deal with childhood trauma and/or stressors. Nevertheless, it is important to recognize that past experiences can have a profound impact upon one's current state of health, including experiences of arthritis and other physical diseases. Seeking professional help from a clinical psychologist or other mental health professional might help to lessen the pain and psychological consequences of past stressors (such as child abuse, child neglect, death of a parent, etc.) that may be having an impact upon one's current life. Moreover, if you are experiencing depression or anxiety, seeking professional mental health services might be of benefit.

Recognizing and resolving psychological issues may have an effect upon, not only your psychological health, but also your physical health. The traumas from the past have a persistent way of affecting one's physical body and psyche in a manner that can impede your successful progress and stifle your enjoyment of life. Sometimes, freeing yourself from the effects of past pain can unlock your ability to heal in ways that would be impossible otherwise.

Some people who experience trauma in childhood may suffer from post-traumatic stress disorder (PTSD). In addition to other maladaptive behaviors, PTSD can also result in anxiety and guilt. Of people experiencing PTSD, more than twice as many are women.[10] Individuals who undergo trauma and suffer from post-traumatic stress disorder may often experience what psychologists call dissociation. This is when a person's consciousness becomes disconnected from what is happening to them. One's memory for the traumatic event is impaired and often inaccessible. It is a protective device that is employed to shield the person from the experiencing of a traumatic event that is too overwhelming for the person to bear at that time. Because of this, the event cannot be integrated into one's sense of self, or one's sense of self within one's environment. Unfortunately, even though the person may not remember the event, the negative impact of the event upon the person remains. It becomes part of a person's enduring "psychobiology," so to speak. It affects many physiological and biological aspects of human functioning to include the extremely important hypothalamic-pituitary-adrenal axis that I referred to above.

This is of much importance when considering chronic inflammatory diseases such as arthritis. The hypothalamic-pituitary-adrenal (HPA) axis functions to both suppress the production of cytokines and to incite the actions of cytokines.[11] The HPA axis, thus, affects the immune system, as well as many of the neurotransmitters that influence mood and pain such as serotonin and endorphins.[12]

The immune system and pain processes are intricately involved in various aspects of diseases such as arthritis. The effects of early stressors in childhood can have an enduring effect upon how one responds to stress and upon one's immune system. Some problems, such as post-traumatic-stress disorder, may be difficult to resolve on one's own. Seeking professional help could assist one in alleviating the impact of adverse events from the past that may result in current dysfunctional behaviors and emotional distress. Not all sources of anxiety in the present run this deep, however. We will look at some anxiety and stress-reducing practices in the latter part of the chapter. Let's turn now, though, to how menopause, anxiety, and arthritis may be related.

Menopause, Arthritis Pain, and Anxiety

As previously summarized in Chapter Six, the current experience of anxiety was found to be significantly associated with self-reported pain with arthritis in postmenopausal women. In this research, the Baltimore Longitudinal Study of Aging, women who reported knee pain (without any evidence of radiographic arthritis) had higher anxiety scores than women who did not have knee pain. Self-reported anxiety was unrelated to knee pain in men.[13]

In another study, the effects of anxiety and depression on weekly arthritis pain in women were explored. It was anxiety that had the most profound effect upon arthritis pain. When all factors were taken into consideration, anxiety accounted for nearly 15% of the variation between women in their experience of pain, whereas depression only accounted for approximately 4%. Anxiety was directly related to a woman's current arthritis pain and to her arthritis pain score within the next week. Depression, however, had no direct effect upon arthritis pain. Anxiety was also indirectly related to pain through negative feeling states. Depression, on the other hand, was only indirectly associated with current arthritis pain through a decrease in positive feeling states.[14]

Even simple interventions (to affect thinking or behaviors regarding one's choice of actions) may help to decrease anxiety and depression. For example, scheduling and participating in pleasant or enjoyable activities may be able to reduce negative feelings and increase positive ones. Activities such as these may be able to help bring about some positive changes, lessening anxiety and depression. Various relaxation techniques could also possibly be of help. Finally, learning coping skills was suggested as another potential way to reduce specific stressors in one's life and so reduce anxiety and depression.[15]

Anxiety and Depression: Are They Connected with Menopause?

Do anxiety and depression increase for women around the time of menopause? Some studies seem to indicate that both do increase, whereas other studies have found depression and anxiety to remain at similar or decreased levels compared with other time periods in life.[16] In an important study of 160 midlife women, the Ohio Midlife Women's Study, some possible reasons for the differing incidences of depression and anxiety found among women in meno-pause were highlighted. This was a longitudinal study in which the women were assessed for anxiety and depression at three time-points over a period of 18 months. These researchers found that two impor-tant predictors of anxiety (in addition to education level) were loss of resources and coping effectiveness. In fact, loss of resources consis-tently predicted anxiety and depression at each assessment over time. Resource losses can include conditions (e.g., a good marriage), energy resources (e.g., time, money), object resources (e.g., car, house), and personal characteristics (e.g., mastery, self-esteem). However, these researchers found that it was the loss of personal characteristic re-sources that was most important and central in predicting anxiety and depression.[17]

These findings point toward the importance of building and maintaining resources throughout menopause and later life, most es-pecially those pertaining to one's sense of self. Maintaining self-esteem and a sense of mastery can be developed and augmented as these researchers have emphasized. They refer to the Conservation of Resources Model of Stress extended by Hobfoll and colleagues. Within this perspective, ways of fostering social support, facilitating mastery, raising self-esteem, and gaining in skills and competence are emphasized.[18]

The Puzzling and Peculiar Nature of Arthritis Pain

If you are unconvinced about the potential effects of the emotions on arthritis pain, consider this: In a most interesting study of brain activity associated with chronic knee osteoarthritis, it was found that the *knee arthritis pain experienced by participants was directly related to areas of the brain linked to the experience of emotion* (e.g., the amygdala and other prefrontal-limbic portions of the brain).[19] The amygdala, located in the brain's medial temporal lobe, is a key junction in the processing of fear. The amygdala works in processing memories that are not regulated by conscious memory; these memories are unconscious and independent of conscious memory.

The memory which stores the fear itself could be termed a "fear memory." Fear memory exists without being attached to any conscious memory. One could also process the fear-producing episode as a parallel, conscious memory. This would take place through other brain structures such as the hippocampus. In this case, it could be termed a "memory of fear."[20] For example, the "fear memory" might consist of an image of a person brutally wielding a weapon directed at oneself and a wave of emotion and of fright. The "memory of fear," in this case might be the person's verbalization "the person came toward me with a weapon, and I was extremely frightened." It is almost as if one memory, the "fear memory" is raw and unprocessed, and the other, the "memory of fear," has been put into words along with an historical perspective.

What is particularly fascinating about the results of the above research on where arthritis pain is processed is that the experience of mechanical pain (in the same participants) was experienced in a different part of the brain than was their spontaneous arthritis knee pain. Again, it was the part of the brain highly implicated in *memory for emotional events* (such as the amygdala) that was involved in the experience of arthritis knee pain.[21]

The research methodology used within this study was as follows: Participants were asked to rate their arthritis pain prior to receiving the mechanical pain stimulation. This spontaneous arthritis pain was defined as the participant's verbal rating on a scale of 0-100,

from "no pain" to the "worst imaginable pain." Brain scans were performed on participants prior to mechanical pain application and
during the mechanical pain application. Thus, there were two types of
pain ratings for each knee (spontaneous pain and mechanical pain)
and a brain scan covering both. I should point out here in discussing
this study, that the researchers had obtained the informed consent of
participants, and the procedures had been approved by the University
Institutional Review Board. The pain induced was delivered through a
custom-made, plastic piston device (driven by pressurized air) designed to apply deep tissue pressure and to sense and record the
pressure measurements. The researchers had originally hypothesized
or speculated that the mechanical pressure pain would affect the same
areas in the brain that were affected by the spontaneous arthritis pain.
This turned out not to be the case; the two pain types had, indeed,
mapped onto *different areas of the brain*. The researchers noted that
the brain structures involved in the spontaneous arthritis pain (the
medial prefrontal cortex and limbic structures) have been identified as
being linked to *the emotional assessment of one's environment in
relationship to the self*.[22]

There are so many anecdotal accounts of people losing a job
or retiring only to find that they have a sudden onset of arthritis. The
research above and the study noted earlier on the loss of personal resources may be relevant here. Certainly, following a downward
change in vocational status and activity, it is possible that some individuals might assess themselves as being less masterful (accompanied
by a lowered self-esteem). If, indeed, the brain structures in arthritis
pain have been linked to the emotional assessment of one's environment in relationship to the self, could this lowered self-esteem and
mastery be in some way related to the arthritis pain? The possibility is
certainly thought-provoking!

Findings conducted by researchers from the University of
Manchester Rheumatic Diseases Centre and colleagues, provided additional support that arthritis pain is processed in the brain structures
related to emotions and fear (e.g., the prefrontal cortex, amygdala, and
other regions). These researchers compared the brain activities of
osteoarthritis patients across three different pain states: (1) arthritis
pain (pain experienced during normal activities reported as

moderately strong), (2) experimental pain (heat pain applied to the knee experienced as moderately painful) and (3) a pain-free state. The experimental pain was applied to patients when they were not experiencing arthritis pain. The researchers had thought that the two pain conditions would activate the same pain areas or networks. What they found was that although both of the pain stimuli activated the pain matrix, *arthritis pain was associated with increased activity in the areas involved in processing emotion and fear* (e.g., the prefrontal cortex, amygdala, and other regions).[23]

Interestingly, there are gender differences in the activity of the amygdala. For the memory of emotional experiences, the left amygdala is preferentially activated in women, whereas the right amygdala is activated in men (for the same type of emotional material).[24] In the University of Manchester study cited above, it was the left amygdala that was more activated in arthritis pain in comparison with the painfree condition.[25] Since the left amygdala is preferentially activated for the memory of emotional experiences in women, might this not suggest a possible linkage between arthritis pain and anxiety in women? Clearly, more research is needed, but these are very fascinating findings.

In a study which included the prevalence of psychiatric disorders among older adults in the United States, it was found that four times as many women as men suffer from a psychiatric disorder. Moreover, women were diagnosed with mood disorders more than men.[26] Importantly, women also have been found to have a higher prevalence of anxiety disorders than men.[27] Since women are more likely to suffer from osteoarthritis than men,[28] it is not clear whether anxiety or other mood or psychiatric disorders contribute to causing this greater prevalence of arthritis. Anxiety (or depression, for example) could result from trying to cope with chronic pain.

In a study of sixty-one women with knee osteoarthritis, it was found that anxiety and depression were significant predictors of pain. Anxiety and depression were found to account for 40% of the differences between women on self-rated pain scores. Interestingly, none of the factors that they had examined (to include pain scores, psychosocial status, and physical functioning) had any definitive relationship with the structural aspects of arthritis measured such as joint erosion, joint space, osteophytes, malalignment, calcifications, etc.[29] This is consistent with the lack of correspondence of radiological osteoarthritis and pain symptoms that we had seen earlier. These researchers stressed that studies are needed to help understand the relationship between personality traits and the development of osteoarthritis. Moreover, they emphasized that research is needed to clarify whether the type of pain experienced with arthritis may lead to emotional dimensions of pain.[30]

Does Anxiety Cause Arthritis Pain?

Although causal relationships among arthritis, anxiety and depression are far from clear, the fact that arthritis is often associated with anxiety in women is evident within the literature. Given the prevalence of anxiety and mood disorders in women, and the association with arthritis and arthritis pain, what can be done to help alleviate anxiety and increase positive mood? We have already mentioned, of course, seeking professional help. Sometimes this may be necessary to resolve anxiety and mood disorders rooted in the past or to handle present anxiety with which you are unable to cope. Notwithstanding, there are other things that you can do as well to try to alleviate anxiety and improve mood. The following activities have research evidence behind them in terms of their positive and beneficial effects. Some of these practices are based in the idea of the interrelationship of the mind and body (mind-body approaches) such as Tai Chi exercise, yoga practice, mindfulness-based stress reduction, and muscle relaxation training.

Mind-body techniques have become more readily incorporated into Western culture over the past thirty years. Indeed, training in techniques such as these is even offered at some major universities such as Harvard Medical School and the University of Massachusetts. In addition, the United States government has set aside ten million dollars for the National Institutes of Health (NIH) to develop centers for learning "Mind/Body Interactions and Health." Meditative and related techniques are increasingly being used by patients to treat anxiety and depression.[31] Perhaps, by lessening anxiety in women and improving mood, arthritis symptoms might be reduced. One of the significant factors that has been shown to protect against lower physical functioning scores in knee osteoarthritis (as reported by patients) was mental health status.[32]

Obviously, research is needed to disentangle the factors of mental health status, pain symptoms, and arthritis. It does seem clear however that stressors (even those from childhood) can affect the immune system and may make diseases such as osteoarthritis more likely in adulthood. Further research is necessary to determine causal connections between anxiety and arthritis pain. Nevertheless, I am including within this chapter some techniques to reduce stress and increase positive mood since they might present a possible way to help augment a personal healing program for arthritis. So, what can some of the mind-body techniques do to quell anxiety and create more positive moods, and are there other benefits as well?

Ways to Alleviate Anxiety and to Improve Mood, Metabolic Syndrome, and More

Tai Chi exercise, as well as yoga practice, has been shown to reduce anxiety and depression.[33] In addition, mindfulness-based therapy has been found to improve anxiety and mood.[34] Even progressive muscle relaxation and massage have been demonstrated to reduce anxiety.[35,36] Research study findings have also suggested that in addition to improved mood, metabolic syndrome risk factors may also be reduced (e.g., insulin resistance and physiological components related to cardiovascular disease) with mind-body interventions such as Tai Chi and yoga.[37] As discussed in Chapters One and Two, the prevalence of metabolic syndrome greatly increases after menopause. It has been associated with leptin resistance in older postmenopausal women. Moreover, as we saw earlier, increased leptin levels within the knee joint cavity are associated with osteoarthritis. The improvement in metabolic syndrome risk factors through Tai Chi exercise and yoga practice could be of much benefit in healing from menopausal arthritis.

So, let's take a look at some of the ways in which these types of mind-body and stress-reducing interventions might be beneficial to include within an overall healing program for menopausal arthritis. Of course, improvements in mental health and psychological factors do not necessarily mean that arthritis symptoms will improve too. Nevertheless, with the close connection between the areas in the brain where both arthritis and emotional pain are experienced, these mind-body approaches seem like possible healing interventions that should not be ignored.

Tai Chi Exercise -- Effects on Metabolism, Mood, Stress, and Other Factors

A very recent review of the literature on the physical benefits of Tai Chi exercise found a decrease in stress and anxiety following Tai Chi classes or interventions. Performing Tai Chi has also been linked with decreased feelings of sadness, anger, and fear as well as increased feelings of happiness.[38] One study found significant changes in the areas of physical and psychological functioning after doing Tai Chi. Compared with functioning prior to Tai Chi, the participants had less tension, depression, anger, and anxiety. Mood disturbances, overall, decreased. The practice of Tai Chi also de-creased cortisol levels.[39] Recall, as noted earlier, that cortisol is a hormone produced in response to stress.

In a pilot study of Tai Chi exercise for stress reduction, measures of both physiological and psychological indicators of stress were obtained. Physiological indicators of general stress such as daily cortisol levels, blood pressure, and heart rate were recorded. Per-ceived mental stress significantly decreased following the trial inter-vention with Tai Chi, as did cortisol levels. There were also significant improvements in mental health and psychological well-being.[40]

In a study conducted out of the Stanford Prevention Research Center in the School of Medicine at Stanford University, the effects of Tai Chi exercise on psychosocial benefits was examined. This was a 12-week intervention with women and men who were an average age of 66 years (the majority of them women). Significant improvements were found in psychosocial status, mood, and perceived stress. There was also a significant increase in the self-efficacy scores with regard to overcoming obstacles in learning Tai Chi and significant increases in confidence in performing Tai Chi.[41]

In studies of osteoarthritis patients specifically, a recent review assessed the effects of mind-body exercises upon outcomes such as self-efficacy in arthritis and depression.[42] It was unclear in the review what scaling measures were used for self-efficacy in the studies; however, as an example of possible content, an Arthritis Self-Efficacy Scale developed at Stanford University contained items such as, "How certain are you that you can decrease your pain quite a bit?," and "How certain are you that you can keep your arthritis or fibromyalgia pain from interfering with the things you want to do?"[43] Two out of three randomized, controlled trials found that Tai Chi exercise improved self-efficacy with regard to arthritis symptoms compared with a control group. Also, of three randomized controlled trials, Tai Chi exercise was found to have positive effects upon psychological outcomes. In the two studies with significant findings, positive psychological outcomes were reported. Symptoms of depression improved in the Tai Chi group in comparison to the control group in one study; and, in the other study, Tai Chi exercise was perceived as providing more benefits with regard to stress management and other health behaviors when compared with a control group.[44]

Yoga Practice -- Important Inroads into Alleviating Anxiety

Yoga practice has been found to have rapid and significant effects on stress and anxiety reduction among women who reported that they were emotionally distressed. Women who engaged in yoga training (two, weekly Iyengar yoga classes) over a period of three months were compared with a non-randomized control group (participants on the waiting list). Compared with the control group that did not participate, women who went through the yoga training had dramatic and significant improvements in perceived stress, anxiety, well-being, and depression. In addition, they also reported significant improvements in physical well-being. Cortisol levels also decreased significantly in the yoga class group.[45]

Another study of the effects of yoga training on depression and anxiety in women yielded some very interesting results. The yoga classes were conducted twice weekly for two months. Participants were randomly assigned to either the yoga class intervention or a control group who was assigned to the wait list and did not attend a yoga class. Compared with the control group, participating in the yoga class did not significantly decrease depression scores. However, participation in the yoga class was associated with a significant decrease in anxiety, both state anxiety (short-term) and trait anxiety (the stable behavior pattern of responding to threatening situations with state anxiety). In fact, the decrease in trait anxiety was pronounced and highly significant.[46] This is very important as oftentimes a stable pattern of anxiety in an individual may not always seem very amenable to change through non-psychological interventions.

A recent review of the literature on the use of yoga training for people with arthritis was conducted out of the Johns Hopkins School of Public Health. Of eleven studies (that included four randomized controlled trials, and four non-randomized controlled trials), positive benefits were found. In addition to reduced symptoms of arthritis (e.g., joint tenderness/swelling and pain), there were improvements in self-efficacy and mental health.[47] Thus, yoga practice seems to offer an important possible pathway for improving mental health and emotional states, and in this case, arthritis symptoms as well.

Mindfulness Meditation - Mixed Findings on Anxiety and Depression

Recent reviews are mixed on whether mindfulness-based techniques have an effect upon anxiety and depression. One review of fifteen studies of mindfulness-based stress reduction (MBSR) on anxiety and depression found no reliable effects. When control groups who did not receive the treatment were used as a comparison, the MBSR was not found to have a significant effect.[48] However, in a more recent and more comprehensive meta-analytic review of 39 studies, much larger positive effects were found and benefits extended to improving anxiety and mood. Nevertheless in this analysis, studies that did not have control groups were included.[49] What might be some factors (other than methodological ones) that could account for the varied outcomes of these studies?

First it would be important to look at just what "mindfulness" means within these types of interventions. It is often defined as a state of consciousness that consists of a focus upon the present moment (rather than the past or future). It involves self-regulation of attention, and a perspective that is non-judgmental and accepting in nature. It has also been conceived of as a kind of "mental balance," which transcends simply a state of awareness or attention.[50,51]

Dr. Jon Kabat-Zinn, a pioneer in the area of mindfulness meditation to reduce stress, began his Stress Reduction Program in 1979 at the University of Massachusetts Medical School. In his book, "Full Catastrophe Living," he described practicing mindfulness as "practicing being."[52] Interestingly, he also provides an account of one woman's experiences in the program that would contradict what one might expect to happen. First, she encountered some difficulties with the "body scan." The body scan is an initial practice used to begin mindfulness meditation. As described by Dr. Kabat-Zinn, it requires that the person spend forty-five minutes mentally scanning through the body focusing upon one body part and then moving on to the next. At the end of the session the entire body has received one's attention and awareness. Optimally, it is supposed to bring one a sense of well-being and timelessness.

However, the woman experiencing difficulty had found that she was feeling "blocked" around her neck and head. To summarize briefly, the exercise made her aware of some repressed, traumatic memories with regard to specific parts of her body. The somewhat puzzling and contradictory results of the stress reduction program for this woman were as follows: Her sleep had improved greatly, as did her blood pressure which had gone down from 165/105 to 110/70. She also had greatly reduced pain in her back and shoulders (she had suffered from many ailments to include lupus, arthritis, and coronary disease). However, what did not improve were distressful emotional symptoms; instead, they increased in number. With assistance from a psychotherapist, she was able to greatly reduce these unsettling emotional symptoms that had occurred as a result of the "flashback" experience triggered by the body scan.[53] It is interesting that many parameters of physical health improved at the same time that her emotional symptoms seemed to "worsen." Perhaps this is not so surprising, since harboring and holding these emotions within the confines of the body, and out of one's conscious awareness, can take a giant toll on physical health.

Does the mindset and attitude toward oneself make a difference in the helpfulness of mindfulness meditation? Some research has suggested that perhaps the outcome of mindfulness-based interventions may be influenced by whether one has a sense of self-compassion. Researchers from the State University of New York at Albany (SUNY) have pointed out that many therapists incorporate an attitude of compassion that they try to demonstrate to their clients. The participants within this study comprised a sample in which approximately 90% had sought help from mental health practitioners, and 82% had been given a psychiatric diagnosis. The concept of self-compassion that they were examining within their study might be thought of as being similar to the therapist's compassion toward the client. Optimally, the client is able to internalize this compassion (or bring this compassionate attitude into his or her own mental functioning as self-compassion). The results of this study suggested that self-compassion more strongly predicted symptoms of depression and anxiety than did mindfulness. It appears that whether one judges oneself harshly, or conversely with compassion, may be of key importance.[54]

When mindfulness-based interventions were looked at with regard to specific effects upon chronic pain conditions, a review of the literature found a limited amount of evidence for their effectiveness.[55] However, in a trial of mindfulness-based stress reduction (MBSR) with rheumatoid arthritis patients (that was included within this review), significant improvement in psychological dimensions was found. After six months of using mindfulness-based stress reduction (MBSR), there was a significant reduction in psychological distress and a significantly improved sense of well-being compared with the control group.[56]

Much more research needs to be conducted to understand the effects of mindfulness-based interventions on rheumatic diseases. In addition, as noted earlier, other psychological factors such as self-compassion may be important in whether mindfulness-based approaches are beneficial in alleviating depression and anxiety. Nevertheless, there has been a growing interest over the past decade in the potential of mindfulness meditation to lessen emotional distress and to help foster improved well-being in many different populations of people. This was emphasized by Dr. Laura Young, of the University of North Carolina School of Medicine, in her recent article "Mindfulness Meditation: A Primer for Rheumatologists."[57] Mindfulness-based stress reduction may offer a healing pathway for some, and further investigation of this possibility is certainly warranted.

Muscle Relaxation and Massage for Improving Mood and Well-Being

One might be doubtful that muscle relaxation and massage would be as effective as the more complex mind-body approaches discussed. However, there are some studies that might suggest otherwise. One study compared the effects of yoga training with the effects of muscle relaxation in reducing anxiety in women (the mean age of the women was 44 years). Participants all had mild to moderate levels of self-reported stress. The yoga intervention was a hatha yoga class and the relaxation intervention was a progressive muscle relaxation class. Ten weekly sessions were conducted which lasted one hour each. Hatha yoga was described as including breath awareness and internal centering (to eliminate external distresses, to become aware of one's internal feelings, and to sharpen focus). The yoga practice was also described as allowing for the release of mental and emotional blockages.[58]

The progressive muscle relaxation intervention involved tensing and relaxing each of the body's muscle groups until whole body relaxation was attained. Both of these interventions were equally effective in reducing stress and anxiety. However, those in the relaxation group had higher scores on social functioning, mental health, and vitality at the end of the 6-week follow-up period compared with the participants who attended the yoga classes. The researchers noted that perhaps the greater effectiveness and use of relaxation may have been because it had been easier to incorporate the relaxation techniques into everyday life, than it was the practice of yoga.[59]

However, because of the focus upon internal feelings and mental and emotional blockages, one might wonder if the yoga practice might have uncovered some unresolved psychological issues. If so, it might make sense that it did not fare as well as the relaxation technique in terms of improving social functioning, mental health, and vitality scores. Recall that the woman who was disturbed by the mindfulness-based stress reduction "body scan" had shown an increase in the number of distressful emotional symptoms. Different types of yoga practice (or emphases within individual classes) may lead to dissimilar outcomes on psychological measures. The findings from the yoga practice in this example are very different from the findings obtained within the other studies of yoga described earlier.

Massage has been shown to have beneficial effects upon anxiety reduction. In a Swedish study, the effects of light pressure massage were explored for patients experiencing severe anxiety. The massage therapy consisted of twice-weekly, full-body massage with ten treatments in all. The massage used strokes with light pressure to the skin, and each session lasted for about 45 minutes. The participants were patients referred by staff from a psychiatric outpatient clinic.[60]

These participants were interviewed following their last massage session and asked to describe their experience of the massage therapy. Participants expressed feeling relaxed in body and mind. They also felt appreciation for receiving unconditional attention (that is, they did not have to perform or achieve something in order to be given this experience of attention and caring from others). The participants had experienced reduced anxiety after the sessions and increased self-confidence. For some, reducing the anxiety with massage allowed them to function better in their lives; they were capable of doing things that they would have found difficult prior to receiving massage therapy (e.g., cleaning the house, taking walks, etc.). These individuals expressed getting more in touch with their own strength, power, and capacity to live fully.[61]

In another study, adults aged 60 years and older were randomly assigned to either a guided relaxation group or a massage therapy group. The massage therapy protocol involved three techniques -- Swedish massage, myofascial massage, and neuromuscular massage. The relaxation sessions involved the participant using visualization and relaxation of muscles while they lay upon a massage table. The massage therapy sessions resulted in significantly better scores on anxiety, stress, depression, and positive well-being than the guided relaxation sessions. The researchers noted that the effects of the massage therapy were most likely not due to simply general relaxation and positive human interaction since both the massage therapy and the relaxation session had these positive elements.[62] The myofascial massage and neuromuscular massage may encompass dimensions that are of particular importance to healing from menopausal arthritis, though. As described in earlier chapters, myofascial pain can lead to joint dysfunction, and neuromuscular factors can lead to problems such as body sway. Although not clear whether these types of factors were involved, it is possible that some of the increases in well-being may have been due to positive changes in myofascial and neuromuscular functioning.

Anxiety and Depression: Whether Causes or Consequences of Arthritis (or Both), Interventions May Help in Healing

There is much that one can do to relieve stress and anxiety and to improve mood. The common pathway for arthritis pain and emotion that research has demonstrated is thought-provoking, and it may lead to a better understanding of arthritis and arthritis pain. I look forward to further research that will clarify how stress reduction and improved mental health may have an effect upon the disease of arthritis. I also hope to see research that will explore whether psychotherapy (and other forms of mental health interventions) can positively change ongoing psychobiological responses to stress that may be rooted within childhood experiences. In particular, can the biological and physiological processes in the hypothalamic-pituitary-adrenal (HPA) axis that were initiated by childhood trauma and stress be positively altered during adulthood? Remember from earlier in this chapter, that the HPA axis acts to both suppress the production of cytokines and to incite the actions of cytokines; it, thus, has a critical effect upon the immune system. Moreover as we saw in Chapter Two, cytokines are integrally involved in the disease processes in osteoarthritis and menopausal arthritis. In addition, the HPA axis has an effect upon the neurotransmitters involved in the regulation of moods and the experience of pain. Understanding how to intervene to correct dysfunctions in the hypothalamic-pituitary-adrenal axis may lead to breakthroughs in the treatment of both mental and physical disorders.

These practices reviewed are but a portion of the therapeutic techniques that might be employed to decrease stress and anxiety, and they seem to hold much promise. With an eye toward possible psychological precursors to arthritis, we can approach healing now from multiple perspectives. So, let's move on to putting this all together in the next chapter and begin to heal from menopausal arthritis.

Notes for Chapter Eleven

[1]Nicolson, N. A., Davis, M. C., Kruszewski, D., & Zautra, A. J. (2010). Childhood maltreatment and diurnal cortisol patterns in women with chronic pain. *Psychosomatic Medicine, 72*(5), 471-480.

[2]Heim, C., Young, L. J., Newport, D. J., Mietzko, T., Miller, A. H., & Nemeroff, C. B. (2009). Lower CSF oxytocin concentrations in women with a history of childhood abuse. *Molecular Psychiatry, 14*, 954-958. doi: 10.1038/mp.2008.112

[3]Ibid.

[4]Insel, T. R. (2010). The challenge of translation in social neuroscience: A review of oxytocin, vasopressin, and affiliative behavior. *Neuron, 65*(6), 768-779. doi: 10.1016/j.neuron.2010.03.005

[5]Viviani, D., Charlet, A., van den Burg, E., Robinet, C., Hurni, N., Abatis, M., Magara, F., & Stoop, R. (2011). Oxytocin selectively gates fear responses through distinct outputs from the central amygdala. *Science, 333*(6038), 104-107.

[6]Insel (2010). Op. Cit.

[7]Von Korff, M., Alonso, J., Ormel, J., Angermeyer, M., Bruffaerts, R., Fleiz, C. de Girolamo, G., Kessler, R. C., Kovess-Masfety, V., Posada-Villa, J., Scott, K. M., & Uda, H. (2009). Childhood psychosocial stressors and adult onset arthritis: Broad spectrum risk factors and allostatic load. *Pain, 143*(1-2), 76-83. doi: 1016/j.pain.2009.01.034

[8]Heim et al. (2009). Op. Cit.

[9]Von Korff et al. (2009). Op. Cit.

[10]Shors, T. J. (2002). Opposite effects of stressful experience on memory formation in males versus females. *Dialogues in Clinical Neuroscience, 4*, 139-147.

[11]Anisman, H., Baines, M. G., Berczi, I.., Bernstein, C. N., Blennerhassett, M. G., Gorczynski, R. M., Greenberg, A. H., Kisil, F. T., Mathison, R. D., Nagy, E., Nance, D. M., Perdue, M. H., Pomerantz, D. K., Sabbadini, E. R., Stanisz, A., & Warrington, R. J. (1996). Neuroimmune mechanisms in health and disease: 2. Disease. *Canadian Medical Association Journal, 155*(8), 1075-1082.

[12]Putnam, F. W. (1997). *Dissociation in children and adolescents: A developmental perspective.* New York: Guilford.

[13]Creamer, P., Lethbridge-Cejku, M., Costa, P., Tobin, J. D., Herbst, J. H., & Hochberg, M. C. (1999). The relationship of anxiety and depression with self-reported knee pain in the community: Data from the Baltimore Longitudinal Study of Aging. *Arthritis Care and Research, 12*(1), 3-7.

[14]Smith, B. W., & Zautra, A. J. (2008). The effects of anxiety and depression on weekly pain in women with arthritis. *Pain, 138*(2), 354-361. doi: 10.1016/j.pain.2008.01.008

[15]Ibid.

[16]Bebbington, P., Dunn, G., Jenkins, R., Lewis, G., Brugha, T., Farrell, M., & Meltzer, H. (2003). The influence of age and sex on the prevalence of depressive conditions: Report from the National Survey of Psychiatric Morbidity. *International Review of Psychiatry, 15,* 74-83. doi: 10.1080/0954021000045976

[17]Glazer, G., Zeller, R., Delumba, L., Kalinyak, C., Hobfoll, S., Winchell, J., & Hartman, P. (2002). The Ohio Midlife Women's Study. *Health Care for Women International, 23,* 612-630.

[18]Ibid.

[19]Parks, E. L., Geha, P. Y., Baliki, M. N., Katz, J., Schnitzer, T. J., & Apkarian, A. V. (2011). Brain activity for chronic knee osteoarthritis: Dissociating evoked pain from spontaneous pain. *European Journal of Pain.* Advance Online Publication. doi:10.1016/j.ejpain.2010.12.007

[20]Debiec, J., & LeDoux, J. E. (2009). The amygdala networks of fear: From animal models to human psychopathology. In D. McKay, J. S. Abramowitz, S. Taylor, & G. J. G. Asmundson (Eds.). *Current perspectives on the anxiety disorders: Implications for DSM-V and beyond* (pp. 107-126). NY: Springer.

[21]Parks et al. (2011). Op. Cit.

[22]Ibid.

[23]Kulkarni, B., Bentley, D. E., Elliott, R., Julyan, P. J., Boger, E., Watson, A., Boyle, Y., El-Deredy, W., & Jones, A. K. P. (2007). Arthritic pain is processed in brain areas concerned with emotions and fear. *Arthritis & Rheumatism, 56*(4), 1345-1354. doi: 10.1002/art.22460

[24]Cahill, L. (2006). Why sex matters for neuroscience. *Nature Reviews Neuroscience, 7.6,* 477 (Academic OneFile). doi: 10.1038/nrn1909

[25]Kulkarni et al. (2007). Op. Cit.

[26]Gum, A. M., King-Kallimanis, B., & Kohn, R. (2009). Prevalence of mood, anxiety, and substance-abuse disorders for older Americans in the National Comorbidity Survey-Replication. *American Journal of Geriatric Psychiatry, 17*(9), 769-781.

[27]McLean, C. P., Asnaani, A., Litz, B. T.,& Hofmann, S. G. (2011). Gender differences in anxiety disorders: Prevalence, course of illness, comorbidity and burden of illness. *Journal of Psychiatric Research, 45,* 1027-1035. doi: 10.1016/j.jpsychires.2011.03.006

[28]O'Connor, M. I. (2007). Sex differences in osteoarthritis of the hip and knee. *Journal of the American Academy of Orthopaedic Surgeons, 15*(Suppl. 1), S22-S25.

[29]Salaffi, F., Cavalieri, F., Nolli, M., & Ferraccioli, G. (1991). Analysis of disability in knee osteoarthritis. Relationship with age and psychological variables but not with radiographic score. *Journal of Rheumatology, 18*(10), 1581-1586.

[30]Ibid.

[31]Arias, A. J., Steinberg, K., Banga, A., & Trestman, R. L. (2006). Systematic review of the efficacy of meditation techniques as treatments for medical illness. *Journal of Alternative and Complementary Medicine, 12*(8), 817-832.

[32]Sharma, L., Cahue, S., Song, J., Hayes, K., Pai, Y. C., & Dunlop, D. (2003). Physical functioning over three years in knee osteoarthritis: Role of psychosocial, local mechanical, and neuromuscular factors. *Arthritis and Rheumatism, 48*(12), 3359-3370.

[33]Innes, K. E., Selfe,T. K., & Taylor, A. G. (2008). Menopause, the metabolic syndrome, and mind-body therapies. *Menopause, 15*(5), 1005-1013.

[34]Hofmann, S. G., Sawyer, A. T., Witt, A. A., & Oh, D. (2010). The effect of mindfulness-based therapy on anxiety and depression: A meta-analytic review. *Journal of Consulting and Clinical Psychology, 78*(2), 169-183. doi: 10.1037/a0018555

[35]Smith, C., Hancock, H., Blake-Mortimer, J., & Eckert, K. (2007). A randomized comparative trial of yoga and relaxation to reduce stress and anxiety. *Complementary Therapies in Medicine, 15*, 77-83.

[36]Billhult, A., & Määttä, S. (2009). Light pressure massage for patients with severe anxiety. *Complementary Therapies in Clinical Practice, 15*, 96-101.

[37]Innes et al. Op. Cit.

[38]Field, T. (2011). Tai Chi research review. *Complementary Therapies in Clinical Practice, 17*, 141-146.

[39]Jin, P. (1989). Changes in heart rate, noradrenaline, cortisol and mood during Tai Chi. *Journal of Psychosomatic Resarch, 33*(2), 197-206.

[40]Esch, T., Duckstein, J., Welke, J., & Braun, V. (2007). Mind/body techniques for physiological and psychological stress reduction: Stress management via Tai Chi training - a pilot study. *Medical Science Monitor, 13*(11), CR488-CR497.

[41]Taylor-Piliae, R. E., Haskell, W. L., Waters, C. M., & Froelicher, E. S. (2006). Change in perceived psychosocial status following a 12-week Tai Chi exercise programme. *Journal of Advanced Nursing, 54*(3), 313-329.

[42]Chyu, M-C., von Bergen, V., Brismée, J-M., Zhang, Y., Yeh, J. K., & Shen, C-L. (2011). Complementary and alternative exercises for management of osteoarthritis. *Arthritis*. Advance Online Publication. doi: 10.1155/2011/364319

[43]Lorig, K., Chastain, R. L., Ung, E., Shoor, S., & Holman, H. R. (1989). Development and evaluation of a scale to measure perceived self-efficacy in people with arthritis. *Arthritis & Rheumatism, 32*(1), 37-44. doi: 10.1002/anr.1780320107

[44]Chyu et al. (2011). Op. Cit.

[45]Michalsen, A., Grossman, P., Acil, A., Langhorst, J., Lüdtke, R., Esch, T., Stefano, G. B., & Dobos, G. J. (2005). Rapid stress reduction and anxiolysis among distressed women as a consequence of a three-month intensive yoga program. *Medical Science Monitor, 11*(12), CR555-CR561.

[46]Javnbakht, M., Kenari, R. H., & Ghasemi, M. (2009). Effects of yoga on depression and anxiety in women. *Complementary Therapies in Clinical Practice, 15*, 102-104.

[47]Haaz, S., & Bartlett, S. J. (2011). Yoga for arthritis: A scoping review. *Rheumatic Diseases Clinics of North America, 37*(1), 33-46.

[48]Toneatto, T., & Nguyen, L. (2007). Does mindfulness meditation improve anxiety and mood symptoms? A review of the controlled research. *Canadian Journal of Psychiatry, 52*(4), 260-266.

[49]Hofmann et al. (2010). Op. Cit.

[50]Toneatto et al. (2007). Op. Cit.

[51]Hofmann et al. (2010). Op. Cit.

[52]Kabat-Zinn, J. (2009). *Full catastrophe living: Using the wisdom of your body and mind to face stress, pain, and illness. (15th Anniversary Ed.)*. New York: Delta Trade Paperbacks.

[53]Ibid.

[54]Van Dam, N. T., Sheppard, S. C., Forsyth, J. P., & Earleywine, M. (2011). Self-compassion is a better predictor than mindfulness of symptom severity and quality of life in mixed anxiety and depression. *Journal of Anxiety Disorders, 25*, 123-130.

[55]Chiesa, A., & Serretti, A. (2011). Mindfulness-based interventions for chronic pain: A systematic review of the evidence. *Journal of Alternative and Complementary Medicine, 17*(1), 83-93. doi: 10.1089/acm.2009.0546

[56]Pradhan, E. K., Baumgarten, M., Langenberg, P., Handwerger, B., Gilpin, A. K., Magyari, T., Hochberg, M. C., & Berman, B. M. (2007). Effect of mindfulness-based stress reduction in rheumatoid arthritis patients. *Arthritis Care & Research, 57*(7), 1134-1142. doi: 10.1002/art.v57:7/issuetoc

[57]Young, L. A. (2011). Mindfulness meditation: A primer for rheumatologists. *Rheumatic Diseases Clinics of North America, 37*(1), 63-75.

[58]Smith et al. (2007). Op. Cit.

[59]Ibid.

[60]Billhult et al. (2009). Op. Cit.

[61]Ibid.

[62]Sharpe, P. A., Williams, H. G., Granner, M. L., & Hussey, J. R. (2007). A randomised study of the effects of massage therapy compared to guided relaxation on well-being and stress perception among older adults. *Complementary Therapies in Medicine, 15*, 147-163.

Chapter Twelve

Putting It All Together for Your Own Healing

     The quintessential message within this book is that menopausal arthritis goes *beyond* just osteoarthritis brought on by menopause, and osteoarthritis goes *beyond* just a "wear and tear" disease of aging! Many of the dynamics and much of the pain involved in menopausal arthritis have to do with muscle and soft tissue disorders that *do not have anything* directly to do with osteoarthritis! And, although osteoarthritis is no doubt part of the picture, osteoarthritis is not even what we once thought it was! It's not simply a "wear and tear" disease of aging. Your cartilage is not just a victim of the ravages of time with cartilage chafing against cartilage, slowly but assuredly wearing itself away. Rather, your cartilage exists within a highly metabolic milieu! Hormones such as leptin set into motion proinflammatory cell-to-cell messengers called cytokines that drive the cartilage breakdown!

     At the time that I began to tackle the problem of menopausal arthritis, I was not aware of either of these two things. I didn't know that menopausal arthritis was driven by a disease process that was characterized by inflammation. Neither did I know that there were "non-arthritis" conditions that could actually cause excruciating knee pain that feels exactly like knee arthritis.

When I began my healing program, I had a persistently aching right knee. Not only did it ache *deep* within the knee joint, but I also had a persistent and unrelenting pain that took hold just below my knee. Also, when I began to try to strengthen my muscles, my front thigh muscles or quadriceps seemed terribly weak. I couldn't quite put my finger on what it was, but there was a muscular or neuromuscular sensation that was completely unfamiliar to me. My body just simply wasn't the same as it was just a few short years ago -- a few short years ago and light-years away. Menopause was having a rapid effect upon not only my joints, but also the muscles that upheld them.

Most of the books that I had come across had emphasized building up your quadriceps to get rid of knee osteoarthritis, and this was a unisex solution! But, what about menopausal arthritis? No one had really addressed the issues that are of specific importance to older women. The recommendations for exercise for osteoarthritis have not really taken into consideration the many differences between older men and women. In Chapters Four, Five, and Seven we have clearly seen that there are important gender differences in cartilage, tendons, and muscles. And, although there are gender similarities too, the differences between men and women may be more important to focus upon here. The reason is that menopausal arthritis is, of course, gender- and age-specific! Exercises to help alleviate and heal from menopausal arthritis should focus on features of primary importance to *women in menopause*. The exercises within this book have been designed to do just that.

Moreover, it is not just differences between men and women in cartilage, tendons, and muscles, but also differences in pain that originates *outside of the joint*! It became very clear to me that the soft tissue disorders, muscle shortening, and even muscle inflammation that may be experienced more markedly in women than men were blocking my initial ability to benefit from muscle strengthening exercises!

Finally, although it is one of the last things that I would have thought of when I was first trying to get rid of my knee pain, it turns out that arthritis pain and emotions may have some common biological pathways!

All of these aspects of healing from menopausal arthritis are explored in depth within this book. So as you come to this last chapter, it's really now a matter of knowing how to put it all together.

The Healing Process

1. Begin with a Good Base

Begin first with good nourishment to your body; this is the most vital thing that you can do at the outset. Start with some of the foods, supplements, and herbs that have been summarized in Chapter Ten. Find out which ones seem to be of particular benefit to you. This can only be accomplished through experimenting with them. Sometimes, one can only tell whether a supplement is helping by first using it and then discontinuing its use. Then you will be able to observe whether you see any differences in your arthritis symptoms. There are some supplements that I would miss immediately, as an increase in symptoms would be obvious. Others I have discontinued, and I do not even notice a difference. Try the supplements in Chapter Ten that do have scientific, evidence-based support.

Most likely, some supplements, foods, and herbs will work better than others for you. We are all different in this regard. Those that I have summarized in Chapter Ten have scientific, evidence-based findings to support their use. My experience is that it takes *many different supplements and herbs* to accomplish the anti-inflammatory effects that I have achieved. And, I cannot overstate this point: *This focus on reducing inflammation is critical to healing from menopausal arthritis!*

Indeed, as I write this chapter, brand new research out of Stanford University School of Medicine has uncovered a critical role that low-grade inflammation plays in osteoarthritis. Dr. William H. Robinson and colleagues, using mass spectrometry, were able to detect proteins within the joint fluid of individuals with osteoarthritis that are not present in the same way in healthy individuals. These proteins are part of what is called the "complement system."[1] The main function of the complement system is to spot "foreign" particles and macromolecules and help to eliminate them. It also clears out damaged, altered or used components such as dead cells or clots.[2]

The findings of Dr. Robinson and colleagues are extremely important to your healing from menopausal arthritis. Their findings suggest the following, and this is very critical: *The low-grade inflammation that has been associated with osteoarthritis may actually play a central role in the development of osteoarthritis.*[3] The powerful anti-inflammatory supplements and herbs described within Chapter Ten help to fight inflammation, and thus, should provide you with invaluable resources to help prevent and heal from osteoarthritis and menopausal arthritis. I know that they have for me. Moreover, research has provided evidence for their effectiveness in helping to reduce inflammation and arthritis symptoms.

Although losing weight is one intervention that research shows can help in reducing leptin levels (and thus, decreasing inflammatory cytokines), foods, herbs, and supplements can be powerful in providing anti-inflammatory effects. Moreover, one important herbal component, curcumin, has been shown to actually *reduce leptin levels*. Thus, you may not actually need to lose an appreciable amount of weight to have an effect upon leptin levels.

The close associations drawn in research between low-grade inflammation and osteoarthritis, leptin and inflammation, and leptin and osteoarthritis, are the reasons that I emphasize a strong, natural anti-inflammatory program base. Establishing this nutritional base with adequate natural anti-inflammatory herbs, foods, and supplements is essential to healing within this program.

2. Move On to Exercise

When you begin to feel like you are decreasing the inflammation and pain in your body through foods, herbs, and supplements, then move on to strengthening your muscles and tendons. When you begin exercising, be sure to retain the strong nutritional and anti-inflammatory base that you have already put into place. When you challenge your body through exercise, it is critical to nourish your body afterwards with protein to repair muscle tissues, and nutrient-rich food, vitamins, and supplements that can help your muscles and tendons recover well. You also need good nutrition to sustain cartilage and build strong muscle-tendon-bone units.

As you begin to work the dynamic, kinetic chains of muscles in your body, you will strengthen not only muscles, but muscle-tendon units (and muscle-tendon-bone units). Feel how the muscles within your body move together in dynamic chains; the exercises within this book are specifically designed to strengthen these muscle chains. Take things slowly, and never overstress your muscles or tendons. These exercises do not have to be performed in any set exercise regime or at any particular frequency. They are designed to help you, and you should benefit within your own timeframe and within your own physical capabilities.

Recovering from exercise and rebuilding muscle is harder as we get older. I have listed in the Appendix some healing creams and gels that I have found to be particularly helpful in assisting muscle and tendon recovery after exercise and other stresses to these tissues.

Also, don't undo the benefits of your exercise by adopting everyday behaviors that work against joint and muscle health! Be sure to use correct posture when you walk (spine erect, body not tilted forward), and *use* your muscles when you ascend and descend the stairs. Wear shoes with flexible soles that allow the muscles, tendons, and bones in your ankles and feet to move freely. Focus on strengthening your muscles, muscle chains, tendons, muscle-tendon-bone units, and building the healthy connective tissues, or fascia, that surround your muscles!

The exercises within this book address menopausal arthritis symptoms that are caused by muscle weaknesses, imbalances, tendon stiffness, and joint laxity. They also help to build strong bone and cartilage. Recall from the research reviewed that in addition to building bone, moderate loading (as within some forms of exercise) on cartilage tissues has also been shown to help stimulate cartilage cell health. The exercises within this book are designed to provide moderate loading on the joints and surrounding tissues. The strengthening of your muscles and muscle-tendon-bone units are essential for healing, and research now shows that cartilage might be included within this functional unit!

3. Heal from the Inside and the Outside

Traditional medicine practices such as Ayurveda and Traditional Chinese Medicine have stressed the importance of approaching the healing of arthritis through *both* internal and external means. For thousands of years, people with diseases such as arthritis have secured benefits from the *combination* of what is taken internally for healing and what is applied externally. Try some of the external applications that have been discussed in Chapter Nine. Experiment with them, and seek to determine which ones are providing positive effects for you. Sometimes, a particular external application may work exceptionally well in enhancing an anti-inflammatory effect that you are obtaining from an herb, food, or supplement taken internally. Try various types of massage and other manual therapeutic techniques, and see which ones work best for you. Some types of massage may be amenable to self-massage and others not (and some may not be appropriate for particular health conditions). As with any of the procedures, therapies, exercises, or other remedies within this book, obtain medical advice.

4. Make Everyday Lifestyle Changes that Promote Your Healing

Something as basic as the type of shoes that you are wearing can have a dramatic effect upon the amount of stress that you put onto your knees. As we have seen, increased knee loads are associated with the severity and progression of osteoarthritis and with pain in osteoarthritis. Clogs and other stiff-soled shoes limit the flexibility of your ankles and feet. Switching from clogs (or other shoes with stiff soles) to shoes that have flexible soles can be an important factor in promoting healing!

In addition to maintaining an erect posture, notice how you place your feet on the steps when you proceed downstairs. Are you placing the weight onto the middle portion of your foot, or are you placing more weight upon the front, toe area of your foot? Just making a fundamental change such as ensuring that your weight is evenly distributed as you descend the stairs can play a significant role in healing.

Be sure to decrease activities that may worsen arthritis or increase your risk for developing arthritis (such as my heavy gardening work involving digging that I had described in Chapter One). As you may recall, the amount of digging that I was doing was associated with the development of medial compartment knee osteoarthritis! Moreover, increase the everyday activities that will promote healing. The exercises within this book can be done so easily at various points during the day, as they require nothing but a doorway for you to perform them (or nothing at all but yourself) and a minute or two at a time. They needn't be done in a full set or in any fixed exercise regime.

As they are all done standing, there is no need to disrupt the flow of your everyday activities by having to get down on the floor or to get a set of exercise props in order. Moreover, for menopausal women with arthritis, props such as bands can be uncomfortable or painful. Getting down onto the floor to exercise and then back up to a standing position can hurt as well, and may stress vulnerable joints. So, in doing these exercises you benefit doubly -- through the exercises *and* through not straining your joints. I choose the exercises that I feel my body needs most at the time. *They have become part of my everyday movements.*

In thinking about your everyday activities that can promote healing, please keep in mind that your feelings and emotions *do* affect and *can* alter immune responses. In your everyday life, cultivate attitudes and behaviors that promote healing, and engage in activities that can reduce stress for you.

5. Be Patient - Some Aspects of Healing Will Come Quickly, Others Will Take Longer

Healing from menopausal arthritis is a process where some parts of healing will come swiftly, while others will take longer to attain. Some of the benefits from the herbs, vitamins, and supplements can be obtained very rapidly. On the other hand, building muscles, tendons, and building muscle-tendon strength take time. When I first began to do the "Body Lowering" exercise the tendons and muscles around my knees and ankles were very weak. It was difficult to do this exercise without feeling some discomfort in my knees and ankles. So I began slowly, but kept working at this exercise for many months. Sometimes I would let a week or so go by without doing the exercise at all if my muscles had not seemed to recover fully yet. Listen to what your body is telling you. If it seems stressed or has not repaired itself from exercise, then stop for a while, and let it fully recover.

Similarly when I began the "Toe Raise" exercise, my right calf muscle was so weak that it would quiver and shake as I raised my toes up and lifted my calves and legs. Now, after keeping at this exercise for many months, my right calf muscle has become strong. This strengthening of the muscles and tendons, to include buttocks, thighs and lower leg muscles has paid off greatly for me! The activation of whole, kinetic muscle chains fosters balance and power. I now relish the "leg power" that I have when I climb up the stairs and the strength and balance I enjoy as I descend the stairs!

Indeed, I am amazed at the strength of my knees, ankles, and the surrounding muscles and tendons. There are many unique exercises within this book such as "Stepping and Holding Your Ground," and "Body Lowering" that along with the other exceptional exercises in this program will build the strength and stability that you need to have well-supported joints that can move with ease. These exercises comprise a comprehensive protocol especially designed for menopausal women.

Healing from Menopausal Arthritis: In Sum

I hope that the information in this book will help you to heal from menopausal arthritis. I also hope that I have been able to convey the potency, strength, and effectiveness of self-healing. That deep ache within my knee is gone, and so too is the once unrelenting ache just below my knee. My muscles are strong, and I can ascend and descend the stairs with ease! I have, in essence, healed from my menopausal arthritis!

I have provided within this book, guidelines and insights that have been helpful to me and research findings that have pointed me in a direction toward my own healing. Take the research findings, and piece them together in your own unique way, from your own unique perspective.

Find and emphasize the aspects of this program that are particularly important in your own personal healing from menopausal arthritis. Add your own research and insights. Be open to how conventional medicine might be able to help you, but wise enough not to engage in anything that does not promote your health and healing! Over and above all, believe in your ability to strengthen and heal your body; your passion and commitment will reap great rewards!

Notes for Chapter Twelve

[1]Wang, Q., Rozelle, A., Lepus, C. M., Scanzello, C. R., Song, J. J., Larsen, D. M., Crish, J. F., Bebek, G., Ritter, S. Y., Lindstrom, T. M., Hwang, I., Wong, H. H., Punzi, L., Encarnacion, A., Shamloo, M., Goodman, S. B., Wyss-Coray, T., Goldring, S. R., Banda, N. K., Thurman, J. M., Gobezie, R., Crow, M. K., Holers, V. M., Lee, D. M., & Robinson, W. H. (2011). Identification of a central role for complement in osteoarthritis. *Nature Medicine*. Advance Online Publication. doi:10.1038/nm.2543

[2]Carroll, M. V., & Sim, R. B. (2011). Complement in health and disease. *Advanced Drug Delivery Reviews, 63*, 965-975. doi: 10.1016/j-addr.2011.06.005

[3]Wang et al. (2011). Op. Cit.

Flying Up the Stairs!

Midway through my program, I had grabbed a shovel and a pot of soil amendment and walked down the flagstone steps that are imbedded in the slick, heavy clay soil. This time, I thought of the chain of actions of my muscles, starting with the gluteus maximus and hip abductors, and I made sure that they were exerted, that I engaged their full force. Then I felt the contractions of the quadriceps and the hamstrings and made sure that they were equally part of the energy being expended. Then the calf muscles. I ensured that I didn't inadvertently and reflexively bend forward to lighten the load on my muscles and knees. Instead, I pulled every muscle in the lower half of my body into the orchestrated, agile actions of gardening. "Glutes, quads, hamstrings, calves," became a litany of sorts in my mind. When I shoveled out two large, carved holes to place the rosemary plants into the soil, I made sure that I was not jarring and injuring my right knee this time. I was carefully digging. Yes, carefully digging, instead of tackling the task at hand with the determinedness of a deckhand. I took a moment to enjoy the springtime air, and the delicate, but wing-strong hummingbird that landed on the flower a breath away. It was exhilarating to be out gardening once again. "Glutes, quads, hamstrings, calves." I was back in the saddle again.

That was six months ago. Now, walking toward my house, I feel something that I haven't felt for a very long time. In fact, it is so foreign to me that at first it does not even seem real. I am moving with ease, without effort. I am simply enjoying moving; enjoying walking. I don't have to think about it. For the first time since menopause, my muscles are strong. My knees don't hurt. I open the door, I walk into the foyer. I take a brief moment, I reflect. Then with a heart full of joy and gratitude, I am flying up the stairs!

Glossary

Adipocyte -- A fat cell; it is a connective tissue cell with the specific function of manufacturing and storing fat.

Adipokines (Adipocytokines) -- Cytokines (Cell-to-cell signalers) produced by adipose (fat) tissue.

Adiponectin – A protein hormone manufactured and secreted by adipose tissue which regulates the body's metabolism of lipids and glucose (and has an effect upon the body's response to insulin).

Adiposity -- Obesity or the state of being fat

Afferent nerve -- Sensory nerve that conveys impulses or information from organs or tissues within the body to the spinal cord and brain (i.e., the central nervous system).

Androgen -- A sex hormone generating male characteristics produced in males by the testes, and in females by the adrenal glands.

Annexin-1 -- Human endogenous (arising from within the human body) anti-inflammatory protein, an important modulator of inflammation.

Anterior cruciate ligament (ACL) -- A major stabilizing ligament in the center of the knee which works together with the posterior cruciate ligament (PCL). These two ligaments cross each other (hence the term "cruciate") to form an "X." This stabilizes the knee and allows it to flex and to extend without moving from side to side.

Antigens -- Elements (such as foreign blood cells, bacteria and viruses) that when introduced into the body produce an immune response stimulating the production of antibodies.

Anti-inflammatory Cytokines -- Molecules which are involved in the immune system regulation through controlling the actions of pro-inflammatory cytokines. Major anti-inflammatory cytokines include IL-4, IL-10, IL-11, and IL-13.

Antioxidant -- A substance which counteracts oxidative damage (damage from oxygen) such as oxidative damage from free radicals within the body. This oxidative process is associated with the progression of diseases such as cancer or age-related diseases within the body.

Arachidonic acid -- An unsaturated fatty acid that is essential to human beings, but cannot be produced by the human body; it must be obtained through diet. It is a basic building block for the biosynthesis of prostaglandins and of leukotrienes.

Arthralgia -- Pain, or severe pain in a joint. The pain extends along a nerve or group of nerves and is experienced in one or more joints.

Arthroplasty -- Surgery to alleviate joint pain and help restore proper joint functioning. Procedures involve either reshaping a joint and adding a prosthetic between the bones of the joint, or joint replacement.

B-cell -- A type of white blood cell that is part of the lymphocyte grouping. It is not dependent upon the thymus for its development, and it is essential in fighting off infections. It functions in the process of immunoglobulin production.

Biomechanics -- The application of mechanical laws to living organisms such as the functioning of the human body, especially with regard to the forces involved in locomotion and the musculoskeletal structures, body positions, and functions.

Blood glucose level -- Concentration of glucose (blood sugar) within the bloodstream. Many factors within the body work to keep blood glucose levels within a normal range (such as insulin and other hormones).

Bone mineral density (BMD) -- A measure of bone mass, in which the amounts of calcium and other minerals within the bone are assessed in order to determine how dense their presence is within a bone segment.

Boron -- A nonmetallic element/mineral which is found in foods such as leafy greens, grains, and nuts. It has estrogen-elevating effects within the body.

Cartilage -- Tough, fibrous, connective tissue composed of chondrocytes (cartilage cells) and various tissue fibers or ground substance.

Cat's Claw -- A South American woody vine (Uncaria tomentosa) in which the root bark is used as an herbal preparation. It has anti-inflammatory, antiviral, and immune system stimulant properties.

Cell adhesion molecules -- Membrane proteins produced by endothelial cells (cells that line the blood and lymph vessels); these membrane proteins regulate the movement of molecules and leukocytes (white blood cells) from the bloodstream to the tissues of the body.

Central Sensitization -- Increased response to stimulation in which activity that would not normally result in a painful response does so due to amplified signaling in the central nervous system (CNS). The neurons had been previously activated due to a noxious stimulus (such as an injury), but now are recruited even when the stimulus is not harmful or injurious.

Chondrocyte -- A cartilage tissue cell within the cartilage matrix.

Chondroitin -- A natural substance within the body that gives cartilage its elasticity. It also exists as a dietary supplement derived from animal cartilage, often in the form of chondroitin sulfate.

Collagen -- The main protein in connective tissue, cartilage, ligaments, tendon, and bone. It provides strength to these structures.

Collagenase -- Any of a variety of enzymes that help to bring about the decomposition of a collagen (and gelatin) through the reaction with water.

Complement system -- A group of approximately 35-40 proteins and glycoproteins that work collectively within the immune system to recognize "foreign" particles and macromolecules (such as immune complexes) and help to rid the body of them. It does this by helping to dissolve and destroy foreign particles and macromolecules and by making them more susceptible to phagocytosis.

Concentric contraction -- A muscle contraction in which the muscle shortens as it contracts. An example would be the upwards movement in a biceps curl (bringing the forearm to the shoulder).

Correlational research design – Study design in which the association between two or more variables is assessed. This research method examines patterns of relationships between variables, but it cannot determine causality.

Creatinine -- The metabolic by-product of creatine, which is found in blood, urine and muscle tissues. Creatine helps the body to produce muscle contractions. Its by-product, creatinine, is removed from the bloodstream by the kidneys and excreted in urine.

Curcumin -- An extract from turmeric. It has antioxidant, chemoprotective, and anti-inflammatory properties. It also helps to reduce leptin levels.

Cyclooxygenase-2 (COX-2) -- An enzyme that produces prostaglandins (strong, hormone-like substances) which is associated with pain and inflammation.

Cytokines -- Regulatory proteins (such as interleukins) that are released by cells within the immune system and carry signals to other cells. They operate as intercellular mediators. Some of the cytokines are proinflammatory, and others are anti-inflammatory.

DHA (Docosahexaenoic acid) -- An essential fatty acid. It is an Omega 3, polyunsaturated fatty acid found in fish such as tuna and bluefish and marine animal oils.

DHEA (Dehydroepiandrosterone) -- Steroid hormone produced by the adrenal glands with a testosterone-like action. It is converted into testosterone and estrogen. Levels of DHEA decline in the bloodstream with aging.

DNA – (Deoxyribonucleic acid) -- A double-stranded molecule that encodes genetic information. It is one of two genetic-encoding molecules with the other being RNA (ribonucleic acid). RNA is derived from DNA in humans.

Eccentric contraction -- Force used as a means of decelerating part of the body, or muscle force used in gradually lowering a load (such as a weight) rather than letting it fall with the force of gravity. The muscle is lengthening: for example, in the downwards motion in a biceps curl.

Eicosanoids -- Signaling molecules (such as prostaglandins) that exert actions in systemic processes such as inflammation and immunity. They are derived from Omega 3 and Omega 6 fatty acids.

Elastase -- An enzyme that acts as a catalyst for the digestion of elastic tissue.

Elastic energy -- The energy created by compressing, twisting and/or stretching of a substance (e.g., a compressed spring, or the compression of the Achilles tendon in running).

Endocrine -- Relating to endocrine glands, which are glands that produce and secrete hormones directly into the bloodstream. Endocrine sites are many to include the pituitary gland, thyroid gland, adrenal glands and fat cells.

Endogenous -- Originates from within an organism

*EPA (*eicosapentaenoic acid) -- A fatty acid found nearly singularly in fish and marine animal oils

Epidemiological – Referring to the branch of medicine that studies the causes, statistical distributions, and control of diseases

Estradiol – The most potent of the naturally occurring estrogens. At menopause, the ovaries stop their production of estradiol.

Estrogen -- Any of a particular grouping of steroid hormones that are produced primarily by the ovaries (also by the placenta), and are responsible for the development and functioning of the female reproductive system.

Estrone – A less active form of estrogen than estradiol; it is a metabolite of estradiol and of androstenedione. It is the major source of estrogen in postmenopausal women.

Exogenous – Originates outside of an organism

Extracellular matrix -- Any substance that is produced by cells and secreted into the surrounding tissue space that is usually noncellular in form. It helps to hold tissues together, and it may contain substances such as collagen, elastin, and proteoglycans.

Fascia -- Sheets and bands of connective tissue that are present throughout the entire body. They surround and provide support to muscles and to organs.

Fibroblasts -- Elongated, flat cells present in connective tissue which are capable of forming collagen fibers. They perform essential functions both during development and within adulthood. In development, they are involved in the formation of organs, and development of different tissues; in adulthood, they appear to have regulatory effects on cells, such as those in the immune system. In disease conditions, they appear to have a role in the growth and functioning of cells such as inflammatory and cancer cells.

Fibromyalgia -- Syndrome in which a person suffers from long-term pain that involves the entire body. Pain and tenderness are felt within the joints, muscles, and tendons, to include soft tissues such as fascia.

Free radical -- An unstable atom or group of atoms due to one or more unpaired electrons. Free radicals can damage cells and may help promote or accelerate diseases such as cancer and cardiovascular disease, among others.

Gait – A characteristic manner of walking; walking motions which would include length of step, speed, rhythm, and cadence.

Gene expression -- The process that allows information from a gene to be converted into mRNA and then into a protein. This process allows for the physical appearance or expression of a gene-derived characteristic inherent within the organism's genetic make-up.

Glucocorticoid – An adrenocortical (derived from the adrenal cortex) steroid hormone that has an anti-inflammatory effect and is active in many body functions such as carbohydrate, protein and fat metabolism. A primary example is cortisol. Glucocorticoids, used in medicine, are also an approved treatment for rheumatoid arthritis and other diseases such as asthma, allergies, etc.

Glucosamine – A derivative of glucose that occurs in many glyco-proteins (see below).

Glucosaminoglycan – Any of the carbohydrates that contain amino sugars that occur in proteoglycans (such as hyaluronic acid and chondroitin sulfate).

Glucose – The body's primary source of energy; it is a type of sugar resulting from the digestion of the sugar and starch in carbohydrates. Glucose is absorbed through the small intestine into the bloodstream.

Glycoprotein – A molecule consisting of a carbohydrate and a protein. They have primary roles in body processes such as the immune system where nearly all central molecules in the immune response are glycoproteins.

Growth factors – A family of biological factors that the body produces to regulate growth and the division and maturation of blood cells by bone marrow (an example would be fibroblast growth factor).

Hamstring muscles – The muscles of the posterior thigh that are used to flex the knee joint, adduct the leg, and extend the thigh. The semimembranosus, semitendinosus and the biceps femoris make up the hamstring muscles.

Heberden's Nodes -- Small, bony growths or nodules, spurs of the articular cartilage, usually found on the distal interphalangal joints (end joints closest to the fingertips).

Hormone -- A chemical transmitter substance produced mainly by the endocrine glands, but that may also be produced by other organs and tissues, as well. Hormones send chemical messages to body organs upon which they exert a specific regulatory effect.

Hyaline cartilage -- Semitransparent, very strong, flexible and elastic cartilage that provides the buffer between articular (joint) bones by reducing friction. It consists of cartilage cells (chondrocytes) that are within a matrix of hyaluronic acid, collagen and protein that exists around the cartilage cells.

Hyaluronic Acid -- A gel-like polysaccharide (substance belonging to a class of long chains of monosaccharides) that serves lubricating and protective functions such as it does within the synovial fluid of joints.

Hydrocolloid – A substance that when mixed with water forms a gel.

Immune complex -- Any of a number of molecular complexes that combine an antigen (a foreign substance that causes an immune reaction) and an antibody (a blood protein that counteracts the specific antigen). Immune complexes often build up in bodily tissue and are associated with various disease conditions.

Immunoglobulins -- Proteins that are manufactured by lymphocytes and plasma cells; they have a vital role in the immune system by fastening onto foreign substances (such as bacteria) and helping to kill or destroy them.

Infrapatellar fat pad -- A pad of fat that is situated behind and underneath the patella.

Insulin – A hormone produced by the pancreas that regulates the amount of sugar (glucose) in the blood; it stimulates body cells, principally the liver and muscle cells, to take in, store, and metabolize sugar.

Insulin Resistance – A condition in which the body has a lowered response to insulin. Because of this, the body produces larger amounts of insulin so that the glucose level within the blood can be maintained at a normal level. Insulin resistance is associated with other metabolic dysfunctions such as Type II diabetes and metabolic syndrome.

Interleukin -- One of a large group of proteins, the cytokines, that are produced for multiple functions within the body and mediate communication between cells. Most interleukins are produced by T cells, but in some cases they are produced by phagocytes (cells that engulf and get rid of harmful material such as waste material or foreign bodies within the bloodstream or tissues) or other cells. They play significant roles in stimulating immune responses such as inflammation.

Interleukin-1 – Any of a group of cytokines that prompt the production of interleukin-2 by helper T-cells stimulating an inflammatory response within the body.

Interleukin-2 – A lymphokine, a substance released by T-cells stimulated by antigens. Interleukin-2 is released in response to an antigen and to interleukin-1, and stimulates rapid growth of helper T-cells.

Interleukin-4 – A cytokine that can induce many activities in the body, such as prompting rapid spread of T cells, and mast cells (connective tissue cells often injured in allergic reactions which releases histamine and other substances). It also induces antibody secretion by B cells (type of white blood cell needed to fight off infection)

Interleukin-6 -- A cytokine with both proinflammatory and anti-inflammatory properties. It is released by T cells and macrophages to stimulate immune response to tissue damage causing inflammation. It has anti-inflammatory actions through its inhibition of TNF-alpha and interleukin-1, and its activation of interleukin 10.

Interleukin-10 – A cytokine with a vital role as a regulator of the immune system. Its two major roles include inhibiting cytokine production by macrophages and inhibiting some of the functions of macrophages during the activation of T cells. Because of this, it is considered to exert primarily an anti-inflammatory action within the immune system.

Interleukin-12 -- A cytokine that has an effect upon many of the biological functions of T-cells and of natural killer cells (or NK cells).

Interleukin-13 – A cytokine activated by T-cells (white blood cells of critical importance to the immune system). IL-13 inhibits inflammatory cytokine production in monocytes (a phagocyte with only one nucleus) located within the blood. Phagocytes surround and absorb harmful waste materials and other foreign bodies in the blood or tissues.

In vitro -- A process that occurs within a laboratory container such as a test tube, or other controlled (non-natural), environment.

In vivo -- A process that occurs within a living organism or natural environment, as opposed to within a test tube or non-natural, controlled environment.

Isometric Contraction -- Muscle stays at the same length as it contracts without movement at the affected joint. An example would be holding a static contraction in the biceps curl at the point in which one achieves the upward concentric contraction, prior to bring the arm down in the eccentric contraction.

Isotonic Contraction -- Muscle force stays constant even though there is a change in the length of the muscle, and there is usually accompanied movement at the affected joint or body parts. (See Concentric and Eccentric contractions).

Iyengar Yoga -- A form of yoga especially characterized by its use of props (e.g., chairs, blocks, straps, etc.) to assist in attaining the yoga positions or poses, and its emphasis on physical alignment.

Joint capsule – An envelope that encloses and seals off the joint. It is comprised of dense connective tissue that forms a casing around the synovial joint (joint lined with a membrane which secretes lubricating fluids). This casing helps to keep in the synovial fluid that lubricates the joint.

Joint cavity – This is the space filled with the synovial fluid that is held in place by the joint capsule.

Joint space – The space between the bones of the joint

Joint space narrowing -- A decrease in joint space, or space between the bones of the joint. This is used as an indicator of existing cartilage loss and/or possible meniscal damage.

Kellgren and Lawrence Classification -- A grading system of knee osteoarthritis severity based upon x-rays; classifications include from Grade 0 (absence of changes indicating disease) to increasing indicators in Grades 1, 2, 3, and Grade 4. Features of osteoarthritis of the knee identified through radiographs and used in this scaling system include: narrowing of joint cartilage, osteophytes, and sclerosis (See Osteophytes and Sclerosis).

Knee valgus moment -- An external load that functions to move the knee into a valgus positioning or posture (knees caved inwards).

Krill oil – An oil derived from small crustaceans, tiny shrimp, semi-translucent and pink in color. They are food for whales and other sea animals such as seals, penguins, and squid. Consumed as food in many cultures, they are often used in some Asian cuisines in dry form in soups and noodle dishes. Krill oil naturally contains phospholipids which facilitate the bioavailability of the omega-3 fatty acids to cells in the body.

L-Arginine – A semi-essential amino acid since many people require more of it than can be supplied by their bodies alone (for example, infections, rapid growth and other conditions would necessitate additional arginine). Arginine is converted into nitric oxide which relaxes the blood vessels producing vasodilation, and it also stimulates the body to manufacture protein.

L-Carnitine -- A substance derived from the amino acid lysine. It helps in the process of transforming fat into energy. It is produced within the liver and kidneys, and stored in tissues such as the muscles, heart, and brain. Dietary sources include red meat and dairy products, as well as fish, poultry, avocados, and peanut butter.

L-Glutamine – A non-essential amino acid found widely in plants and animals; it has a significant role in protein metabolism.

Leptin – A protein hormone secreted by adipose tissue that regulates hunger and eating behavior in humans. It also has been found to be associated with obesity and some chronic disease conditions, such as osteoarthritis.

Leptin resistance -- Abnormally elevated leptin levels (hyper-leptinemia) associated with a reduction in leptin receptors, as well as a reduced signaling capacity of leptin.

Leukocyte – A white blood cell that can compress its way through intracellular spaces. It protects the body by acting as a destroyer of bacteria, fungi, and viruses, and as a detoxifying agent for toxic proteins resulting from allergic reactions and injuries to cells.

Leukotriene -- Chemical compound within the body that helps to maintain inflammatory reactions (such as hay fever or asthma, for example). These compounds are derived from arachidonic acid.

Ligament -- A band of fibrous tissue that holds bones together, and strengthens and stabilizes joints by preventing excessive movement of the joint.

Lipid -- Any of the major fats circulating within the body such as cholesterol and triglycerides. (See serum lipoprotein)

Lipid homeostasis -- A process which allows for the maintenance of a steady, internal state of lipid within either a cell or an organism.

Lipid metabolism -- The physiological, metabolic processes that function to take in and assimilate lipids from dietary sources and to synthesize and break down lipids or fats within the body.

Lipoprotein -- (See Serum Lipoprotein)

Low-Grade Inflammation -- Type of inflammation that is not acute in nature, but rather can be prolonged with inflammatory markers that are not as pronounced as in other forms of inflammation. Serum High-sensitivity C-reactive protein (hs-CRP) levels are used as a marker for low-grade inflammation.

Lymphokine -- Considered to be a sub-group of cytokines, they are soluble protein mediators that have been released by T-cells that are responding to an antigen. They affect the behavior of other cells such as increasing the production of macrophages within the immune response.

Maca (Lepidium meyenii) -- An herbaceous plant, with the common name of "Maca," it is native to Peru and Bolivia, and is consumed as a root vegetable and used as an herbal medicine.

Macrophage -- A large white blood cell that helps in fighting off infections by destroying foreign antigens such as bacteria and viruses. Usually immobile, they become vigorously mobile when inflammation is present.

Magnetic Resonance Imaging (MRI) -- An imaging technique that is able to directly depict all of the tissue structures of the most common and movable joints; that is, it is able to visualize the cartilage, ligaments, bone, menisci and other tissues. It shows anatomical structures in three-dimensional form, thus allowing for quantification of cartilage characteristics (e.g., thickness, volume).

Matrix metalloproteinase -- A protease (enzyme that breaks down proteins) that is capable of degrading a variety of extracellular matrix proteins.

Mechanoreceptor -- Nerve ending that is receptive to mechanical pressures (such as produced by touch, sound, and muscle contractions).

Medial compartment of knee -- Anatomical part of the knee that contains all of the supporting structures and layers of fascia located at the medial area (inner middle side), to include the medial collateral ligament.

Menopausal arthritis -- Arthritis associated with the menopause; it was first explored scientifically and identified as a clinical syndrome (within a major medical journal) by Dr. Russell L. Cecil and Dr. Benjamin H. Archer. In 1925, they published the article, "Arthritis of the Menopause: A Study of Fifty Cases" in the Journal of the American Medical Association (See Chapter One). Also, the specific conceptualization of menopausal arthritis put forth in this current book is a collection of symptoms that may or may not have their origin within the disease of osteoarthritis. (See Chapter Six)

Menopause -- The time when menstrual periods permanently cease. It is commonly defined as the time when 12 consecutive months have passed without having a menstrual period (with no other identified biological or physiological reasons for menstrual cessation).

Metabolic syndrome -- Also called insulin resistance syndrome, and Syndrome X, it is the term for a group of co-occurring risk factors that increase the risk for coronary artery disease, Type 2 diabetes, and stroke.

Metabolism – The overall process through which cells produce the necessary substances and obtain the energy needed to sustain life. Within this process, organic compounds are broken down to provide heat and energy (*catabolism*), and molecules are used to build more complex organic compounds to help grow and repair tissues (*anabolism*).

Metalloproteinase -- A family of enzymes from the group of proteases (enzymes that break down proteins). The catalytic acceleration of chemical reactions occurring within this protease family involves a metal, with most metalloproteinases being zinc-dependent.

MMP-13 (Matrix metalloproteinase-13) -- One of the collagenases that exist between cells (interstitial) that function to degrade or break down Type II collagen in cartilage. Also known as collagenase-3, it is usually manufactured solely by cartilage and bone during a person's development, and by cartilage cells in the disease of osteoarthritis. It serves a primary function in the progression of both rheumatoid arthritis and osteoarthritis. (See collagenase above)

Monocytes -- Largest of the white blood cells within the body, they are found within the bone marrow and the bloodstream. They turn into macrophages when they move into the tissues of the body. (See macrophage)

Myalgia -- Muscle pain that characteristically is diffuse (spread throughout various parts of the body) and is non-specific in nature. There may also be a feeling of associated malaise.

mRNA (messenger RNA) -- A molecule of RNA that is a complement to one of the DNA gene strands. It moves out of the nucleus of the cell into the cytoplasm (surrounding gel-like substance where most cellular processes take place) and carries with it the coding information for synthesizing protein. This process of transporting RNA molecules from the cell's nucleus to its cytoplasm is essential for gene expression to occur. (See Gene expression)

Muscle -- Contractile tissue that generates force causing movement of the joints (through skeletal muscle) and movement of internal organs (through cardiac and smooth muscles).

Muscle cell (myofiber) – A single muscle cell; it is densely filled with contractile proteins, energy stores, and signaling structures. It is the smallest contractile muscle unit and requires subsystem facilitation for contraction and metabolism.

Muscle fibrils (myofibrils) – Each myofiber, or muscle cell, contains a network of myofibrils; these fibrils contain the contractile proteins that generate and produce force.

Muscle hypertrophy -- Growth of muscle cells and an increase in their size; enlargement of muscles. In non-pathological conditions, this usually occurs as a result of exercise such as weight lifting.

Muscle-tendon junction (myotendinous junction) -- A specialized region of the muscle-tendon unit where the muscle fibers and the collagen fibers of the tendon meet with each other; it is here that muscle force is transmitted between muscle and tendon.

Muscle-tendon unit -- The main component of force generation during athletic and other activities involving active movement of the body. Force is generated through a combination of the muscle actions (that can include concentric, eccentric and static muscle activity) and the release of elastic energy from the unit's tendon. (See concentric, eccentric and static contraction)

Natural killer cell -- A cell that can kill another cell without needing to have been sensitized to it; they are small lymphocytes that are formed within the bone marrow. A "first line of defense" against cells infected by viruses or by cancer cells, they develop in their entirety without any function of the thymus gland, and have no markers of origins from T-cells or B-cells.

Neutrophil -- A type of white blood cell that contains little sacs of enzymes used to help the neutrophil kill and digest or assimilate bacteria and other microorganisms. It does this through the process of phagocytosis (in which the neutrophil envelopes and digests micro-organisms and cellular debris in order to remove them from the bloodstream).

Nerve cell (or neuron) -- A specialized cell for sending and receiving electrical signals within the body. Motor neurons send electrical signals from the brain and spinal cord to muscle neurons and other neurons, while sensory neurons receive electrical signals from sensory cells (sensory neurons) and from other neurons and transmit these signals to the spinal cord and brain.

Nitric oxide (NO) -- A toxic compound which, nevertheless, plays significant roles within the body. These roles include the transport of oxygen to tissues, transmission of nerve impulses, and the killing of tumor cells and cells infected by viruses.

Nociceptor – A nerve cell ending that acts as a sensory receptor and receives painful stimuli or messages; it picks up the stimuli that damaging stresses (e.g., mechanical, chemical or other) are acting upon tissues within the body and provides the first step in the process of pain sensation.

Non-sagittal motion -- Motion that deviates from the vertical plane of the body (the sagittal plane that splits the body into right and left sections). Examples of non-sagittal motion include frontal and transverse plane motions such as internal rotation of the hip as well as knee valgus positioning.

Omega-3 fatty acids -- Essential fatty acids (not formed by the body, but necessary for normal metabolism). Omega 3 fatty acids include α-linoleic acid (ALA), eicosapentaenoic acid (EPA), and docosahexaenoic acid (DHA). Common dietary sources include fish oils and flaxseed oil.

Omentum -- A fold of the peritoneum (the membrane that lines the abdominal cavity). The greater omentum is attached to the lower edge of the stomach and extends down over the intestines attaching at the transverse colon. The lesser omentum is attached at the upper edge of the stomach and stretches to attach to the liver.

Osteoarthritis -- A disease in which the cartilage that protects the joints begins to deteriorate, and in its later stages, begins to disappear. It also degrades subchondral bone and leads to bony overgrowths.

Osteoarthritis, Primary -- Form of arthritis associated with aging.

Osteoarthritis, Secondary -- Form of arthritis caused by factors other than those associated with aging (e.g., injuries, congenital disorders).

Osteophyte -- An abnormal bony outgrowth (or bone spur). The bony outgrowth is usually around a joint and can cause pain when there is friction with adjacent nerves.

Patella -- Commonly called the kneecap, it is a small bone at the front of the knee.

Peak external knee flexion moment -- A biomechanical term referring to the greatest dynamic forces at the knee involved in flexing the knee, for example, at various points of flexion during walking.

Peak external knee adduction moment -- A biomechanical term referring to the greatest dynamic forces at the knee involved in rotating the knee during walking and other movements. With the external knee adduction moment during walking, there is an ordinary tendency for "varus" rotational angle or torque; that is the portion of the leg below the knee would tend to rotate inward. This knee adduction moment has been considered to represent or indicate the loading on the medial knee compartment.

Perimenopause -- The time period prior to menopause when a woman is going through the transition from regular menstrual cycling and ovulation to cessation of ovary functioning or menopause.

Pes anserinus -- The location of insertion for the tendons of sartorius, gracilis, and semitendinosus. It was given the Latin name pes anserinus (which means "goose foot") because of its similarity to the webbed foot of the goose. It is located at the medial side of the tuberosity of the tibia.

Pes Anserine Bursitis -- A painful condition in which the bursa of the pes anserinus becomes inflamed through overuse or injury. It can be a cause of chronic knee pain and often involves pain and tenderness at the site.

Phagocyte -- A cell that surrounds and consumes foreign bodies such as harmful bacteria and microorganisms.

Phagocytosis -- The process by which a phagocyte surrounds, engulfs and absorbs harmful microorganisms and cells.

Placebo -- In medical research, a substance that does not contain any medicine (a sham therapy) that is used as a "control," in comparison with the substance that does contain medicine (an authentic therapy). This is done to control for the patient's expectation that an intervention will work, with a resulting significant effect due simply to the patient's positive expectation (called the "placebo effect").

Polyarthritis -- Arthritis involving inflammation in several (two or more) joints.

Postmenopause -- All of the time period after the experience of menopause, or the end of menstrual cycles.

Premenopause -- The time before menopause, which includes peri-menopause but is not limited to it.

Progestin -- Generic term for any of a group of steroid hormones that is consistent with the effects of progesterone; it produces some or all of the biological effects of progesterone. Synthetic progestin, however, is not the same as progesterone produced within the body; they are different in molecular composition with different effects upon the body.

Proinflammatory Cytokines -- Cytokines that are produced primarily by immune cells that have become activated; they are involved in the extension and strengthening of inflammatory reactions. They include IL-1, IL-6, and TNF-α.

Prostaglandins -- Any of a number of substances that have hormone-like qualities (such as controlling blood pressure and the contraction and relaxation of smooth muscles) They are also involved in modulating inflammation. Prostaglandins are derived from arachidonic acid.

Prostaglandin E2 (PGE2) -- The most common prostaglandin, it is also the most biologically active. PGE2 is considered to be a primary factor involved in the progression of the disease of osteoarthritis through promoting cartilage degradation.

Proteoglycan – Any of a group of glycoproteins that are found principally in connective tissue. Hydrated forms comprise the very viscous (thick and sticky) fluid of mucus, and the matrix of the ground substance of connective tissue such as cartilage.

Proteoglycan Aggregate -- A large aggregation or clustering of proteoglycans that are bound to an elongated molecule of hyaluronic acid. It is integral to the cross-linking of collagen fibrils within the cartilage matrix.

Proinflammatory adipokines -- Proinflammatory cytokines produced by adipose tissue. (See adipokines and proinflammatory cytokines)

Protease -- Any enzyme that helps facilitate the breakdown of proteins into amino acids or peptides (compound containing two or more amino acids). Amino acids are known as the "building blocks" of proteins; and hence, protease is an enzymatic agent involved in the disassembly of the built protein structure.

Proteome -- The entire set or full complement of proteins that are expressed by either a genome (all of the DNA within a human being), a cell, a tissue (specified type of cell or tissue), or an organism.

Proteomics -- The study of the full range and complement of an organism's proteins; analysis of how the organism's proteins are structured, and how they function within the biological processes of the body (e.g., how they function within metabolic pathways).

Quadriceps -- The quadriceps femoris, often termed the "quads," is a group of four muscles that perform knee extension. The rectus femoris, the vastus intermedius, vastus medius, and vastus lateralis all act together to extend the leg.

Radiographic -- Usually refers to X-rays; referring to an image produced on radiosensitive material by radiation, not produced by visible light.

Radiography (Plain Radiography) -- Primary imaging technique used in the assessment of osteoarthritis. It is able to detect bony abnormalities and indirect indicators of damaging cartilage changes. It cannot directly view the menisci and other soft tissue structures such as tendons, ligaments and bursae.

Randomized, controlled trial (RCT) -- A study in which participants are allocated at random (by chance alone) to be in a group that receives a clinical intervention or treatment, or to a group that receives no intervention/treatment or acts as a comparison group (control group). The control group may receive a placebo (e.g., "sugar pill," "sham therapy"), no intervention, or may receive what is considered to be standard practice. This quantitative, experimental method allows for greater determination of causality than other less rigorous methods.

Range of motion (ROM) -- The difference between the angle of a joint in its fully extended position and the angle of the joint at its maximum flexion. Each individual joint in the body has its own normal range of motion.

Range of motion exercises -- Exercises used in physical therapy (and in many arthritis exercise programs) to improve joint mobility and function by gently and gradually increasing the range of motion of individual joints. These exercises are believed to help decrease pain and stiffness.

Reactive oxygen species (ROS) -- Molecules or ions of oxygen that have an unpaired electron making them highly reactive; they include peroxides and hydroxyl radical. ROS play a part in the destruction of microbes by phagocytes and in oxidative damage to proteins and lipids within the body.

Resistin -- Considered to be an adipocytokine (although some research has suggested that it is not expressed in human fat cells, or only abnormally at very low levels). Its role in sensitivity to insulin in humans remains controversial and undetermined at this point in time.

Resveratrol -- A natural compound (polyphenol), it is produced by a plant's defense system as a response to invasion by harmful agents such as fungus, injury or infection. Red wine, grapes, raspberries and peanuts are examples of good sources of this compound. It may have protective effects against cancer, cardiovascular and other diseases through antioxidant and anti-inflammatory actions.

Rheumatoid arthritis -- A type of inflammatory arthritis and an auto-immune disorder; synovitis that is persistent in nature, systemic inflammation, and the presence of autoantibodies (e.g., rheumatoid factor) are characteristics of this disease.

Rose hips (Rosa canina) -- The round part of the rose flower that is located just underneath the petals. The hips are considered to be the fruit of the plant. An herbal product used for many disorders such as arthritis and gout; it is a diuretic and an antioxidant.

Sarcopenia -- The decline in muscle mass and loss of muscle strength that occurs as a result of the aging process.

Sclerosis -- A hardening or thickening of tissues or other parts of the body, particularly from excess formation of fibrous tissue.

Serum lipoprotein -- A lipid and a protein in combination which comprise the form in which lipids move through the blood -- examples would be high density lipoprotein (HDL) and low density lipoprotein (LDL).

Sex hormone binding globulin (SHBG) -- A protein (glycoprotein) that binds to estrogen and to testosterone. It has a role in the transport of sex steroids in plasma.

Signaling cascade -- Proteins and other molecules involved in converting one type of stimulus or signal into another are involved in a process that escalates. The number of molecules involved increases, as a process that began with an initial signal or stimulus results in a "cascade" in which a large response (or whole series of reactions) is brought forth through a single trigger stimulus.

Signaling molecules -- A chemical or substance produced by cells to carry out extracellular communication between cells

Skeletal muscle -- Muscle under voluntary control (as opposed to cardiac and smooth muscle which contract without conscious, voluntary control). It functions to provide skeletal movement and to maintain an upright stance or posture.

16 alpha-hydroxyestrone -- An estrogen metabolite; a breakdown product of estrogen. It is metabolized in one of two mutually exclusive pathways (the other pathway yields 2-hydroxyestrone). The biological activities of the two metabolites within the body are very different in terms of estrogenic and other biological actions. (See 2-hydroxyestrone)

Static contraction -- An isometric contraction; the muscle is activated but there is no movement of a joint and no change in muscle length. Examples of static or isometric contractions would include holding a dumbbell weight in place with a bent arm, or pushing against a wall. (See isometric contraction)

Subchondral bone -- The bone that is just below the cartilage that cushions the joint; cartilage degeneration in osteoarthritis is associated with subchondral bone thickness and abnormalities in the formation of bone proteins.

Subcutaneous nodule -- A small solid mass or lump underneath the skin. These nodules are commonly seen in rheumatoid arthritis patients, but may also occur in other types of rheumatic disorders to include systemic lupus erythematosus.

Synergistic effect -- An effect or outcome based in the combined action or joined operation of two or more things which would not be achievable without their combination. The presence of one thing (for example one chemical substance) is able to enhance the effects of the second thing (another chemical substance). In this sense they are working together, or demonstrating "synergism" (combined action) to produce an effect not possible by either chemical substance independently.

Synovial fibroblasts -- Cells present in the synovial tissue of individuals with rheumatoid arthritis and osteoarthritis, as well as individuals with healthy synovial tissues. When they have been subjected to certain cytokines and other proinflammatory agents, these cells appear to contribute to chronic inflammation by releasing mediators such as cytokines and matrix metalloproteinases contributing to tissue damage. Much focus has been directed toward their possible role in the development of rheumatoid arthritis; a unique synovial fibroblast cell type has been identified in rheumatoid arthritis research.

Synovial fluid -- A viscous fluid that lubricates the joints and provides nutrients to joint cartilage; it is secreted by the membranes within the joint cavity, as well as by tendon sheaths and bursae.

Synovial lining (synovium) -- The lining of the joint; the innermost lining of the synovial membrane is one to two cells thick and contains specialized cells that have been described as having phagocytic actions. Synovial membrane cells (along with joint cartilage cells) produce lubricants. The synovial lining is semi-permeable, but sufficiently restrains outflow of the lubricating synovial fluid.

Synovial sac -- The capsule that surrounds the entire joint; it includes both the synovium or synovial membrane and lining and the synovial fluid.

Synovitis -- Inflammation of the synovial membrane that is characterized by effusion or increased fluid in the synovial sac; swelling, pain, and or joint motion restriction may result.

Systemic Lupus Erythematosus (SLE) -- A chronic, inflammatory autoimmune disease that may target any part of the body to include the skin, joints, and internal organs such as the heart and brain. Lupus is a disease that may have periods of flares (with worsening symptoms) and remissions (improving symptoms). The disease can range in severity from mild to life-threatening.

T-cells -- A type of white blood cell that is part of the white blood cell grouping known as lymphocytes (other lymphocytes include B cells and natural killer cells). They are called T cells because they become mature cells within the thymus.

Tai Chi -- An ancient Chinese exercise system that continues to be practiced today with many reported health benefits (such as stress and blood pressure reduction). The formal exercise consists of a series of between 18 and 37 very slow, gentle movements of postural positions.

Tendon -- The tissue structures between bones and muscles that transmit force generated within muscle to the bone (thus, making it possible for the joint to move).

Tensile strength -- The maximum amount of tensile stress (stress from tension) that a material or biological entity (such as a tendon) can take or withstand from being stretched before it fails (e.g., breaks, ruptures).

Tibiofemoral -- Of or pertaining to the tibia and the femur bones.

TIMP-2 -- A member of the family "Tissue Inhibitor of Metalloproteinases," TIMP-2 inhibits activity of metalloproteinases which play a role in degrading the extracellular matrix.

TNF-alpha (Tumor necrosis factor-alpha) -- A cytokine that is produced primarily by activated macrophages (and also T-cells). It brings about the expression of other cytokines and cell adhesion molecules. It also activates macrophages, T-cells and B-cells.

Type II collagen -- Structural basis for articular (joint) cartilage and hyaline cartilage (the smooth-surfaced cartilage which reduces friction between the bones of a joint.

2-hydroxyestrone -- An estrogen metabolite; a breakdown product of estrogen. It is metabolized in one of two mutually exclusive pathways (the other pathway yields 16 alpha-hydroxyestrone). The biological activities of the two metabolites within the body are very different in terms of estrogenic and other biological actions. 2-hydroxyestrone is sometimes considered to be the "good" estrogen metabolite.

Ultrasonography (high frequency MSK ultrasonography) -- An imaging modality that is able to show many articular or joint structures within and around affected joints. Importantly, it is able to depict tendons, ligaments and bursae and the outside characteristics of the menisci.

Valgus knee alignment -- Commonly referred to as "knock-kneed," this alignment of the knee causes an increase in stress at the lateral compartment or outside compartment of the knee.

Valgus positioning -- Knees cave inward.

Varus knee alignment -- Commonly referred to as "bow-legged," this alignment of the knee causes increased stress on the medial or inner compartment of the knee.

Vasomotor -- This refers to actions that cause dilation or constriction of blood vessels and the regulation of their diameter (accomplished through nerves and muscles).

Visceral adipose tissue -- Visceral fat that surrounds the internal organs; the fat is located within the abdominal cavity.

Visfatin -- A protein that has been said to have functions that are like a cytokine; it has also been viewed as a hormone derived from visceral fat, and has been categorized as an adipokine. Some research suggests that it may mimic some of the effects of insulin.

Vitamin K -- A fat soluble vitamin that is needed by several proteins involved in forming blood clots. The natural plant form of vitamin K is known as phylloquinone.

Whey -- The part of milk that is watery and is able to be separated from the portion that forms a solid or semi-solid state (i.e., curd); this is a process that occurs during cheese-making. Whey provides lactose and many vitamins and minerals.

White adipose tissue (WAT) -- The most common type of fat tissue found within the body; it functions in various ways, such as storing food energy reserves and providing insulation to the body. It is one of two types of fat, the other being brown adipose tissue.

Resources

Readings and Informational Websites That I Have Found Helpful in Healing Menopausal Arthritis:

Diet and Nutrition with a Focus upon Leptin:

Richards, B. J., & Richards, M. G. (2009). *Mastering leptin (3rd Ed.)* Minneapolis, MN: Wellness Resources Books.

Rosedale, R.. & Colman, C. (2004). *The Rosedale diet.* New York: HarperCollins.

Herbal Remedies:

Ingram, C. (2001). *The cure is in the cupboard: How to use oregano for better health.* Buffalo Grove, IL: Knowledge House.

Muscle Anatomy:

Dimon, Jr., T. (2008). *Anatomy of the moving body.* (2nd Ed.) Berkeley, CA: North Atlantic Books.

Jarmey, C. (2008). *The concise book of muscles.* (2nd ed.). Berkeley, CA: North Atlantic Books.

Website: GetBodySmart.com An Online Textbook About Human Anatomy and Physiology

(This is a website that provides visuals and interactive animations to understand the human body)

Orthopedic Massage and Manual Therapy:

Hendrickson, T. (2003). *Massage for orthopedic conditions.* Baltimore, MD: Lippincott Williams & Wilkins.

Weintraub, W. (1999). *Tendon and ligament healing: A new approach through manual therapy.* Berkeley, CA: North Atlantic Books.

Trigger Points and Trigger Point Therapy:

DeLaune, V. (2010). *Trigger point therapy for foot, ankle, knee, and leg pain: A self-treatment workbook.* Oakland, CA: New Harbinger Publications.

Finando, D., & Finando, S. (2005). *Trigger point therapy for myofascial pain. The practice of informed touch.* Rochester, VT: Healing Arts Press.

Niel-Asher, S. (2008). *The concise book of trigger points.* Berkeley, CA: North Atlantic Books.

Product and Resources That I Found Helpful in Self-Healing of Menopausal Arthritis

Topical Creams/Oils/Lotions:

---For Muscle and Arthritis Pain & to Help Heal Tissues:

Traumeel (anti-inflammatory analgesic)

Heel, Inc.

Albuquerque, NM 87123

www.heelusa.com

1-800-920-9203

Arniflora – Arnica Gel

Distributed by: Boericke & Tafel

Green Bay, WI 54311

A division of Nature's Way Products, Inc.

Topricin

Topical BioMedics, Inc.

P.O. Box 494

Rhinebeck, NY 12572

Phone: 1-845-871-4900

Fax: 1-845-876-0818

www.topricin.com

---*Mineral-Rich Topicals & Healing Oils*

Dead Sea Mud

San Francisco Bath Salt Company

33231 Transit Avenue

Union city, CA 94587

1-800-480-4540

customerservice@sfbsc.com

Mahanarayan Oil

Banyan Botanicals

 6705 Eagle Rock Ave. NE, Albuquerque, NM 87113

541-488-9525 1-800-953-6424

 info@banyanbotanicals.com

---*Vitamins, Food and Herbal Supplements*

New Chapter - *Ginger force*

90 Technology Drive

Brattleboro, VT 05301

888-874-4461

www.newchapter.com

New Chapter - *Turmericforce* (Dual extracted Turmeric)

90 Technology Drive

Brattleboro, VT 05301

888-874-4461

www.newchapter.com

New Chapter - *Zyflamend softgels*

90 Technology Drive

Brattleboro, VT 05301

888-874-4461

www.newchapter.com

Vitality Works - *Oregano Oil - Carvacrol 70*

Jennifer L. Baca-Morris
Customer Service Manager
Vitality Works, Inc.
8409 Washington Street NE
Albuquerque, NM 87113
Toll Free: (800) 403-HERB (4372)
phone: 505-268-9950
fax: 505-268-9952

jenniferm@vitalityworks.com

PomeGreat Pomegranate (4x Juice Concentrate)

Jarrow Formulas

P.O. Box 35994

Los Angeles, CA   90035-4317

www.jarrow.com

Source Naturals - Niacinamide B3 -100 mg.

Source Naturals, Inc.

P.O. Box 2118

Santa Cruz, CA 95062

(800) 815-2333

www.sourcenaturals.com

Index

A

patella
    and infrapatellar fat pad, 24
        and cytokines, 24
        and leptin, 25
    and knee pain, 64
    and medial plica syndrome, 105
tibia
    and menisci, 81
    and passive manual mobilization, 162
    and pes anserine bursitis, 102
    keystone in extensor sling, 57
Bursae, 6, 61-62, 100-101, 154
    and muscle shortening, 6, 154
    of semimembranosus tibial collateral ligament, 100-101
    pes anserine bursa and pes anserine syndrome, 61-62
Bursitis
    bursitis of sartorius, 102
    pes anserine bursitis, 59, 62, 100-103, 105, 136, 154, 202, 258, 356
    prepatellar bursitis, 100
    semimembranosus -TCL (tibial collateral ligament) bursitis, 100, 142
    superficial infrapatellar bursitis, 100

C

Carbohydrates, 236, 237
    restriction and rebound effect, 237
Cartilage, articular
    and calcifications in matrix, 84
    and emerging hypotheses on cartilage breakdown, 84, 93-94
    and estrogen receptors, 86
    and gender differences, 86
        decreased patellar thickness in women, 86
        greater cartilage volume loss in women, 86
    and genetic differences, 83
    and ground substance (extracellular matrix), 16, 81, 83
    and regeneration in special strain of mice, 85
    menisci, 81-83, 93, 256
        lateral meniscus, 81-82
        medial meniscus, 81-82
Central sensitization, 7-8, 102, 342
    and osteoarthritis, 7-8
Cecil, Russell, 4-6, 14, 18-20, 29, 40, 94, 139, 352
Chinese Traditional Medicine
    and arthritis as impediment condition, 251-252
    and massage (tui na), 263
Chingford Study, 41

Prostaglandins, 20, 27, 40, 133, 293, 341, 343, 344, 357
Proteoglycans, 16, 22, 81, 83, 85, 255, 261, 284, 345, 357
Proteomics, 118-119, 358
    proteomic overlaps between rheumatoid arthritis and osteoarthritis, 118-119
Psychoneuroimmunology, 108, 110

Q
Quercetin, 230, 281-282, 284, 293

R
Radiographic findings, 23, 41-42, 89, 100, 102, 106-108, 112, 116, 136,
    268-269, 309
    lack of correspondence to self-reported arthritis symptoms, 106-107
Reiter, Russell J., 254
Research on Osteoarthritis Against Disability (ROAD) Study, 110
Resistin, 27, 91, 118, 357
    and ischemic stroke, 27
    and ligament laxity, 91
Rheumatoid arthritis, 7, 38, 100, 107-108, 110-111, 113-121, 256, 359
    and gender differences in treatment effects, 115-117
    and inflammation, 7, 117-118, 256
Resveratrol, 230, 280-282, 288, 359
    synergistic effect with curcumin, 282
    synergistic effect with genistein, quercetin and vitamin D, 230
Robinson, Dr. William H., 332-333
Robert Wood Johnson Medical School, 68
Rooster comb injections (see Hyaluronic acid - injections)

S
Satellite cells, 163, 254, 284
Selye, Hans, 7
Skeletal fluorosis, 295
Sowers, MaryFran, 23
Stair climbing, 51, 52-53, 55-57, 60, 64-65, 135-140, 144, 155-157,
    161, 202
    Stair ascent, 52, 54, 64, 140
        and body height, 138-139
        and flexor moments, 64
        and force on the patella, 64
        and knee flexion angle, 138-139
    Stair descent, 54, 64, 139-140, 143, 148
        and decreased activation of vastus medialis muscle in women, 139
        and delays in activating muscles in women, 139
        and less knee flexion in early stance with osteoarthritis, 64
StairClimbingSport.com, 53
Stanford University, 155, 317

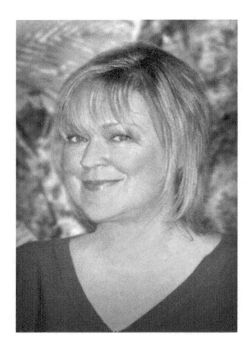

Phyllis Rickel-Wong is a researcher and writer in the fields of health, medicine and psychology. She received her Bachelor's Degree from the University of Michigan and her Master of Arts Degree in Psychology from San Francisco State University. She has a long-standing interest in alternative and complementary medicine, and more recently, in integrative medicine. She resides in Northern California, and her work base is her company, Life Span Research and Consulting Group located in San Ramon, California.

Contact

To Contact Phyllis Rickel-Wong, please send letters to:

Phyllis Rickel-Wong, Director

Transforming Menopause, Inc.

111 Deerwood Road, Suite 200

San Ramon, CA 94583

or please visit her website:

www.transformingmenopause.com